WEIGHT MANAGEMENT THE FITNESS WAY

The Jones and Bartlett Series in Health Sciences

Aging, Health and Society
Kart/Metress/Metress

Basic Law for the Allied Health Professions
Cowdrey

Basic Nutrition: Self-Instructional Modules
Stanfield

The Biology of AIDS
Fan/Conner/Villarreal

The Birth Control Book
Belcastro

Contemporary Health Issues
Banister/Allen/Fadl/Bhakthan/Howard

Drugs and Society, Second Edition
Witters/Venturelli

First Aid and Emergency Care Workbook
Thygerson

Fitness and Health: Life-Style Strategies
Thygerson

Health and Wellness, Third Edition
Edlin/Golanty

Interviewing and Helping Skills for Health Professionals
Cormier/Cormier/Weisser

Introduction to Human Disease, Second Edition
Crowley

Introduction to Human Immunology
Huffer/Kanapa/Stevenson

Introduction to the Health Professions
Miller-Allan

Medical Terminology (with Self-Instructional Modules)
Stanfield/Hui

The Nation's Health, Second Edition
Lee/Estes/Ramsay

Principles and Issues of Nutrition
Hui

Sexuality Today
Nass/Fisher

Teaching Elementary Health Science, Third Edition
Bender/Sorochan

Weight Management the Fitness Way
Dusek

Writing a Successful Grant Application, Second Edition
Reif-Lehrer

WEIGHT MANAGEMENT THE FITNESS WAY

EXERCISE • NUTRITION • STRESS CONTROL
EMOTIONAL READINESS

Dorothy E. Dusek, Ph.D.

JONES AND BARTLETT PUBLISHERS
BOSTON PORTOLA VALLEY

This book is dedicated to the N.O.B.: Lorrie, Donnie, Jean, Bud, Lee, Mot

Editorial, Sales, and Customer Service Offices

Jones and Bartlett Publishers
20 Park Plaza
Boston, MA 02116

Printed in the United States of America
10 9 8 7 6 5 4 3 2 1

ISBN 0-86720-416-8

Library of Congress Cataloging-in-Publication Data

Dusek, Dorothy.
Weight management the fitness way : exercise, nutrition, stress control, emotional readiness / Dorothy Dusek.
p. cm.
Includes bibliographies and index.
1. Health. 2. Physical fitness. 3. Exercise. 4. Nutrition. 5. Stress management. I. Title.
RA776.D94 1989
613—dc20 89-8102
CIP

Cover photos

Front, jogging, H. Armstrong Roberts, Inc. (A. Teufen); bicycling, Camerique; vegetables and fruit, FPG, Int. (Margerin Studios). *Back*, cross-country skiing, FPG, Int. (E. Gebhardt).

PREFACE

THE FIRST EDITION of this book was designed exclusively for those who wanted to "lose weight." Through the years of using the book in university programs and in my private counseling practice, it has become apparent that when students or clients enroll in a weight management practicum or enter a health counseling program with an obvious or spoken goal to get rid of unwanted pounds, behind that presenting problem there are other target goals that are unspoken, perhaps not even realized on a conscious level. Among these less obvious targets are wanting to be strong, agile, attractive, popular, happy, and healthy in all aspects of their lives. The areas of personal strengths, confidence, and self-esteem are rarely addressed immediately by clients, but emerge as vital areas of change during the program. Because all health behavior change is most effective when approached in a holistic manner, I have changed the focus of the book slightly to give greater emphasis to the importance of physical fitness, coping ability, eating behavior, and interpersonal relationships. The target behaviors for health behavior change expand from that of weight management to a total increase in fitness: physical, mental, emotional, social, and what we might even call spiritual. Those who are used to the first edition will note the subtle shift in emphasis, while new users can immediately begin to use the expanded focus.

Most of the clients who come to me suspect that I have a magic program to give them that will cause them to shed pounds, become more fit, be less stressed, and thereby be healthier and happier.

Instead, clients are introduced to a plan for changing their lifestyles—a plan that includes the successful parts of many different weight management, fitness, and general health counseling programs.

In helping people of all ages and both sexes work through their weight, fitness, and health problems, I have found that their basic needs are to understand themselves and to obtain information that will help them find their own strengths and personal power to change themselves into the persons they wish to be. The success of any program depends on each client's meeting those needs. Research follow-up one year after this program has elicited comments such as: "I think that part of the reason for my ability to control my weight this past year was due to a real rethinking about my whole life." "Since your program I have gradually lost pounds and inches . . . I feel so much better about myself." "This has changed my whole life!" These statements of past students and clients help illustrate that this method does work.

The program is a holistic mixture of assessing personal goals and values and then embarking on a lifestyle-changing program that will enhance the likelihood of weight loss and fitness that can be maintained throughout a lifetime. This change in lifestyle includes some exercise, some relaxation, good nutrition, a lot of self-responsibility, and a new awareness of how this package affects a flow of positive energy all around.

This book presents all the aspects of the program that have been tried and proven to be helpful to former and present students and clients. The book systematically illustrates how you can set goals suitable to *you* and compile a profile of the factors in your present lifestyle that motivate your specific eating, exercise, and coping behaviors. Then with this understanding of yourself, you can choose from among several exercise, nutrition, and stress-management options to incorporate them into a healthy lifestyle that supports the image that you require of yourself.

If you comply with the full treatment as summarized in the last chapter, you will enjoy a new dimension of your life and will thank yourself for that gift of growth.

Winter Park, Colorado DOROTHY E. DUSEK

CONTENTS

INTRODUCTION

BECAUSE weight management tops the list of reasons why individuals (especially women) engage in fitness programs and become students of nutrition, we offer two beginning profiles. One reflects your medical history, and the other reflects your weight history. Both are important to anyone contemplating a health lifestyle change, especially if it is motivated by a desire to take off unwanted pounds and get your body into shape. So before you begin reading the rest of the book, fill in the following forms.

MEDICAL HISTORY PROFILE

NAME ____________________ BIRTH DATE / / S.S. # ________

NAME OF LOCAL PHYSICIAN(S) ____________________

DATE OF LAST M.D. VISIT / / Reason ____________________

Results ____________________

In the last year, how many times have you seen a physician for health problems? ____________________

In the last year, how many days did you miss work/school due to illness? ____________________

Ever hospitalized? Y N When? / / Reason ____________________

Results ____________________

WEIGHT PROFILE

Consider each question carefully and don't kid yourself. You have picked up this book for a purpose—probably because you perennially try to shed weight and have never quite been able either to get rid of it or to keep it off. Each of the questions that follow will draw comment somewhere in the following chapters, so take time to put your answers down—you'll want to reflect on them throughout the book.

1. My present weight is 135 pounds. My height is 4'10".
2. I want to weigh 105 pounds.

   My basis for determining this weight is when I was down to 100 lbs. I felt good about myself.
3. If I were at this ideal weight (complete the following sentences where they apply):

   I would feel good about myself.

   My parents would ______.

   My sister(s)/brother(s) would ______.

   My partner or closest friend would ______.
4. I eat at least three nutritious meals a day (Yes or No) ______.
5. I spend most of my time sitting (Yes or No) ______.
6. I have tried the following diets:

   ______.
7. I have tried the following weight control program(s):

   Weight Watchers ____ TOPS ____ Diet Workshop ____

   Overeaters Anonymous ____ Hypnosis____

   Fitness Program(s) ______.

   Others (name them) ______.
8. The most weight I ever lost on a diet/weight reduction program was ______ pounds on ______ diet/program.
9. After that diet/program, I regained ______ pounds to this date.
10. I started having a weight problem when I ______.
11. There are others in my immediate family with a weight problem: sister(s) ____ brother(s) ____ (Yes or No, how many of each); mother ____ father ____ (Yes or No).

12. I live with at least one overweight person (Yes or No, who) ________.
13. I like to exercise ____ (Yes or No.) My usual activity (or activities): ____ ____.
14. When I'm upset about a stressful incident or situation, I ______.
15. I feel like I'm ready to reduce to my ideal weight and stay there for the *rest of my life* ______________________ (YES or NO in *big* letters).

The Holistic Concept of Health and How it Controls Your Weight, Fitness, and Stress Levels

If you've tried to reduce your weight before and couldn't reach your goal—or couldn't stay there once you achieved it—perhaps it was because you see your weight as an isolated part of your health.

Actually, the health of an individual hinges on at least four aspects of lifestyle:

1. Physical activity
2. Nutrition/eating patterns
3. Relaxation or centering ability
4. Relationships and communication with self and others

Today's maladies—such as the problem of being overweight, ulcers, headaches, low back pain, or even cold sores—reflect a less than optimum caretaking of each of the four aspects given above, and to eliminate a malady, *all* aspects must be "treated" at the same time. This is the concept of *holism* or holistic health.

The ancient Oriental philosophies and philosophers recommended the concept of holism, and Eastern medicine still holds that treatment for any aspect of health must be arrived at through a holistic method. Westerners have recently been exposed to the idea of holism, and bookstores have ever-expanding sections of "self-health care" books on topics from autogenics to psychometrics. The idea of holistic health is old and simple: Help yourself become the best person you can become and your health will take care of itself.

The concept of holism symbolizes the interaction among all aspects of the body and the mind—one aspect cannot carry out good health by itself, and the disorder of one aspect will eventually become noticeable in all the other aspects as well.

Figure I.1 shows that all aspects of the body are interrelated: If an individual causes a structural, physical malformation of the body, the psyche suffers when the individual realizes that appearance and physical ability are deteriorating, and biochemical imbalance will eventually occur.

For example, if you let your abdominal muscles lose their tone (See Figure I.2), the pelvic girdle rotates forward and the buttocks protrude to counterbalance the protruding stomach.

When this happens, the spinal column at the lumbar (or low back) area becomes cramped and over a period of time pain increases in this area as nerves coming off the spine are pinched. Low back pain is familiar to most American adults; this malady not only costs the labor market loss in work hours but also psychologically affects those who cannot work or play as usual. The mental aspect can then cause biochemical imbalance by calling forth stress products, which in turn cause more physical or structural disease such as rashes, headaches, or other stress-related maladies. Thus, the causes and cures of all disease in the body are of a holistic nature.

Many people involved in the weight control business think that weight control is surely a main aspect of health. But as one matures into a holistic lifestyle, it becomes apparent that weight control is only a "puppet" of the major health aspects. If you are physically active, feed yourself nutritiously and at optimum times during the day, are mentally well balanced, and spend a few minutes each day centering yourself, then your weight will normalize.

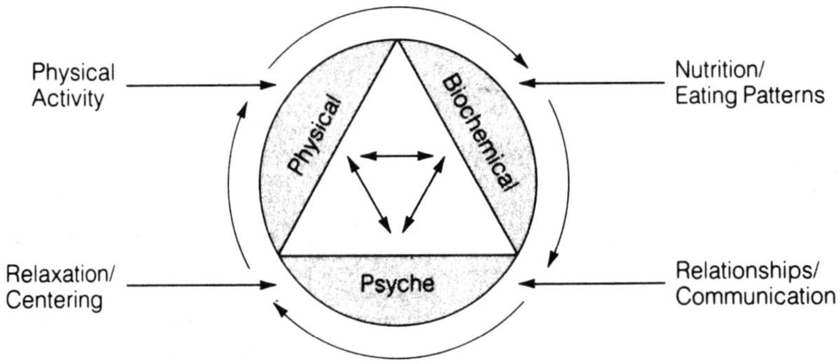

FIGURE I.1 The Holistic Concept of Health

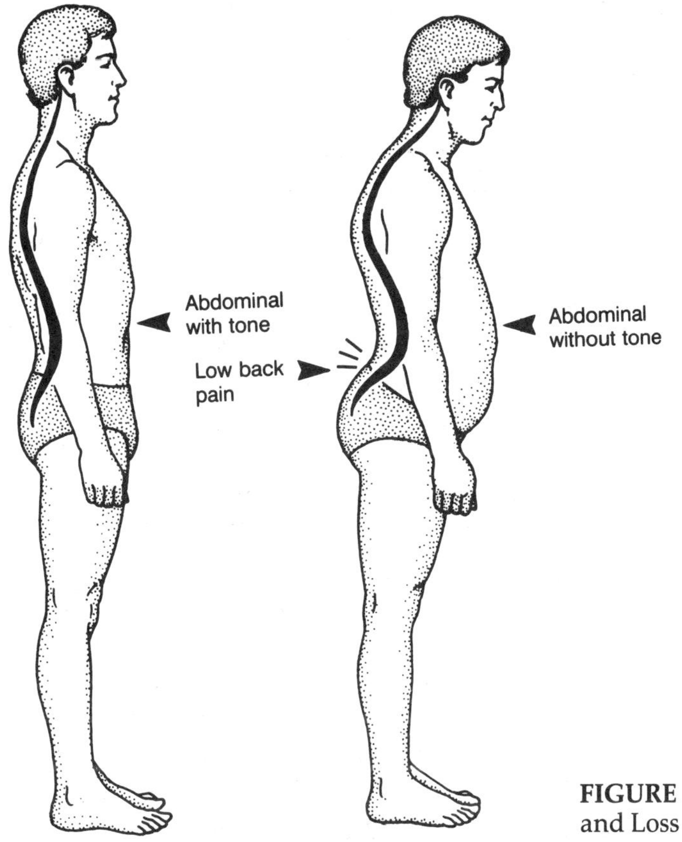

FIGURE I.2 Abdominal Tone and Loss of Tone

One way of looking at the dependence of weight control on each of the four major components of health is through the concept of *energy*, since weight loss and gain are dependent upon the use of energy: energy expenditure and energy consumption. The first two aspects of health given here, physical activity and nutrition/eating style, are inherently and obviously involved in controlling one's weight. The other two aspects, centering and relating/communicating, although perhaps not so obviously involved with body weight, do in fact exert a strong influence. Anxiety, worry, suppressed anger, guilt, depression, and fear are emotions that block your energy. How and what you think about yourself and how you relate to others has much to do with eating, exercise, and relaxation habits. And how you handle stress may directly relate to eating also. A study at the University of Maryland (Mann, 1979) clearly showed a significant positive correlation of stressful life situations with body weight and percentage of body fat; that is, the college students who had the most stressful life events in the past year weighed the most and had the highest percentage of body fat.

Do You Have a Holistic Lifestyle?

How many diets have you been on? Were they nutritionally sound? Even if they were, you were trying to correct a whole health problem using only a partial treatment program. Have you tried *only* behavior modification? Or *only* hypnosis? Or *only* a fitness program? Or *only* yoga? Trying to reduce weight by focusing on only one aspect of health is like trying to gain your balance sitting on a chair with only one leg, or running a four-cylinder car on only one cylinder. The *only* way to deal with a problem that has many causes is to treat the whole problem, and that is what this book is all about—a holistic program that focuses especially on nutrition and eating patterns, exercise and physical activity of all sorts, stress management, and psychological-social relationships and communication with yourself and others that, in this book, is called self-responsibility and readiness.

As you read through the book you will realize how these factors mesh together to form a total lifestyle. Chapter 1 presents a readiness/self-responsibility profile whereby you can study your independence, spontaneity, assertiveness, and other characteristics. Chapter 2 will help you set your weight goal, and Chapter 3 provides a method of calculating how much physical energy you expend. Chapter 4 will take the mystery out of how you become fat or thin, and Chapter 5 offers a new eating plan geared toward taking fat out of storage and keeping it out. Chapter 6 suggests some reasons why you eat: psychological, social, physiological. Chapter 7 offers a stress protection program that ties into your diet, exercise, and self-responsibility. Chapters 8 and 9 offer you a means of analyzing the food that you're eating and how you go about eating it. Chapters 10 through 13 give many exercise options that you may incorporate into your own lifestyle. Chapter 14 will help you plan your commitment to a totally, healthy lifestyle.

Reference

Mann, Patricia H. "Assessment of Personality Traits in the Overweight." Master's thesis, University of Maryland, 1979.

1 VALUES AND READINESS

DO YOU FEEL you're ready for change? Can you close your eyes and see yourself at your ideal size and weight? Is that image a reality for you? Or are you only dreaming, only wishing, telling yourself that you should diet, that you should get out and get more physical exercise, that you should learn how to control your anxiety? If you are "shoulding" yourself, it's a sign that you're not serious, and health behavior change at this time is not a high priority on your value list. But if you heard that little voice inside you saying, "Yeah, yeah, I'm ready; I can see myself at my ideal size and weight," then you are ready for the program. By picking up this book and reading it, you automatically show that you do value a stronger, slimmer, healthy body.

Valuing

You learn your values from many different sources—from your parents, peers, and society in general, especially early in life before you build your own internal support system. Some people, however, never really shift to an internal system and throughout life are controlled by expectations, desires, demands of others. It's pretty hard to do what you want to do and make yourself happy when you let yourself be externally controlled. Sometimes striking your own internal beat is difficult when some external band is marching by, beating a social cadence that rings in your ears and reverberates through your body. This is part of the pain of seeking autonomy as a teenager.

As you experience life's challenges and learn to succeed while listening to your internal dialogue, a self-support system grows and your motivations for behavior originate from your own values rather than the values of others. This shift in support system is sometimes a rending experience, as it may call for more autonomy and, thus, less reliance on those around you. And those around you may have become quite accustomed to their motivational power over you and not want to give it up!

Getting to your ideal size and weight and then maintaining—like such other health behaviors as quitting smoking or learning to relax—require that you be the motivator of your behavior, that you change a behavior because *you* want to, because you will be the recipient of the rewards. It's wonderful if others reap the benefits, too, but they cannot initiate the program without your cooperation, willingness, and readiness. You know what this means if you have ever tried to *make* someone quit smoking, learn to relax, shed some weight, or stop drinking. If the other person didn't choose to do it, then he or she didn't succeed in your program, no matter how perfectly you planned it.

I like to try to separate those who are not ready to change from those who are, so that my students and I don't waste each other's time and effort. I have counseled students who tried to shed weight for their spouses, for their parents, and for me. When I'm the one they are trying to please, I turn the gift back to them—if it is not a gift to themselves first and foremost, I choose not to accept it either. Prognosis for weight maintenance at ideal weight is poor when pounds are taken off for somebody else.

One method I use to determine readiness in clients is the personal interview. A related method puts the interview questions in written form. So in larger groups, where personal interviews are impractical, a checklist of characteristics can indicate how spontaneous the students are, how much they depend on approval from others, how much they worry about the future or feel guilty about the past, how social convention might govern them, how much they demand justice, how they feel about conscious control over their emotions, if they enjoy independence, and if they tend to procrastinate a lot. This tells me a good deal about how well equipped each person is to begin a self-help program in weight control. The following profile is the one I use.

The Readiness Profile*

I include this readiness profile here so that you may derive some insights into your readiness and your self-support system. Check

*The Readiness Profile presented throughout this chapter is reprinted with permission of the author (*The Readiness Profile*, Dorothy E. Dusek, Paradox Publishing. Winter Park, CO. 80482).

yourself on these items throughout the chapter. As you answer them, put down your "gut" response—don't deliberate. Your first, automatic response is probably the most truthful.

You versus Them. The first part of this scale concerns how important social convention and the opinion of others are to you. Give yourself one point for every "yes" answer you put down. Write your total for these ten questions at the end.

	YES/NO
1. I attend weddings, funerals, graduations, baby showers, and so on (any of these) when I don't want to.	______
2. I always read a book from front to back cover.	______
3. I try to dress according to the current fashions.	______
4. I applaud even when I haven't particularly enjoyed a performance.	______
5. I tip for all services where a tip is expected, even if I don't feel a tip is deserved.	______
6. I change my position when others I respect show signs of disapproval.	______
7. I feel put down when someone I respect voices opinions contrary to my own.	______
8. I do things for others and later feel resentful about not being able to say "no."	______
9. I eat food the way it is served at a restaurant rather than ask the waiter to correct a mistake.	______
10. I apologize for myself often.	______
TOTAL	______

Becoming aware of these traits in yourself is the first step toward enjoying or not liking them as part of you. If you feel uncomfortable about answering "yes" to any of these questions, you are experiencing conflict between how you act and how you feel you really want to act or think you *should* act. For instance, if you don't enjoy weddings and go to them anyway, you should ask yourself how do you benefit from going to weddings. In tipping someone who, according to *your* feelings, doesn't deserve a tip, do you find yourself resenting someone you're with, the waiter, the management, the "system" that invented tipping? Throughout this first set of items you will note that a "no" answer is saying "I act on my own feelings, not because the system or someone else dictates that I do it." A "no" answer is just that—ability to say no to outside motivation—while "yes" is the answer of the proverbial "yes person."

How do you break out of the "yes" pattern? *Observe yourself.* When the opportunity arises to choose between doing what you feel is right and doing what someone else wants you to do, *become aware* that a "choice" situation is at hand. At first you might want simply to observe. Give yourself a limited time to do this—one day, two days, a week at the longest. With each observation, write down the choices that you see are possible and also write down how you feel about them. After your observation period, make a contract with yourself to choose in your behalf at least once a day for a week. Then gradually increase the number of such choices until you feel that you are making the majority of your decisions from *your* point of interest.

Justice for All? The next five questions evaluate your sense of justice. Use the same scoring—one point for each "yes" answer.

	YES/NO
1. It bothers me when I see others break the law and get away with it.	______
2. I like to treat people in the same manner they treat me.	______
3. When others invite me to dinner, I always take a bottle of wine and/or am sure to invite them in return.	______
4. When someone gives me a gift, I try to return a gift that costs about the same as the one I received.	______
5. If a person takes advantage of me, I feel I have the right to take advantage of that person.	______
TOTAL	______

Expecting justice can get you into trouble. To spend your day looking for and demanding justice is to burn a lot of energy that could be used for greater returns. Demanding justice is setting up expectations that usually cannot be met; then you are forced to be unhappy about injustice. It isn't fair that 100 people die in a plane crash, that a child is retarded, or that someone bought $10 tickets for a bowl game and is selling them for $40! But justice is not something you can demand, much less control. Concentrate on what you can control—*your* wishes, *your* emotions, *your* behavior, *your* lifestyle.

There's a little book called *How to Make Your Life Work* (Keyes and Burkan, 1974) that offers an alternative to demanding justice: Instead of saying, "It isn't fair," say, "I'd prefer. . . ." Then if you get a speeding ticket and the guy who passed you didn't get one, you can say you'd prefer that he also get a ticket for his misdeed. But if he doesn't, it won't force you into unhappiness. Preferring something doesn't oblige you to *expect* an outcome—you don't demand, you merely prefer.

If your motivation for your actions is based on justice rather than what you really want to do, give yourself a break and do the latter! Give a gift when you feel like it and let the cost be governed by how much you can or want to spend. Take a bottle of wine as a statement of love and the knowledge that your friend is a connoisseur of good wine, not as an exchange for dinner. And, of course, the flip side of acting on your preferences is that you drop your expectations of others, letting them be free to make their own choices.

Do It Now. These four items deal with your willingness to tackle things *now*. Same scoring—one point for each "yes."

	YES/NO
1. I tend to put off boring, hard, or menial tasks until the last moment.	______
2. I avoid confrontation with others.	______
3. I characteristically put off changing a poor health habit such as quitting smoking or taking off weight.	______
4. I put others' happiness before my own.	______
TOTAL	______

I used to be a procrastinator, and every time I said it, it gave me license to put something off. What is at the root of putting something off until tomorrow? Probably not laziness, but instead some insecurity about your ability to do this job or finish that project. Or perhaps some reticence about hurting someone's feelings because what you must do or say would hurt your feelings if the roles were reversed, or if it hurts others' feelings, you run the risk of losing their love or friendship.

Superficially, it is easy to say, "Well, I'm just lazy," or "I'm tired now, I'll do it later," but when things are put off until another time, an honest look at the motivation to "put off" may reveal a much deeper aspect of the personality that it is important to recognize.

The first thing you can do for yourself if you didn't score well on these questions is get rid of the label. And to do that, you begin to act where you formerly did not act. Start as I did by saying, "I *used* to be a procrastinator. . . ."

Then sit back, close your eyes, and think back to a time, a specific incident, when you did indeed procrastinate. Rummage through your mind and see if you can recognize the motivation behind that specific act. Somehow your procrastination protected you from something. What did it protect you from? What did it do for you? Did it protect you from rejection, from risking a friendship, from fear of inability to do the project? Then with your eyes still closed, think of three different solutions to how you could have obtained the same reward through some other behavior. Work through that same situation up to the time of your procrastination, then slip in one of your new solutions.

Let's take a hypothetical case: Pat asks me to call five people on campus to ask them to come to a meeting, and I put it off until the day before the meeting. So I close my eyes and see Pat asking me to call these people, and I try to remember the feelings I had at the time about (1) Pat, (2) calling strangers on the phone, (3) my dislike of telephoning anyone, (4) the nature of the meeting, and (5) how Pat would react if I didn't accept the task. From these feelings I determine that the reward of procrastinating was relief from the fear of being turned down on the phone by a stranger. And so I begin to reconstruct the scene from the moment of Pat's request. The first alternative might be to refuse to do tasks that don't appeal to me. This might be considered avoidance, but it might also be considered honest and assertive behavior. My second alternative to procrastinating is that I immediately do a task I've accepted before I get a chance to put it off or to consider the fear element. Definitely an anti-procrastinatory move. My third choice of action might be to work actively and constructively to relieve my fear of rejection. The next time action is called for, instead of putting off the task, I will use one of my alternatives.

There may be many different, immediate reasons why a procrastinator puts things off, but there is always some reward for postponing an action. Examine how you have kept yourself from slimming down or getting fit until now. You've been putting it off for some reward. Look for that reward. And then create for yourself some ways to reduce your weight or increase your fitness, but still get the reward that procrastination has been giving you.

Spontaneity. The next questions deal with your spontaneity—the ability to laugh, cry, sing, or hug when you feel like it. Score it the same, one point for each "yes" answer.

	YES/NO
1. I don't open up to new experiences very easily.	______
2. I think it's foolish and dangerous to try new things or have new and different experiences just so I can say, "I've tried that and I like (or dislike) it."	______
3. I feel foolish breaking into song in public.	______
4. I have trouble expressing my laughter, love, or tears any time I want to—I usually hold them back.	______
5. I tend to stay away from people, things, and ideas that are unknown and potentially troublesome.	______
6. I usually don't allow myself to meet and deal with new people and ideas.	______
7. I strive to do tasks exactly how others want them done.	______
8. I demand perfection of myself.	______
9. I'd rather stay at a job I don't particularly like than risk finding a new job that may be worse.	______
10. I wear my watch all the time—even to bed.	______
TOTAL	______

Remember the Broadway musical or the movie where someone breaks out into a happy song and dances down a public street? And did you smile inside and wish that you had the nerve even to whistle a little tune aloud as you walk home?

Our formal education and the messages from our elders when we are young and full of spontaneity teach us: Be seen and not heard; don't try new things because you'll get hurt; don't cry in public; don't laugh loudly in public; accept the prejudicial beliefs of your parents, teachers, or community. Before we know it, the natural, spontaneous "player" in each of us is boxed up in fear of reprimand.

It's an interesting paradox that maturation means returning to an open childhood—feeling self-assured enough to learn new things and accept new ideas, allowing tears or laughter whenever they are felt, and enjoying the wonder of life. Carl Rogers (1961) points out some characteristics of people who can "be themselves." Rogers's list of characteristics for "becoming a person" are:

Rejection of facades
Rejection of submissiveness
Rejection of cultural expectations
Ability to trust
Movement away from trying to please others
Movement toward being open to experiences
Movement toward being a person in flux
Movement toward completeness of self
Movement toward acceptance of others

In order to become yourself, you need to recognize, know, and like yourself for who you are. You are the *perfect* you. Each person is perfect in being himself or herself. Pick up a handful of stones on a river bank and look carefully at them. Each is a perfect stone. There may be one you like better than the others because it appeals to your taste in color, texture, or shape, but each *is* a perfect stone. Or think of the announcer at a football game yelling that the extra point was "perfect!" What is an imperfect extra point? There is none. And so each of us is perfect in who we are and each of us can be only an imperfect form of someone else we try to imitate. In trying to be someone else or trying to be someone your family members, authority figures, partner, or others want you to be, you can be *at best* only second best.

And if you compare yourself to others who have particular skills that you don't yet possess (or may never possess), then you will be spending much time berating yourself. Suppose as you're playing racquetball you completely miss the ball! You can laugh and play on, or swear quietly at yourself, or shout a self-destructive obscenity loudly so that everyone will certainly know you're not at all happy with your imperfect imitation of the local racquetball champion. Demanding perfection is good if you're talking about being a perfect you—that's easy. But demanding that you make no mistakes at any time is unneeded pressure on yourself (and will also probably annoy your friends).

If you describe yourself as nonspontaneous, ever striving to be the best, and always demanding perfection of yourself, then choose one new activity to try this week and do it. Then accept how you do it. Next week introduce yourself to a clerk who walks up to help you in a store: "Hello, my name's Terry Jones and I'm looking for a sports shirt." Start to notice the times that you feel as though you aren't being you, when you're doing things the other person's way, when you dress uncomfortably to please others, instead of how *you* play, when you suppress your emotions, and so on. Write down these instances in a notebook or diary and then also write how you could have done things more the way *you* would have liked. The next time a "non-you" situation arises, be assertive and do it *your* way. Perfect!

Self-Declaration. Another set of questions relates to how you view your degree of independence. Give yourself one point for each "yes" answer and record your score.

	YES/NO
1. If I know that a person wouldn't like what I have to say, I never tell that person what I think.	______
2. I have certain expectations for how my parents/spouse/lover/friends/children/others should act or be.	______
3. I am often embarrassed by the actions of my family or others close to me.	______
4. My actions are mainly governed by orders or expectations of others.	______
5. I generally ask advice from someone I respect before making decisions.	______
6. I don't smoke/drink/swear in front of the important people in my life if I know they would not approve.	______
7. I try not to "rock the boat" so others in my life won't be upset.	______
TOTAL	______

Declaring your independence depends on your being your own spontaneous self and realizing that others are trying to do the same—to be themselves. One of the basic tenets in Zen Buddhism is that sorrow stems from desire. In other words, when you don't get what you want (desire), you're going to be unhappy. In a *Playboy* magazine many years ago, someone gave this formula for happiness:

$$\text{happiness} = \frac{\text{what you get}}{\text{what you expect}}$$

If you get \$100 and you expected only \$10, your happiness score is higher than if you expected \$100 and also got \$100, or if you expected $100 and got nothing! Life situations work very much in the same way—we set ourselves up to expect to be pleased or happy *if* we get that new car for graduation, *if* we get that job we want, *if* we get that raise. When the new car doesn't arrive, someone else gets the job, or we don't get the raise, we make ourselves unhappy.

Expectations also appear in what might be called a "power trip," that is, expecting and forcing others to do things in a certain way. When a friend expects you to help her with her homework and you don't comply, she's displeased. When someone wants you to do things *his* way, and you don't, he's displeased. Parents, teachers, mates, nearly everyone you know all try their power trips at various times. And guilt is usually your reward for noncompliance.

Declaring independence, then, is not only to sidestep or abort the power trips of others, but also to give up the need for power over anyone else. To have expectations of how your family, partner, or friends should act or what they should wear, or to be embarrassed when they don't do as you expect—these are feelings about others' behaviors that you cannot control. Such feelings are a sure way to set up unhappiness for yourself.

In situations where you're tempted to accept only one course of action from someone else (that is, expect the other to do it your way), remember the little trick of "preferring" something rather than expecting it. If you just prefer that your friend not play the radio so loudly, you can either be happy with your friend and the loud radio or choose to go. But if you are addicted to shutting off loud music, your friend's habit will drive you berserk in no time.

If you are allowing others power over your life, reread the section on spontaneity and be sure to read your assertiveness rights later in this chapter.

Guilty or Not. The next few questions deal with guilt and worry. Use the same scoring—one point for each "yes"—and record your total.

	YES/NO
1. I label myself as a worrier, a procrastinator, shy, clumsy, a poor speller, poor at math, or some other descriptive term, and then act out the label.	______
2. I would be a much better person if I could change some of the things I have done in the past.	______

	YES/NO
3. Most of my actions and behaviors are pleasing and productive for others rather than for myself.	______
4. I feel guilty about not leaving a tip, even after poor service.	______
5. If my actions are contrary to what those who are important to me want me to do or be, I worry about it.	______
6. I worry about my ability to get a job.	______
7. I worry about my interpersonal relationships.	______
8. If I'm worried in the morning, I usually carry the worry with me all day.	______
9. I find myself worrying about future events often.	______
10. I catch myself avoiding some activity because I'd worry too much about its outcome if I engaged in it.	______
TOTAL	______

Dr. Wayne Dyer in his best-seller, *Your Erroneous Zones* (1976), outlined two useless emotions: guilt and worry. These two phenomena have many times prevented every one of us from being ourselves and doing what we thought was right for us.

Guilt is how we are kept "in line" by those we care for, or are afraid of, or don't want to risk possibly alienating. The words *should, must, ought to,* and *if* all derive from guilt. Have you heard from someone close to you, "If you loved me, you would . . ."? If you do love this person and don't do what is wanted, you are likely to feel guilty. And so in this way you may be coerced into doing something you don't want to do. How often do you say, "I should be studying," or "I ought to go on a diet," or "I must go see my mother"?

However, guilt is often not so plainly spoken. How large a tip do you leave when the service has been poor? The same as usual? How do you feel when you drive past a hitchhiker, or refuse to donate to the flower-bearers at the airport, or refuse to buy Girl Scout cookies? Claude Steiner in *Scripts People Live* (1974) proposes that some (or all) people have a "guilt script," that is, their parents made them feel guilty so often that guilt is a basic motive throughout life. If you identify this in yourself as you answer these questions, you are probably recognizing also that you are ready to start giving up guilt as a motive.

Worry, the other useless emotion, identified by Dr. Wayne Dyer, is sometimes related to guilt, but many people can successfully worry without guilt as the motive. Worry and guilt may be related if you refuse a dinner date because you would worry about how your partner would feel if you had dinner with someone else. A good way to check the guilt-worry motive is to accept a dinner date when your partner is also engaged for dinner or is out of town. If you don't worry about your partner's feelings of being threatened, of being alone, and so forth, then you can recognize that guilt is your motive for not going when your partner would be left alone.

Worrying is basically telling yourself "mind stories" about what evil thing might occur in your future. For example, while driving back to a store to return an item, you may begin a mind story about what will happen when you ask the store clerk to take the item back. In your story the clerk says that it is not the policy of the store to take back items once they are sold. Then you start to worry that you'll be stuck with an item that is too small. So in your mind you argue with the clerk, who then calls the manager. The manager coldly states that it is impossible for the store to comply with your wishes. You become even angrier. By the time you actually reach the store you are furious and stomp up to the nearest clerk and demand that the store take the item back. The clerk calmly replies that it's just a routine matter and fills out a return form for you to sign. So you suffered all that worry and upset your system for no cause! Out of such fear that the unpleasant would happen, that your ego might be hurt, you work yourself into a very stressful, unhealthy state.

"What if he doesn't like me?" "What if I get on the wrong bus?" "What if I'm late to class?" "What if that big dog up the block bites me as I run by?" Gestalt therapy offers a good substitute for worrying—enjoy being where you are *right now*: Feel the feelings, hear what's going on, see what and who are in your visual field and taste all of it, savor it, because this moment will never be here again. Enjoy preparing yourself right now for physical and psychological "survival," and every moment will not only take care of itself, it will be savored for its uniqueness. Know that the future will be more moments of learning, growing, and experiencing, and let go of some of your power to shape them—because you can shape the actions of others only through manipulation and guile, thus imposing guilt and worry on them.

If you could control everyone else and everything else that concerns your being, you might be able to worry constructively. But such control is not possible, so you might do as a friend of mine does: Set aside a half hour each day to do nothing but worry, and then take a nap during that half hour!

If you worry excessively, learning and practicing meditation may be helpful to you. The art of meditation teaches you to rid your mind of ego-involved stories, especially ego-threatening stories. Chapter 7 on how to protect yourself from stress will introduce other methods of controlling the stress of worry.

Emotions. These few questions deal with anger and other emotions in general. Use the same scoring—one point for each "yes" answer.

	YES/NO
1. Joy, fear, anger, and pain happen to me at certain times, and I cannot control when they will occur.	______
2. In situations I find difficult to handle, I get angry.	______
3. I spend much of my time being depressed.	______
4. When I am unhappy, I just have to wait until something good happens to me to change my mood.	______
5. When I am angry at someone, I generally keep it to myself.	______
TOTAL	______

It is apparent that after a period of time in life people often *choose* their emotions to match the expectations of others. When you miss the sure shot in tennis, you become angry. When you break up with a partner—even if it was not a particularly good relationship—you may cry and mope around sadly. When you brake suddenly to avoid hitting someone, you usually experience a fear reaction later. And when you win something, whether you like the winning or not, you probably show joy; the supreme example of this is the game show contestant—the more unrestrained the contestant's joy, the more pleased are the sponsor, the emcee, the audience, and the producer!

Our emotions of pain, anger, fear, and joy are conditioned by a lifetime of consequences, and we have all succumbed to unhappiness merely because it was expected. When children learn that crying after scraping a knee will bring them much sympathy, a kiss on the knee, and a badge of courage in the form of a Mickey Mouse bandage, why should they simply pick themselves up and go happily on their way?

In his book, *Love Is to Be Happy With* (1977), Barry Neil Kaufman points out that every time you are unhappy, you ought to examine your unhappiness because it is your prerogative to be happy or unhappy. He calls his method of self-examination of unhappiness the

"Option Method." In Kaufman's method, when you are unhappy, you examine your situation by asking yourself three questions:

1. What am I unhappy about?
2. Why does that make me unhappy?
3. Why do I believe that?

If there are rewards in unhappiness, you may indeed choose to linger in unhappiness rather than to move on to new, fulfilling experiences.

In feeling pain, fear, or anger (usually considered the "negative" emotions) you must recognize them and act on them at the time of sensation. Usually these emotions are related to a particular person in your life, and in such a situation assertiveness can be the exorcist of the emotion. When you're angry with someone's behavior, tell them so and do it in a posture of anger. If you laugh and say, "Hey, I'm really angry about how you just put me down in front of Susan," who would believe that you're truly angry? Anger can be stated in an angry way, just as joy can be related in an ecstatic way. Some people set up a pattern of violence to show that they're angry because they have never been able to talk about their anger in an angry way (without, for example, throwing something).

Assert Your Rights. These questions regarding assertiveness should be scored by assigning one point for each "yes" answer.

	YES/NO
1. I assume others are upset with me when they walk by and don't speak to me.	______
2. I find it difficult to ask someone for a hug or other show of affection.	______
3. I have noticed that I use the terms *dumb* and *stupid* for people who don't agree with my likes or dislikes.	______
4. Once I make a decision with someone else, I feel that I shouldn't change my mind.	______
5. I would rather use a subtle or roundabout way to get what I want if asking directly might hurt someone's feelings.	______
6. I feel guilty when I say "no."	______
TOTAL	______

Assertiveness is honest communication – stating how you feel and saying what you want in a straightforward manner. Sometimes assertiveness is confused with *aggressiveness*. Being aggressive connotes demanding what you want or stating how you feel in an intimidating and threatening manner. Aggressiveness usually involves being disagreeable but not accepting disagreement from others. And someone who does disagree with the likes or dislikes of the aggressive person is usually called "dumb," "sick," "crazy," or some other derogatory term. The aggressive person builds self-esteem at the expense of others. No doubt you can picture some aggressive persons in your life. Are you comfortable around them?

In being *assertive*, you state aloud your likes and dislikes and you say them in a manner that doesn't deride someone else. You can dislike a behavior in a person without disliking the person. In telling others that you would appreciate their silence in the theater, you are not saying that they have poor personalities with no redeeming qualities; you're merely saying that you would like to hear the soundtrack of the movie, not them.

In a recent assertiveness training class, the following characteristics were listed by the participants to describe an assertive person. If you don't consider yourself assertive, you might relate each of these characteristics to yourself. In the space after each characteristic, rate yourself on this basis: A = "No, this characteristic doesn't generally describe me"; B = "This characteristic fits me as well as most other people I know"; and C = "I recognize this as a well-developed characteristic in myself." After you have finished testing yourself, total your scores and see which answer predominates. The results should be self-explanatory.

THE ASSERTIVE PERSON

______ Honest	______ Direct	______ Tactful
______ Confident	______ Open	______ Mellow
______ Objective	______ Calm	______ Cheerful
______ Sincere	______ In control	______ Articulate
______ Empathetic	______ Positive	______ Nonvindictive
______ Self-aware	______ Decisive	______ Self-disciplined
______ Flexible	______ Constructive	______ Flowing

______ Competent	______ Responsive	______ Risk-taking
______ Nonabusive	______ Energetic	
______ Considerate	______ Responsible	

Totals: A = ______ B = ______ C = ______

Reflect on Rogers's list of characteristics for "becoming a person" that were listed earlier. It should be clear that all these characteristics appear in those people who are being themselves, making their own decisions, and allowing others to do the same in their lives.

I have found that people in assertiveness training classes tend to be nonassertive when they don't want to risk the consequences of telling someone how they feel or what they want. Any relationship suffers when both people have to guess the other person's emotions. And when honest communication is missing, aggressiveness or manipulation must be used.

Manipulation—subtle, roundabout ways of getting what is wanted—is used by those who can't say directly what they want or what their likes and dislikes are. If someone doesn't like to be near a particular person, he or she can make subtle innuendos so that friends would not like that person either. Or he or she can simply say, "I don't care to be around so-and-so," and let the friends decide whether they want to or not. If you have ever been manipulated, you know the demeaning aspect of trickery or of being maneuvered. The dialogue usually sounds like the following after someone has been manipulated and is being assertive with the manipulator:

> *Assertor*: You know, you could have just told me what you wanted rather than maneuver around me.
> *Manipulator*: I didn't want to hurt your feelings.
> *Assertor*: The manipulation hurt my feelings.

What has the manipulator circumvented? Nothing. If you think your actions will hurt others' feelings, ask them. Checking with them is the only way you'll know. Telling them how you feel is the only way they'll know. Asking for what you want is your best chance for getting it.

In *The Assertiveness Option* (1978) Jakubowski and Lange give a list of basic assertive rights that may be helpful to you on your path to greater assertiveness and the benefits that accrue from that behavior. These rights are:

1. The right to act in ways that promote your dignity and self-respect as long as others' rights are not violated in the process
2. The right to be treated with respect
3. The right to say "no" and not feel guilty
4. The right to experience and express your feelings
5. The right to take time to slow down and think
6. The right to change your mind
7. The right to ask for what you want
8. The right to do less than you are humanly capable of doing
9. The right to ask for information
10. The right to make mistakes
11. The right to feel good about yourself

I have found in my work with those who are overweight and obese that as a group, they have lower body images and lower self-images than do individuals with normal weight (Girdano and Dusek, 1977). Body image refers to the feelings one has about his or her physical body, while self-image refers to the feelings one has of his or her psychological and spiritual self. (Chapter 6 contains a self-test on body image.) It would be difficult to prove a cause-and-effect relationship here, but I have also found that after 15 weeks of the program offered in this book, participants' scores on self- and body image improve significantly. So it is possible that strengthening your personality characteristics may make fat elimination easier, just as it is possible that the elimination of fat from your body may enhance how you feel about yourself.

How does a person become more assertive? Following some of the suggestions in all sections of this chapter should help. Taking an assertiveness training class is not only informative but also extremely supportive as your assertiveness grows. And there are some excellent books on the subject: *The Assertive Option* (Jakubowski and Lange, 1978) provides a step-by-step method for developing assertiveness skills. *Your Perfect Right* (Alberti and Emmons, 1987) has some good advice on how to overcome obstacles to assertive behavior. *STAT: Special Techniques in Assertiveness Training* (Chenevert, 1983) is very readable and informative as it provides realistic options and encouragement to use them. *Your Erroneous Zones* (Dyer, 1976) is an enjoyable book on how to take charge of your life. These are just a few of the books recommended for self-help in this area; others are listed under "Suggested Readings" at the end of the chapter.

LOOKING AT YOUR SCORE

Now that you have a score for each of the eight sections of the Readiness Profile, total them here.

You versus Them	______ out of 10
Justice for All?	______ out of 5
Do It Now	______ out of 4
Spontaneity	______ out of 10
Self-Declaration	______ out of 7
Guilty or Not	______ out of 10
Emotions	______ out of 5
Assert Your Rights	______ out of 6

GRAND TOTAL ______

Commitment to Change

In Table 1.1, write in your scores for the categories of your Readiness Profile. The rest of the table is for scheduling specific change techniques. Choose an area you need to work on and write down the technique(s) that you will use each week. At the end of the week, write down your results and how you feel about them. This chart-style diary will help you reflect on your growth.

WHAT DOES IT ALL MEAN?

The higher your score on the Readiness Profile, the less ready you probably are to shed that extra weight unless you are very strongly motivated by *other* people and that external reward system is very strong and lasting.

A score below 10 indicates that you are internally motivated and you act independently by nature. This makes you a good candidate for successfully eliminating fat and maintaining your lower weight once achieved. A score over 40 indicates the opposite—it reflects a general picture of control by others that makes you quite dependent upon praise or other rewards to accomplish a task. Once you recognize this characteristic of yourself, you can learn to be more internally motivated.

TABLE 1.1 Readiness/Self-Responsibility

Area	*Score*	*Technique(s)*	*Dates Used*	*Results*	*How I Felt*
You vs. Them (social convention)	_/10				
Justice for All (your addiction to justice)	_/5				
Do It Now (procrastination)	_/4				
Spontaneity (freedom of expression)	_/10				
Self-Declaration (independence)	_/7				
Guilty or Not (guilt and worry)	_/10				
Emotions	_/5				
Assert Your Rights (assertiveness)	_/6				

If you scored between 11 and 28, your internal system of support generally overrides an external support system, and the opposite is true for a score of 29 to 40. If your score was high, your task along with your regimen to reduce weight will be to work on those personality characteristics on which you scored high—if in fact you choose to perform both tasks at once. Lowering your score enhances your probability of long-term weight maintenance at your lower weight because it reflects a more spontaneous, independent, self-assured attitude of acting from an internal set of values. Then you will do what you choose to do.

Another effective way to work on readiness and self-responsibility is to buy a small notebook or a blank book at a bookstore and keep a daily diary of situations dealing with any of the areas covered in the Readiness Profile. In the front of your book write down the types of situations you want to improve your behavior in:

Social convention—Do you behave in a certain way because someone else wants you to?
Addiction to justice and power—Do you want things done your way or how you expect them to happen?
Procrastination—Do you postpone actions?
Spontaneity—Do you stifle your impulses to laugh, cry, sing, hug, and so on?
Independence—Do you act on your own ideas or on those of others?
Guilt and worry—What do you worry about or feel guilty about?
Emotions—Do your emotions control you?
Assertiveness—Do you say what you feel?

At the end of each day write down the situations, how you handled them, how you felt about the way you handled them, how you wish you would have responded if you don't feel good about your response, and how you will respond next time. Make a commitment to change your response if it will make you feel better about yourself.

References

Alberti, Robert, and Michael Emmons. *Your Perfect Right*, 5th Edition. New York: Impact Publishers, 1987.
Dyer, Wayne. *Your Erroneous Zones*. New York: Funk and Wagnalls, 1976.
Chenevert, M. *STAT: Special Techniques in Assertiveness Training*. St. Louis: Mosby, 1983.

Girdano, Daniel, and Dorothy Dusek. "Performance-Based Evaluation," *Health Education* 8 (1977): 13–16.
Jakubowski, Patricia, and Arthur Lange. *The Assertiveness Option: Your Rights and Responsibilities*. Champaign, IL: Research Press, 1978.
Kaufman, Barry Neil. *Love Is to Be Happy With*. New York: Fawcett Crest, 1977.
Rogers, Carl. *On Becoming a Person*. Boston: Houghton Mifflin, 1961.
Steiner, Claude. *Scripts People Live*. New York: Bantam Books, 1974.

Suggested Readings

Astrachan, A. *How Men Feel*. Garden City, N.Y.: Doubleday, 1986.
Eichenbaum, L., and S. Orbach. *What Do Women Want?* New York: Berkeley Books, 1984.
Gawain Shakti. *Living in the Light*. Mill Valley, CA: Whatever Publishing Co., 1986.
Glasser, William. *Taking Effective Control of Your Life*. New York: Harper & Row, 1984.
King, Serge. *Mastering Your Hidden Self*. Sheaton, IL: Theosophical Publishing House, 1985.
Maslow, Abraham. *Toward a Psychology of Being*. New York: Van Nostrand Reinhold, 1968.
Padus, Emrika. *The Complete Guide to Your Emotions and Your Health*. Emaus, PA: Rodale Press, 1986.
Ram Dass. *Be Here Now*. Albuquerque: Modern Press, 1978.
Shainess, N. *Sweet Suffering: Woman as Victim*. New York: Wallaby, 1984.

2 GOAL SETTING: WHERE DO YOU GO FROM HERE?

THROUGHOUT THIS BOOK you will be encouraged to set goals because goals serve as both motivators and milestones. Many people only vaguely know what they want, so they never know success by reaching stated goals. There is an ancient Egyptian formula for success that has six steps that must be accomplished. According to this formula, success is dependent upon these steps:

1. You must be able to clearly state what you want.
2. You must be willing to approach your goal step-by-step rather than wanting it *all*, right now.
3. You must stay in your own authenticity and truth—be who you are rather than trying to be those who are models to you.
4. You must be willing to follow a path that has heart and passion for you. If your plan of action doesn't feel right to you, you won't succeed.
5. You must be able to give your plan constant energy, rather than big or small spurts of energy. Many begin a program going like gangbusters and then fizzle out for lack of energy.
6. You must be willing to be flexible, open to new options and opportunities, new ways of doing things, even resetting goals.

Although this is an ancient formula, you can clearly see that it still applies to present-day quests.

In Chapter 1, you were asked to set self-responsibility goals for yourself and begin an action plan there. Go back and look at what you need to work on and apply the six steps given above to your goals there. This chapter illustrates how to set a weight goal, Chapter 7 asks you to set stress management goals, Chapter 9 gives opportunity to set eating plan goals, and Chapters 11, 12, and 13 ask you to set exercise goals in the areas of strength and muscular endurance, flexibility, and aerobic exercise. As you set your goals and plan your program to meet those goals, keep in mind the six steps to success.

Finding Your Ideal Weight

Now that you have decided some of this body-not-so-beautiful must go, you must decide how much should go. This chapter will present a number of ways to help you determine what your weight should be. It proceeds from very simple height/weight tables to some scientific methods that require skills of trained professionals. Determine your ideal weight through whatever methods you can here and compare all the results. Then, if possible, ask a trained professional to calculate your percentage of body fat (what percentage of your body weight is fat), because *fat* reduction (rather than just weight reduction) is really what you are working toward. Finally, make a goal chart for yourself at the end of the chapter.

Many people have a concept of their ideal weight tucked away in their minds—how much they weighed in high school or at peak athletic performance, or what weight will allow them comfortably to fit again into some favorite clothes. If this "ideal" weight is rationally possible for you, it may indeed be what you could and should weigh *for the rest of your life* (become used to this concept). But if there is only a very slim chance that you can attain such a stringent goal, then perhaps a formula derived from research or actuarial tables may be what you need in order to set a weight goal.

The MLI Formula

One of the oldest printed guides to what you should weigh is the Metropolitan Life Insurance height-weight tables seen in Tables 2.1 and 2.2. These have been derived from insured individuals, and the weights are determined by mortality risk rates according to height and frame size. Each height is given a weight range—the lower end is the ideal and the upper end is the easiest to attain. To add a bit of stringency, I recommend using the lowest weight for your frame to the midpoint weight as the usable range for setting your goal.

The main benefit of using height/weight tables such as the Metropolitan Life Insurance tables is the simplicity with which these

TABLE 2.1 Metropolitan Life Insurance Height/Weight Table for Men

Height	*Small Frame**	*Medium Frame**	*Midpoint**	*Large Frame**
5′ 2″	112–120	118–129	124	126–141
5′ 3″	115–123	121–133	127	129–144
5′ 4″	118–126	124–136	130	132–148
5′ 5″	121–129	127–139	133	135–152
5′ 6″	124–133	130–143	137	138–156
5′ 7″	128–137	134–147	141	142–161
5′ 8″	132–141	138–152	145	147–166
5′ 9″	136–145	142–156	149	151–170
5′10″	140–150	146–160	153	155–174
5′11″	144–154	150–165	158	159–179
6′ 0″	148–158	154–170	162	164–184
6′ 1″	152–162	158–175	167	168–189
6′ 2″	156–167	162–180	171	173–194
6′ 3″	160–171	167–185	176	178–199
6′ 4″	164–175	172–190	181	182–204

*Desirable weights given in pounds for men age 25 and over wearing indoor clothing. Midpoint added by author.

TABLE 2.2 Metropolitan Life Insurance Height/Weight Table for Women

Height	*Small Frame**	*Medium Frame**	*Midpoint**	*Large Frame**
4′10″	92–98	96–107	102	104–119
4′11″	94–101	98–110	104	106–122
5′ 0″	96–104	101–113	107	109–125
5′ 1″	99–107	104–116	110	112–128
5′ 2″	102–110	107–119	113	115–131
5′ 3″	105–113	110–122	116	118–134
5′ 4″	108–116	113–126	120	121–138
5′ 5″	111–119	116–130	123	125–142
5′ 6″	114–123	120–135	128	129–146
5′ 7″	118–127	124–139	132	133–150
5′ 8″	122–131	128–143	136	137–154
5′ 9″	126–135	132–147	140	141–158
5′10″	130–140	136–151	144	145–163
5′11″	134–144	140–155	148	149–168
6′ 0″	138–148	144–159	152	153–173

*Desirable weights given in pounds for women age 25 and over wearing indoor clothing. Midpoint added by author.

measurements can be made. Also, many researchers use them to determine whether a person qualifies as clinically obese or not. *Clinical obesity* according to Metropolitan Life Insurance has been set at 20 percent or more above ideal (or desirable) weights given in the tables. In addition, the overweight percentage figures derived from these tables are used by some to categorize patients, clients, or subjects and then compare them to other studies or individual weight loss program results.

A definite drawback to these MLI tables is that they are only two-dimensional (height and frame size) and so do not deal with the amount of actual fat a person may have. For instance, a person could be in a normal weight range in the tables but have excessive fat, just as a very muscular person might appear overweight but not be excessively fat. As an example of the latter case, many professional players encountered difficulties in buying life insurance—they appeared to fit into the overweight range, therefore they were considered greater insurance risks. For the person who *is* overly fat, yet fits complacently in the "normal" weight range, other devices discussed later can enable them to discover their body compositions, that is, how much of their body is fat. Because the MLI tables do not give body composition, many people in the weight control business consider the tables a hindrance rather than a help in goal setting. Other sources described later will add the important component of body fat percentage.

YOUR WEIGHT RANGE ACCORDING TO MLI

To begin your search for your ideal or desired weight, determine your weight range and percentage overweight (or underweight) on the worksheet in Figure 2.1. Frame size can be determined by an old "rule of thumb." Wrap your thumb and index finger around the opposite wrist. If the thumb and finger don't meet, consider that you have a large frame. If they just meet or barely overlap, you probably have a medium frame. If the thumb and finger overlap, you probably have a small frame. More scientifically, you can measure your wrist with a tape measure. For men, 5.6 to 6.7 inches indicates a small frame; 6.8 to 7.4 inches indicates a medium frame; and 7.5 inches or more indicates a large frame. For women these measurements are: 4.6 to 5.5 inches for a small frame; 5.6 to 6.2 inches for a medium frame; and 6.3 inches or more for a large frame (Hockey, 1977). To determine frame size, another scientific formula takes

EXAMPLE			*YOUR WORKSHEET*	
Subject height	= 5′4″ + 1″	= 5′5″	Your height	=____ + 1″ =____
weight	= 150 lbs.		weight	=____ lbs.
Frame size	= medium		Frame size	=____
Ideal range (low to mid)	= 116–123		Ideal range (low to mid)	=____
Percentage overweight:			Percentage overweight:	
at low end	= 29% [(150–116)/116 = .29]		at low end	=____
at midpoint	= 22% [(150–123)/123 = .22]		at midpoint	=____

FIGURE 2.1 Ideal Weight Range: Example and Worksheet

height and the width between the inside and outside bones of the elbow into consideration. For men 6′2″ to 6′3″ tall, the elbow measurement for a medium frame is between 2½ and 2⅞ inches; for those 6′4″ to 6′7″ it is 2⅝–2⅞ inches; for those 6′8″ to 6′11″ it is 2¾ to 3 inches, for those 7′ to 7′3″ it is 2¾ to 3⅛ inches, and for men taller than 7′3″ it is 2⅞–3¼ inches. For women 4′8″ to 5′3″ the elbow measurement for a medium frame is 2¼ to 2½ inches, for those 5′4″ to 5′11″ it is 2⅜ to 2⅝ inches; and for women 6′ and taller it is 2½ to 2¾ inches.

Since the heights and weights given in the MLI tables are determined for clothed subjects, add an inch to your barefoot height; remember also that your weight range includes the weight of your indoor clothing. Once you find your range, determine how you compare to the low and midweights in this range. To calculate your overweight percentage, subtract the low figure of the range from your actual weight. Then divide that difference by the same low figure of the range. After the division, multiply by 100 and you will have the overweight percentage:

(Actual weight − low end of range in MLI table)/low end of range × 100
(Actual weight − midpoint weight)/midpoint weight × 100

The example in Figure 2.1 is of a woman of medium frame standing 5 feet 4 inches barefoot, weighing 150 pounds. On the MLI table for women her height of 5 feet 5 inches (give her an inch for shoes) shows a range of 116–130 with the midpoint of 123 pounds. According to the midpoint rule of stringency, her range is 116–123. For the high figure of the range she is 22 percent overweight:

(150 pounds actual weight − 123 midpoint pounds)/123 pounds = .22 or 22%

For the lower weight figure she is 29 percent overweight:

(150 pounds actual weight − 116 low point pounds)/116 = .29 or 29%

These figures are important because according to the MLI tables clinical obesity is considered to be any percentage over 20 percent. This individual would be considered clinically obese using either the low or the midpoint figure. By using the figure at the top of the range, however, she is only 15 percent overweight and not considered clinically obese:

(150 pounds actual weight − 130 high point pounds)/130 = .15 or 15%

The use of overweight percentage offers comparability among individuals, aids in categorization (if, indeed, you wish to be categorized!), and may act as motivation for weight loss *now* if you fall in the obese category. Many people can tolerate being overweight, but abhor being obese!

Other Height/Weight Methods

Few who choose to help themselves lose weight have access to more sophisticated methods of assessing their fat status. In knowing how tall you are, you can do some educated goal estimations. So, in addition to using the MLI tables, you can follow the simple rule that desirable weight for women is 100 pounds (45 kilograms) for the first 60 inches (5 feet) and then for each inch over 5 feet, 5 pounds are allowed (Bray, 1976). In the example in Figure 2.1, the desirable weight for the woman who is 5 feet 4 inches tall (64 inches) would be 120 pounds according to this method.

This rule for men allows them 106 pounds for the first 60 inches and then 6 pounds for each inch over 5 feet. Thus, a man 6 feet 1 inch tall would have a desirable weight of 106 pounds for the first 60 inches and then 6 pounds for each of the 13 inches beyond that (6 × 13 = 78). Therefore, his weight should be around 184 pounds.

The body mass index (BMI) is another height-weight measure often used to determine the health risk of being overweight. The formula is: weight in kilograms divided by height in meters squared.

An average adult BMI is between 20–25, with an excess of 26 being an indication of increasing health risk (Frankel, 1986).

$$BMI = \frac{wt}{ht^2}$$

The Height/Waist Index

One more simple test for determining obesity uses the measurement of the waist. If the circumference of the waist subtracted from the height in inches is less than 36, the individual is probably overweight. For example: A subject's waist measures 33 inches and the height is 5 feet 4 inches (64 inches).

$$64 - 33 = 31 \text{ (less than 36)}$$

This person would qualify as obese using this method.

The Mahoney Formula

Another formula offered for determination of ideal weight is a little more stringent but nonetheless can be a valuable guideline for ideal weight. In addition to height, the Mahoney formula uses physical activity as an indicator of what your weight should be. It is also a guideline for calorie intake until you achieve your desired weight and the calories needed to maintain desired weight.

This formula (Mahoney and Mahoney, 1978) requires that women multiply their height in inches by 3.5 and then subtract 110 to find their desired weight. Men multiply their height in inches by 4 and then subtract 130. The 150-pound, 5 feet 4 inches woman would have a target weight of 114 pounds:

$$(64 \times 3.5) - 110 = 114$$

A 150-pound, 5 feet 4 inches man would have a target weight of 126 pounds:

$$(64 \times 4) - 130 = 126$$

The Mahoneys take their formula a step further and ask you to rate your activity as shown in Table 2.3.

TABLE 2.3 The Mahoney Activity Rating Scale

Very inactive (sedentary)	13 points
Slightly inactive (occasional physical activity)	14 points
Moderately active (frequent physical activity)	15 points
Relatively active (almost always on the go, physically active)	16 points
Frequent strenuous activity (at least one daily hour of running or other physical activity)	17 points

Once you determine your activity level (in a rational, honest manner—walking to work once a week doesn't win you 15 points), multiply that rating by your ideal weight and the result is the number of calories per day needed to maintain that ideal weight. The sample woman, if sedentary (13 points), would need 1,482 calories per day to maintain 114 pounds; the sample man, if sedentary, would need 1,638 calories per day to maintain 126 pounds.

To find how many calories you need to maintain your present weight, multiply your activity rating by your present weight. Again, in our example, the woman, to maintain 150 pounds, would take in 1,950 calories per day (150 × 13). The theory behind this formula says that if she is consistently taking in more than 1,950 calories per day, she is gaining weight. The difference between actual weight maintenance intake and ideal weight maintenance intake is 468 calories (1,950 minus 1,482). This is the number of calories of energy that she will need to cut back each day to arrive at and maintain her ideal weight.

Determining Body Composition

One more important bit of information you must include in your calculations in your goal-setting efforts concerns not just weight, but the amount of *fat* you have accumulated on your body. It appears that Americans continue to get fatter and fatter. Current records show that the *average* percentage of body fat of college-age females is between 20 and 25 percent. An *excellent* range that not many females achieve is 10 percent or below. The average percentage of body fat of college-age males is between 15 and 20 percent, with the excellent category at 12 percent or below (Allsen, et al, 1980). The excellent ranges are reached mainly by endurance athletes. A *realistic* range for adult females to aim at would be 15 to 20 percent, and for adult males the range of 10 to 15 percent should be realizable.

As we grow older we tend to store more of our energy rather than burn it up—a product of waning psychological motivation rather than predestined physiology, although after the age of 30 the body metabolism decreases about 5 percent per decade.

THE UNDERWATER FORMULA

In our laboratory we have a large, stainless steel tank in which we have our students take a little dip. While they're underwater forcing as much air out of their lungs as possible, we weigh them. Now, this weight pleases most participants because underwater (with a 10-pound weight around the waist) even the heaviest subjects weigh only 20 to 30 pounds. Unfortunately, here a lower weight means more fat because fat floats and buoys up the body. The heaviest candidates underwater are those with large muscle mass because muscle is heavier than water and sinks.

Because not everyone has access to underwater weighing facilities, the scientists who study body composition have arrived at correlational formulas that compare skinfold measurement or body circumferences with body densities derived from underwater weighing. Since weight control is just the nice name for "fat control," it cannot be stressed enough here that the *measurement of body fat is of prime importance* and *a weight goal must certainly be based on the amount of fat that must be lost.*

In dealing with amount of body fat, the currency is percentage of body fat. Jean Mayer, noted nutritionist and body composition researcher, long ago put a "clinical obesity" label on a certain maximum amount of body fat. The Seltzer-Mayer (1965) chart commonly appears in weight control logs, and from this early work these researchers determined that about 39 percent body fat would be considered clinical obesity. Thirty-nine percent body fat would mean that a 200-pound person would have 78 pounds of fat and 122 pounds of lean body mass.

An excellent attribute of the determination of percentage of body fat is that it gives the all-important calculation of how much fat a person is carrying around. It also allows for comparability among research subjects and groups. Currently, figures as low as 20 percent for men and 28 percent for women are often being considered as clinical obesity (Allsen, Harrison, and Vance, 1980).

SKINFOLDS

Although body composition can be more accurately determined through the use of underwater weighing or with high-tech methods such as x-ray, bioelectric impedence, or ultrasound, one of the most expedient ways to determine percentage of body fat is to use skinfold measurements. This, however, involves a trained professional who will measure the skinfolds and apply the proper formula.

Dr. John Burt, exercise physiologist, in research with colleagues in the Marine Corps, weighed underwater a number of college-age women and took various skinfold measurements all over their bodies (Sloan, Burt, and Blyth, 1962). Then these researchers correlated body density with skinfold measurements and found that two measurements in women and three measurements in men have a high correlation with body density derived from underwater weighing. Again, statistics provided formulas to determine percentage of body fat—this time using millimeter skinfold measurements. The two areas that gave the highest correlation measurements for women were subcutaneous tricep (back of upper arm) fat and the fat just above the hip bone. Sloan and Weir (1970) later found that the two skinfold areas that gave the highest correlation for men were midthigh and subscapular. Formulas by Sloan, Burt, and Blyth, and Sloan and Weir are given in Appendix A and are designed to be used with college-age males and females. If you are of college age and know your skinfold measurements given here, you can determine your percentage of body fat. There are also a number of other skinfold areas and formulas in use that will give good predictions of percentage of body fat.

If you are looking for access to such measurements, your best bet is a local college or university that has a health education or physical education program in weight control or physical fitness. Other possibilities may be YMCA's or YWCA's, health centers, physical fitness testing centers, and so forth that have professionally trained health or physical educators. Physicians and health spas characteristically do not employ measurement tools other than a scale and/or a tape measure.

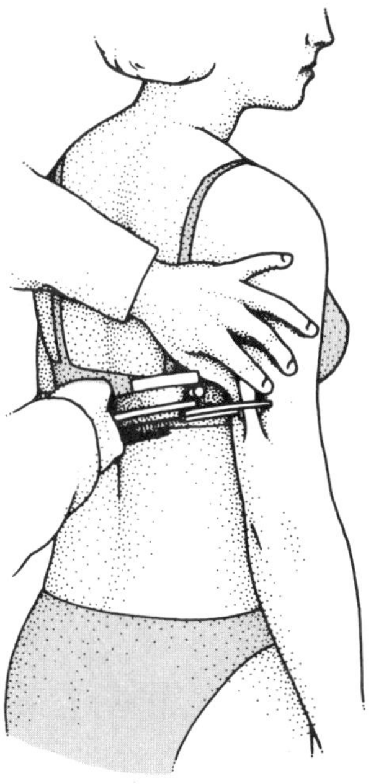

Measuring skinfolds

BODY FAT PREDICTIONS USING CIRCUMFERENCES

There are do-it-yourself techniques that utilize circumferences of various specific parts of the body, usually the waist, hips, arms, thigh, and/or chest. The body sites vary according to age and sex, thus the formula any one person would use depends on those variables. Separate tables of constants are also used according to age and sex (Katch and McArdle, 1983).

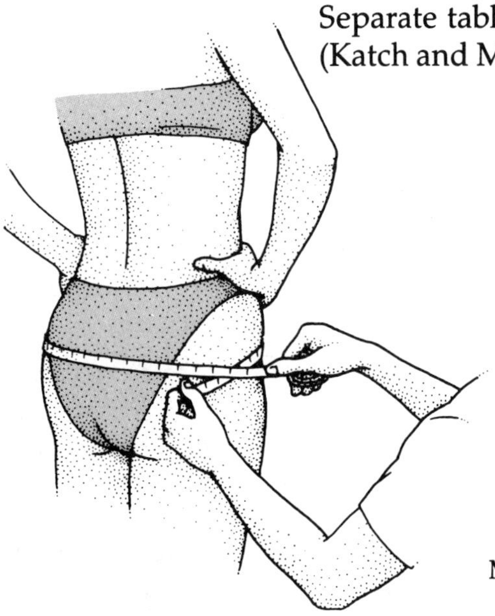

Measuring hips

Summary of Methods

With the methods given here, plus your feelings of how much you should weigh, you should be able to arrive at a magic number that you can work toward. You *will* get varying results from all the different formulas here. For example, a friend of mine applied some of them to herself and according to the MLI method, she was 10 or more pounds overweight; according to the waist measurement formula, she was within normal limits; and according to the Mahoney formula, she was 16 pounds overweight. Through knowledge about herself, her activity, and her diet, she judged that she should maintain her present weight, as her "excess" weight was musculature rather than fat.

A combination of mathematics and your feelings about your body weight and body composition will help you understand what you should weigh and/or how much fat you need to remove. If you are still unsure of what your goal should be, consult an expert.

When you choose your goal weight, it should become your lifetime weight. If you make a commitment to *get* there, also make the commitment to *stay* there. Taking off weight is not a short-term deal—it involves changing your lifestyle so that you can first achieve the percentage of body fat and the weight that you want, then maintain it for the rest of your life.

Take Your Time

A problem often encountered by my students in goal setting is one of overestimating their enthusiasm to lose weight and underestimating the time it will take to achieve the target weight. A rule of thumb in weight loss is to lose not more than two pounds or 1 percent of your current weight per week. At the maximum of two pounds per week, a 7,000 calorie deficit must be attained—about 1,000 calories a day. Extending weight reduction over a period of time seems to help in keeping the weight off, even though gratification is not so immediate. Don't be impatient with your fat—with even a small, constant calorie deficit, weight will gradually be discarded.

Other important factors in goal setting relate to your personality and value structure. As you decide to tackle weight loss, determine what the motivating factor is. Why *now* rather than last year or next month? What is the intensity of your purpose—enough to sustain you in weight reduction and then in maintenance for the rest of your life?

If you are a large percentage overweight and have been for a long period of time, consider the possibility that there will be changing relationships in your life. One student of mine was 50 pounds overweight and very good-looking. When she had lost about 30 pounds, she began to acquire admirers and had trouble in dealing with these new relationships because she still had a "fat personality" rather than a "thin, I-love-my-body-and-thus-myself personality." Some counseling, self-study, and practice in accepting herself as a lovely new person changed her whole outlook on how much fun life can be. Extending the change over a long enough period of time may help in the self-discovery process.

One of the standard miracles that seems to occur with reduced weight (especially when it's more than 10 pounds) involves enhanced self-concept and a more positive energy to share with the world. But this is caused not only by the weight reduction itself, but also by the acceptance of a healthy, holistic lifestyle change that includes increased self-responsibility, physical activity, good nutritional habits, and some stress management. And this feels so good you are willing to keep it for a lifetime!

Making Your Goal Chart

Now that you have considered changing your weight for a healthier, happier you and worked through some estimations of what your ideal or desired weight would be (hopefully also including in your calculation your percentage of body fat), use the chart in Figure 2.3 to set a goal and a path for yourself. Figure 2.2 shows a chart that was filled in by a prospective thin person. Note that actual weight was given on the earliest date and target weights were plotted for each week through 19 weeks. You can set up your chart for a month, many months, or years. By adding the line on the chart to show how you are going to achieve your weight plan, you give yourself daily or weekly goals and also long-term goals. If you have a birthday, a special holiday, or some date on your chart that will probably be calorie-laden, give yourself a break and don't expect any more than holding the weight you have achieved. Try not to add weight at that time, but if it would be too much to expect that you would take off another pound or two that week, *don't* expect it beforehand.

The person who plotted the chart in Figure 2.2 planned to work on the program through Christmas and New Year's Day. This is a brave person! Note, though, that the person planned just to hang on during Christmas and New Year's weeks, and aimed for a greater weight loss in November to compensate for those holidays.

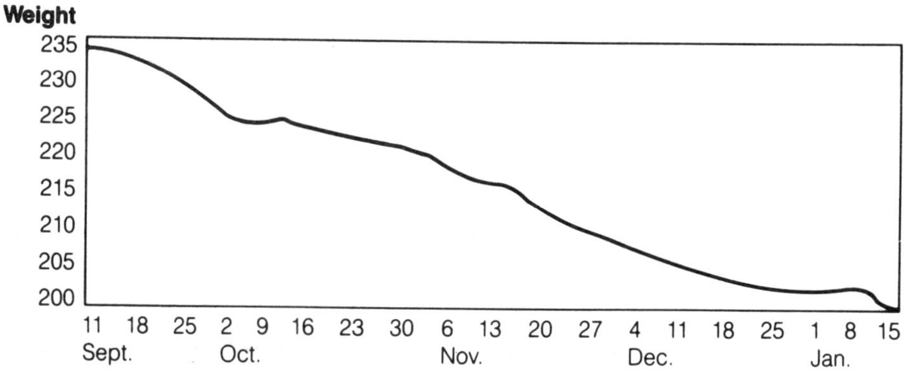

FIGURE 2.2 Sample Goal Chart

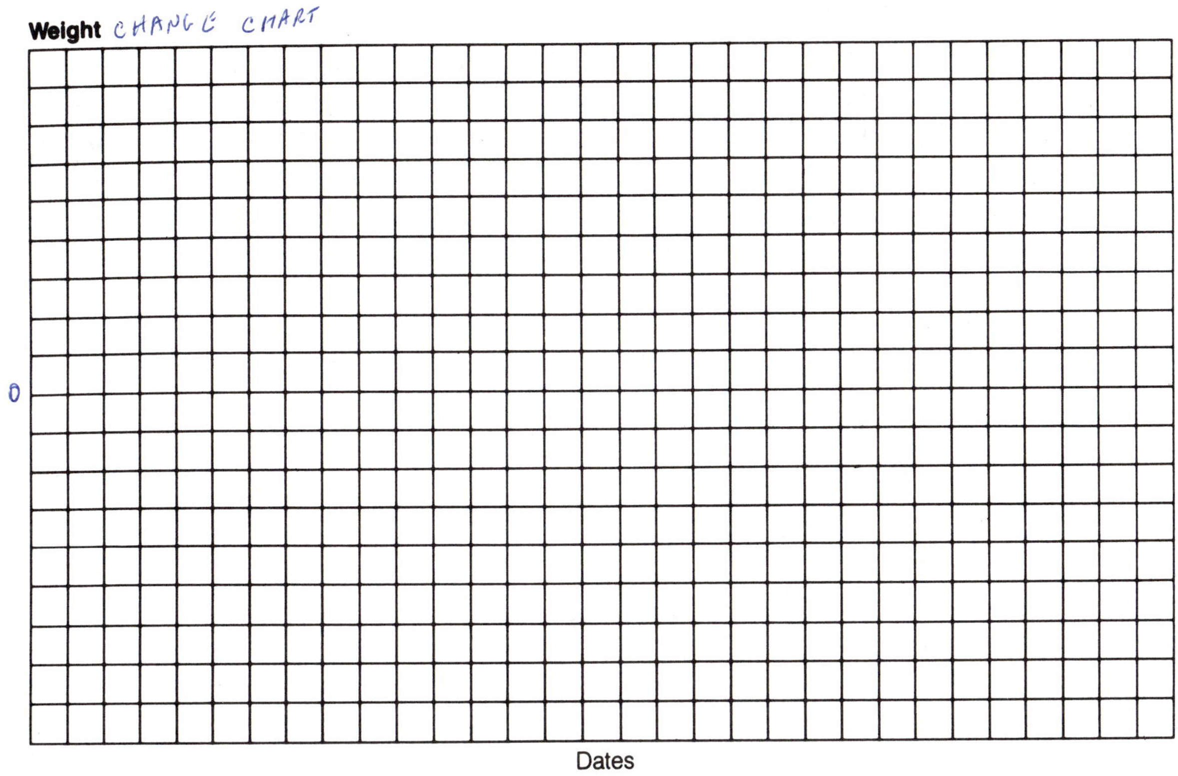

FIGURE 2.3 Your Goal Chart

On the chart in Figure 2.3, plot your present weight, your goal, and draw your path from start to finish. Add the dates that you wish to work with. Tack or tape your chart up somewhere so that you will see it every day and perhaps several times a day. Sight of the chart will be positive reinforcement for you, and you will be more likely to reach your goal and then stay there. Add a maintenance line after your goal weight and put a date on it for the year 2000 or more!

Your goal chart tells you more than just the obvious (where you are and where you are going in what amount of time), it also tells you how many calories you have to cut back or expend. In the example in Figure 2.2 the target was to lose 35 pounds between September 11 and January 15 (126 days). In order to burn one pound of fat, about 3,500 calories must be left out of the diet or expended:

$$1 \text{ pound of fat} = 3{,}500 \text{ calories}$$

So the person who plotted Figure 2.2 plans a deficit of 3,500 calories times 35 pounds, or 122,500 calories. Over a period of 126 days this is a deficit of 973 calories per day. By cutting 400 to 500 calories out of the daily menu and increasing activity to expend 500 to 600 more calories each day, this person can attain the planned goal by January 15. For detailed information on how to attain your goal, read Chapter 3.

References

Allsen, P. E., J. M. Harrison, and B. Vance. *Fitness for Life*. Dubuque, Iowa: William C. Brown, 1980.

Bray, George. *The Obese Patient*. Philadelphia: W. B. Saunders, 1976.

Frankel, H. "Determination of Body Mass Index." *Journal of the American Medical Association* 255 (1986)10:1223.

Hockey, Robert. *Physical Fitness*. St. Louis: Mosby, 1977.

Katch, Frank, and William McArdle. *Nutrition, Weight Control and Exercise*. 2nd ed. Boston: Houghton Mifflin, 1983.

Keys, A., et al. "Indices of Relative Weight and Obesity." *Journal of Chronic Diseases* 25 (1972): 329–343.

Mahoney, Michael, and Kathryn Mahoney. "How Much Should You Weigh?" *Psychology Today* (May 1978) 43.

Seltzer, C. C., and J. Mayer. "A Simple Criterion of Obesity." *Postgraduate Medicine* 38A (1965): 101–107.

Sloan, A. W., J. J. Burt, and C. S. Blyth. "Estimation of Body Fat in Young Women." *Journal of Applied Physiology* 17 (1962): 967–972.

Sloan, A. W., and J. B. de V. Weir. "Nomograms for Prediction of Body Density and Total Body Fat from Skinfold Measurements." *Journal of Applied Physiology* 28, 2 (1970): 221–222.

Suggested Readings

Conn, H., et al. (Eds). *Health and Obesity*. New York: Raven Press, 1983.

Curtix-Prior, P. (Ed). *Biochemical Pharmacology of Obesity*. New York: Elsevier, 1983.

Greenwood, M. (Ed). *Obesity*. New York: Churchill Livingstone, 1983.

Hansen, B. *Controversies in Obesity*. New York: Praeger, 1983.

Pollock, M., and A. Jackson. "Research Progress in Validation of Clinical Methods of Assessing Body Composition." *Medicine and Science in Sports and Exercise* 6 (1984): 606–613.

3 THE CALORIE CONCEPT

MANY PEOPLE entering a fitness program would like to think that there is a magic trick or sleight-of-hand manipulation that can turn them into "the body beautiful" overnight. That's why gadgets, pills, diets, and "easy weight-off" plans gross millions of dollars each year. All of this gadgetry and trickery for the general public is ineffective because removing fat from adipose tissue and shaping the body the way you want it depend upon a caloric imbalance between the food you eat and the amount and kind of physical exercise you engage in.

There are, in fact, a number of factors that determine body shape, how much weight you shed, when you get rid of it, and how easy (or hard) it is. Some of the factors are: (1) what kinds of exercise you get; (2) how often you eat; (3) what you eat; (4) what your eating history is (poor eating habits may have to be straightened out before the principles of weight reduction can work; for example, in coming off a high-sugar diet the body may take some time to get back to normal); (5) how much you eat; and (6) how much food energy you burn through energy output. The first four factors are discussed in other chapters. The last two factors will be the topic of this chapter.

The Calorie Concept

Even if your body is crazed from eating one meal a day consisting of five boxes of Cracker Jacks, your weight will drop if you eat nothing else and do some physical activity. Why? Because you have taken in fewer calories than you have burned. This is the first law of thermodynamics, or the calorie concept. This concept says that weight is reduced if caloric output (exercise) is greater than caloric input (food). This law or concept must be considered the fundamental element in changing body composition. All the other factors may embellish this one, but this is the central feature. Research is replete with studies showing that when the caloric intake and the caloric outputs of students, soldiers, and other subjects are summed over a week's time (or longer), the subjects' weights remain the same when there is a balance between input and output (Van Itallie, 1983).

The calorie concept consists of two sides of an equation as shown in Figure 3.1. One side concerns the food eaten or energy input, and the other side concerns energy output (how much physical activity is performed plus metabolic rate). It is obvious, then, that when the two sides are equal, weight is maintained; but when they are unequal, weight is gained or lost.

Undomesticated animals are examples of how nature tries to provide the innate balance of this equation so that each animal maintains weight rather than continues to gain or progressively reduce weight throughout life. However, the cerebral override of *homo sapiens* has made it possible for learned behavior to set aside nature's plan.

The Calorie, or kilocalorie, is the amount of energy it takes to heat one liter of water one degree centigrade. A kilocalorie contains 1,000 calories. Since the word *calorie* (with a small *c*) is commonly used to report the energy content of foods (for example, an 8 oz. glass of whole milk contains 150 calories), it will be used throughout this book in that manner.

The calorie is the basic currency in weight-reducing regimens. To burn off one pound of fat, approximately 3,500 calories of energy must be expended in addition to what is taken in. Conversely, for every 3,500 extra calories taken in (that are not counterbalanced by energy expenditure), there is a weight gain of one pound.

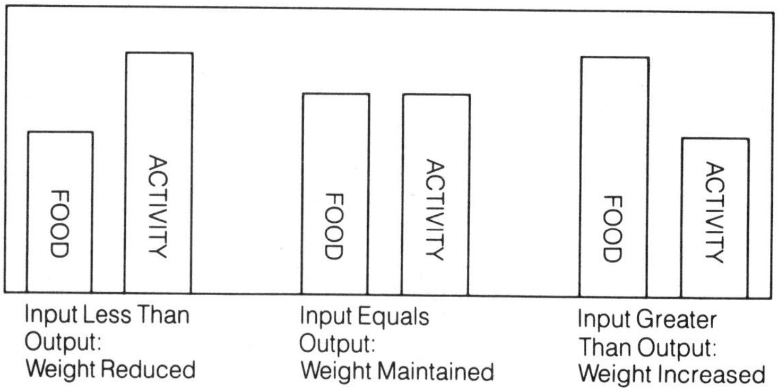

FIGURE 3.1 The Calorie Concept

The attempt at weight reduction will be no more than a frustrating experience unless the prospective weight reducer accomplishes one or more of these necessities: (1) expending more energy while maintaining usual caloric intake; (2) maintaining basic energy levels and reducing food intake; or (3) expending more energy *and* decreasing intake at the same time. What I see in the histories of most of my students is the second option—reducing intake or, in more common terms, "going on a diet," usually to a dangerously low caloric input (sometimes as low as 400 to 500 calories per day!). Very few try the first suggestion (some have such a high caloric intake that they would have to exercise all day to counterbalance it). Using only a diet or using only physical exercise to effect a caloric deficit may be discouraging and perhaps unhealthy, so the answer to weight reduction should be the third option.

Let me give you an example of weight change based on the calorie concept. One of my students, Lisa, was not an exerciser but had tried many diets in her 18-year life. She entered this program weighing 130 pounds and set a realistic goal of 120 pounds. She had to rid herself of 10 pounds (or 35,000 calories). She was maintaining her weight well, so she set an average 500-calorie deficit per day (or 3,500 calories per week) to be accomplished by reducing 250 calories in her diet and increasing her activity by 250 calories.

There are many different activities that will enable a person to expend an extra 250 calories per day (just as 250 food calories can be excluded from any food simply by reducing the portion size). But Lisa had to find an activity she could persuade herself to do at first and finally, through familiarity, enjoy later. Many students, especially those who were not encouraged to exercise or participate in sports when they were young, have found it difficult to enjoy exercise. At first they must force themselves to exercise, but they really learn to love physical activity when they discover how good it feels to control their own bodies.

So Lisa joined a three-days-per-week square dancing class that spent at least 30 minutes each class period actually dancing. Using the figures based on an average energy utilization of a 130-pound woman, Lisa figured that she burned 150 calories in her dance class per session. To expend the other 100 energy calories, she started parking her car in the farthest parking lot at school so she had to walk an extra 10 minutes from her car to her classes and back. Twenty minutes of brisk walking (usually carrying books) meant an extra 100 calories of energy output each day. Lisa had school classes five days a week and her dance class three days a week, so her classes helped her expend 500 calories and 450 calories, respectively, each week. This total of 950 calories added expenditure plus 1,750 fewer calories eaten each week brought her deficit for the week up to 2,700 calories. Needing 800 more calories of expenditure, Lisa started a running program with several friends four days per week, running 20 minutes per day with warm-up calisthenics and stretching and a five-minute cool-down walk. Each 20-minute run (at about five miles per hour) was worth about 180 calories while the warm-ups and cool-downs expended about 25 calories. So her four-times-a-week running program meant she was expending an additional 820 calories (approximately) each week. See Table 3.1 for Lisa's entire program.

At the end of each day Lisa would sit down and give herself credit for her food deficit calories and write down how much activity she had engaged in and what its caloric worth was to her. Each day did not add up to the 500 per day she had set out to accomplish, but the week's total gave her a 3,500-calorie total deficit (3,520 calories, actually). Her pound of fat per week came off almost perfectly as reflected by her scale (which she ignored except for her weekly weigh-in). There were two weeks out of the ten where the scale seemed to fool her a little due to water retention just before her menstrual period, but afterward her weight would jump down two pounds instead of one.

Lisa is a good example to study here because she accomplished her purpose almost perfectly. She didn't try to take the weight off too

TABLE 3.1 Lisa's Program of Caloric Intake and Expenditure

Name ________	*Week of* ____	____ *Week of Program*		*End Weight* ______	
	Diet Deficit	*Dancing*	*Walking*	*Running*	*Warm-up Cool-down*
Monday	250	150	100		
Tuesday	250		100	180	25
Wednesday	250	150	100		
Thursday	250		100	180	25
Friday	250	150	100		
Saturday	250			180	25
Sunday	250			180	25
Column Total	1750	450	500	720	100
Cumulative Total	1750	2200	2700	3420	3520

quickly: She reduced her food intake only a little (to 1,250 calories per day); she added some activities that were fun for her, fit her time schedule, and in which she had group support (especially at first—now she runs five times a week and likes to run alone to enjoy the early morning solitude). Needless to say, Lisa's running program has helped maintain her weight at 120 pounds for the last few years. And you might say that her running program is feeding her right, too, because in becoming aware of her body and being in control of it, she has become highly conscious of not putting low-quality foods into her diet.

Lisa's problem in mathematical terms was this:

$$\text{10 lbs. of fat} \times \text{3,500 calories} = \text{35,000 calories}$$
$$\text{(1 lb. fat} = \text{3,500 calories)}$$

Her contract with herself was to produce a 500-calorie deficit per day: 250 of those calories would be taken from her normal diet and the other 250 calories would come from extra energy output. In one week she would effect a 3,500-calorie deficit, or one pound of fat:

$$\text{500 calories} \times \text{7 days} = \text{3,500 calories or 1 lb. of fat}$$

By staying with her program Lisa took about 10 weeks to reach her goal of 120 pounds.

How did she do it? There are two critical steps Lisa had to take before she could set up her program. One step was learning how to count how many calories she ate (as seen in the Diet Records in Chapter 8), and the second was learning how to count how many calories she burned each day.

Lisa found counting calories eaten per day to be an easy task once she learned the calorie content of some basic foods and found that there were some foods that she ate almost every day. After a short while she could sit down at the end of the day, jot down the foods she had eaten, and assign them the calories she had memorized for most of them. Each day that she had to look up a new food, she would remember the caloric value. The guide to nutritive value of foods became her bible for about 10 weeks!

The system Lisa learned in order to count the approximate calories she burned each day is given on the following pages of this chapter.

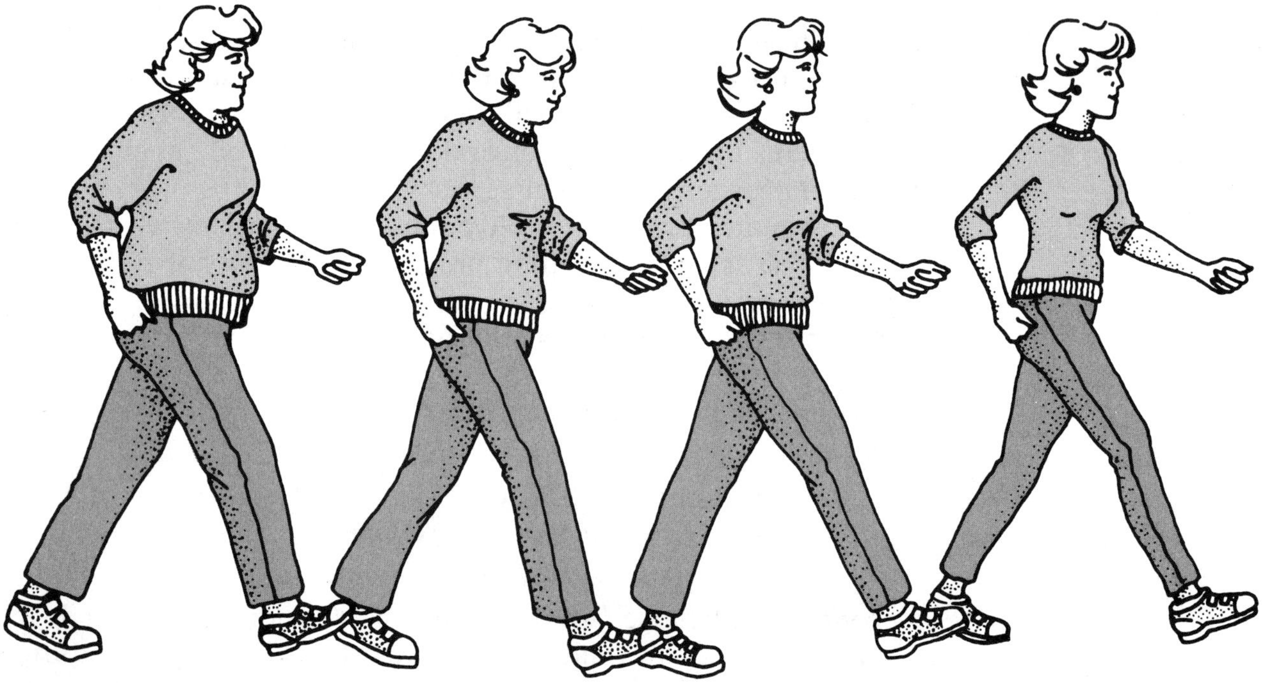

The Activity Record

Almost everyone who reads this book knows how to count calories and/or carbohydrates eaten, but the simple method of counting how many calories you expend in different activities has probably eluded you.

The system presented here is individualized and easy to work—all you have to do is record what you do in a day, assign caloric value to it, and add. The Activity Record should be kept by the *week* so you can look at your total activity pattern rather than the one day that you shovelled dirt for six hours!

On the Activity Record, fill in each quarter hour with what you did during that time. See Figure 3.2 for a sample from Lisa's Activity Record. Lisa got up about 6:30, walked a few steps to the bathroom, and took a shower. Then she stepped out of the shower, dried, and dressed for her classes. Your life won't divide into distinct 15-minute periods, but try to organize your Activity Record this way. It will be easier than a minute-to-minute record. Once you know the system, though, you *can* apply it with more precision if you wish.

If recalling your activities in 15-minute segments appears to be too difficult for you, you might begin by recording 30-minute periods or even one-hour periods if your activities do not vary a great deal during those longer periods of time. Recognize that you will be losing

FIGURE 3.2 Sample from Lisa's Activity Record

A.M.

6:00 Sleep ☐ 6:15 Sleep ☐ 6:30 Shower ☐ 6:45 Dress ☐

some information this way, though. When you start assigning calories to your activities you will have to double or quadruple the 15-minute figure that this chapter works with.

Your first step then is to begin filling out the Activity Record in Table 3.2. If you slept eight hours last night, just block out those eight hours with the word *sleep*. You can do the same thing with blocks of work or play.

THE MET SYSTEM OF ASSIGNING CALORIES TO ACTIVITY

In 1972 the American Heart Association published a booklet called *Modern Concepts of Cardiovascular Disease* that presented the MET system. The MET is a name given to a unit of human energy expenditure while the body is at rest or in its basal state (but not asleep). As energy expenditure increases, the metabolic rate increases accordingly. The metabolic cost of physical activities can be measured through direct calorimetry, and then these activities can be grouped on a scale of 1 to 10 or more METs. Ten METs is 10 times the metabolic cost of 1 MET.

The Basis of the MET. Everything we do uses oxygen. Each person burns about five calories (actually, 4.825 calories if on a mixed diet of fats, protein, and carbohydrates) for every liter of oxygen used in the body. By measuring the oxygen that the body uses in a given period of time, a caloric use can be assigned to that time also.

$$1 \text{ liter of oxygen} = 4.825 \text{ calories used in the body}$$

The process of measuring oxygen use in the human body involves sophisticated electronic equipment that is not usually available in the average home, so extensive laboratory testing has produced the norms seen in the MET tables (Tables 3.3 and 3.4).

The MET system states that at rest, the average person uses about 3.5 milliliters of oxygen per kilogram body weight per minute. This average was determined by studying the results of thousands of individual laboratory oxygen utilization tests. By using this average

TABLE 3.2 Your Activity Record

Name		*Wt.*		*¼-hr MET*		*Date*		
	¼ MET		¼ MET		¼ MET		¼ MET	Total METs per hour
A.M. 6:00		6:15		6:30		6:45		
7:00		7:15		7:30		7:45		
8:00		8:15		8:30		8:45		
9:00		9:15		9:30		9:45		
10:00		10:15		10:30		10:45		
11:00		11:15		11:30		11:45		
12:00		12:15		12:30		12:45		
P.M. 1:00		1:15		1:30		1:45		
2:00		2:15		2:30		2:45		
3:00		3:15		3:30		3:45		
4:00		4:15		4:30		4:45		
5:00		5:15		5:30		5:45		
6:00		6:15		6:30		6:45		
7:00		7:15		7:30		7:45		
8:00		8:15		8:30		8:45		
9:00		9:15		9:30		9:45		
10:00		10:15		10:30		10:45		
11:00		11:15		11:30		11:45		
12:00		12:15		12:30		12:45		
A.M. 1:00		1:15		1:30		1:45		
2:00		2:15		2:30		2:45		
3:00		3:15		3:30		3:45		
4:00		4:15		4:30		4:45		
5:00		5:15		5:30		5:45		
							Total METs per day (add down)	
							Multiply by your ¼-hour caloric expenditure	
							Total calories burned this day	

TABLE 3.3 Calories Burned per Quarter-Hour, per Hour, and per Day According to Weight

*Weight**	*Cal./Hour*	*Cal./Day*	*Cal./¼ Hr.*	*Weight**	*Cal./Hour*	*Cal./Day*	*Cal./¼ Hr.*	*Weight**	*Cal./Hour*	*Cal./Day*	*Cal./¼ Hr.*
75	34.4625	827.1	8.62	114	52.383	1257.19	13.10	153	70.3035	1687.28	17.58
76	34.922	838.128	8.73	115	52.8425	1268.22	13.21	154	70.763	1698.31	17.69
77	35.3815	849.156	8.85	116	53.302	1279.25	13.33	155	71.2225	1709.34	17.80
78	35.841	860.184	8.96	117	53.7615	1290.28	13.44	156	71.682	1720.37	17.92
79	36.3005	871.212	9.08	118	54.221	1301.3	13.55	157	72.1415	1731.4	18.04
80	36.76	882.24	9.19	119	54.6805	1312.33	13.67	158	72.601	1742.42	18.15
81	37.2195	893.268	9.30	120	55.14	1323.36	13.77	159	73.0605	1753.45	18.27
82	37.679	904.296	9.42	121	55.5995	1334.39	13.90	160	73.52	1764.48	18.38
83	38.1385	915.324	9.54	122	56.059	1345.42	14.01	161	73.9795	1775.51	18.50
84	38.598	926.352	9.65	123	56.5185	1356.44	14.13	162	74.439	1786.54	18.61
85	39.0575	937.38	9.76	124	56.978	1367.47	14.24	163	74.8985	1797.56	18.73
86	39.517	948.408	9.88	125	57.4375	1378.5	14.36	164	75.358	1808.59	18.84
87	39.9765	959.436	9.99	126	57.897	1389.53	14.47	165	75.8175	1819.62	18.95
88	40.436	970.464	10.11	127	58.3565	1400.56	14.59	166	76.277	1830.65	19.07
89	40.8955	981.492	10.22	128	58.816	1411.58	14.70	167	76.7365	1841.68	19.18
90	41.355	992.52	10.34	129	59.2755	1422.61	14.82	168	77.196	1852.7	19.30
91	41.8145	1003.55	10.45	130	59.735	1433.64	14.93	169	77.6655	1863.73	19.41
92	42.274	1014.58	10.57	131	60.1945	1444.67	15.05	170	78.115	1874.76	19.53
93	42.7335	1025.6	10.68	132	60.654	1455.7	15.16	171	78.5745	1885.79	19.64
94	43.193	1036.63	10.80	133	61.1135	1466.72	15.28	172	79.034	1896.82	19.76
95	43.6525	1047.66	10.91	134	61.573	1477.75	15.39	173	79.4935	1907.84	19.87
96	44.112	1058.69	11.02	135	62.0325	1488.78	15.50	174	79.953	1918.87	19.99
97	44.5715	1069.72	11.14	136	62.492	1499.81	15.62	175	80.4125	1929.9	20.10
98	45.031	1080.74	11.26	137	62.9515	1510.84	15.74	176	80.872	1940.93	20.22
99	45.4905	1091.77	11.37	138	63.411	1521.86	15.85	177	81.3315	1951.96	20.33
100	45.95	1102.8	11.79	139	63.8705	1532.89	15.97	178	81.791	1962.98	20.45
101	46.4095	1113.83	11.60	140	64.33	1543.92	16.08	179	82.2505	1974.01	20.56
102	46.869	1124.86	11.72	141	64.7895	1554.95	16.20	180	82.71	1985.04	20.68
103	47.3285	1135.88	11.83	142	65.249	1566.98	16.31	181	83.1695	1996.07	20.79
104	47.788	1146.91	11.95	143	65.7085	1577	16.43	182	83.629	2007.1	20.91
105	48.2475	1157.94	12.06	144	66.168	1588.03	16.54	183	84.0885	2018.12	21.02
106	48.707	1168.97	12.18	145	66.6275	1599.06	16.66	184	84.548	2029.15	21.14
107	49.1665	1180	12.29	146	67.087	1610.09	16.77	185	85.0075	2040.18	21.25
108	49.626	1191.02	12.40	147	67.5465	1621.12	16.89	186	85.467	2051.21	21.37
109	50.0855	1202.05	12.52	148	68.006	1632.14	17.00	187	85.9265	2062.24	21.48
110	50.545	1213.08	12.64	149	68.4655	1643.17	17.11	188	86.386	2073.26	21.60
111	51.0045	1224.11	12.75	150	68.925	1654.2	17.24	189	86.8455	2084.29	21.71
112	51.464	1235.14	12.87	151	69.3845	1665.23	17.35	190	87.305	2095.32	21.83
113	51.9235	1246.16	12.98	152	69.844	1676.26	17.46	191†	87.7645	2106.35	21.94

*Weight is given in pounds.
†If your weight is more than 191 pounds, divide it by 2, find that weight on the chart, and then double the calorie figure.

TABLE 3.4 Relative Metabolic Cost of Common Activities

MET Cost	*Activity*
1 MET	Awake, resting quietly, post-absorptive state (not digesting food), reading, watching TV
.85 MET	Sleeping
1.5 METs	Any moving, sitting activity such as eating, writing, sewing, typing, knitting, desk work, driving; also, stationary standing such as showering, dressing
2 METs	Light, moving, standing activity, such as cooking, strolling, and light housework
3 METs	Level walking 3 mph, cycling 6 mph, social dancing, sailing, volleyball, bowling, and heavy housework
4 METs	Walking 3.5 mph, cycling 8 mph, badminton singles, tennis doubles, ballet, many rapid calisthenics
5 METs	Walking 4 mph, cycling 10 mph, ice or roller skating, digging garden, shoveling light earth
6 METs	Walking 5 mph, cycling 11 mph, snow shovelling, tennis singles, light downhill skiing
7 METs	Jogging 5 mph, cycling 12 mph, basketball, paddleball, touch football, mountain climbing, ice hockey
8 METs	Running 5.5 mph, cycling 13 mph, vigorous basketball, social handball or racquetball.
9–10 METs	Competitive handball or racquetball, running 6 mph

Adapted from Samuel M. Fox, et al. "Physical Activity and Cardiovascular Health." *Modern Concepts of Cardiovascular Disease*. American Heart Association. June 1972, p. 27.

figure, then, you can determine how many calories you use at rest. For an example, let's return to Lisa. She weighed 130 pounds when she entered the program. To find her weight in kilograms, divide her weight in pounds by 2.2.

130 lbs./2.2 = 59 kg.

Multiply that figure by 3.5 to determine how much oxygen Lisa used at that weight.

59 kg. × 3.5 ml. of oxygen = 207 ml. oxygen (or .207 liters of oxygen)

Lisa used .207 liters of oxygen as she sat at rest each minute. To find out how many calories she expended in a minute at rest, multiply the liters of oxygen by the number of calories that can be burned by one liter of oxygen (4.825 calories).

$$.207 \times 4.825 = 1 \text{ calorie per minute}$$

If Lisa sat reading quietly for 15 minutes, she would use 15 calories (one calorie per minute at rest). If Lisa didn't do anything else but sit quietly all day, she would burn 1,440 calories.

$$1 \text{ calorie per minute} \times 60 \text{ minutes} = 60 \text{ calories per hour}$$
$$60 \text{ calories per hour} \times 24 \text{ hours} = 1{,}440 \text{ calories per day}$$

Your Caloric Utilization at Rest. To relieve you of such mathematical chores, Table 3.3 will give you your calories per quarter hour, per hour, and per day at a glance. Find your weight in pounds in the left-hand column of the appropriate section, then look at the third column of that section for your *quarter-hour* caloric expenditure. You will be working with calories burned per quarter hour because you will record your activities by the quarter hour on your Activity Record. If you wish to record your activity by the half hour, double your quarter-hour calorie figure.

Remember this figure, because it is the basis of the whole system of calorie expenditure that this program works with. This figure will change as your weight changes, so for each five pounds that you reduce, find what your new quarter-hour caloric usage is and use that new figure in your calculations.

ASSIGNING MET (CALORIE) VALUES TO YOUR ACTIVITIES

After you have listed your day's activities by quarter-hour periods on your Activity Record, your next step is to assign a calorie value to every quarter-hour activity throughout the day. Study Tables 3.4 and 3.5 to get an idea of what values are given to different activities. They range from restful, sitting activities (1 MET) to a competitive game of handball (10 METs). Not every activity you engage in will be listed, so you will have to approximate values for some activities. You will soon be able to estimate accurately which MET value to assign to your own activities.

After studying Tables 3.4 and 3.5, go back to your Activity Record, and for each 15 minutes of activity, assign an appropriate MET for it in the box provided. See Figure 3.3 to see how Lisa filled in her Activity Record. Since your metabolism drops to about 85 percent of awake basal rate when you sleep, assign the value of .85 to each of your sleeping quarter hours.

TABLE 3.5 Approximate Metabolic Cost of Activities

MET Value	*Occupational Activities*	*Recreational Activities*
.85 MET	Sleep	
1 MET		Sitting reading, watching TV
1½–2 METs	Desk work Auto driving Typing (electric) Electric calculating machine operation	Standing Walking (strolling 1 mph) Flying an airplane Motorcycling Playing cards Sewing, knitting
2–3 METs	Auto repair Radio and TV repair Janitorial work Typing (manual) Bartending	Level walking (2 mph) Level bicycling (5 mph) Riding lawn mower Billiards, bowling Shuffleboard, skeet shooting Light woodworking Powerboat driving Golf with power cart Canoeing (2½ mph) Horseback riding (at walk) Playing piano and playing many musical instruments
3–4 METs	Brick laying, plastering Pushing wheelbarrow (100 lbs.) Machine assembly Driving trailer-truck in traffic Welding (moderate load) Cleaning windows Pushing light power mower	Walking (3 mph) Horseshoe pitching Cycling (6 mph) Volleyball (6-person, noncompetitive) Sailing (handling small boat) Archery Fly fishing (standing in waders) Horseback riding (sitting to trot) Badminton (social doubles) Playing music energetically
4–5 METs	Painting, masonry Paperhanging Light carpentry Raking leaves Hoeing	Walking (3½ mph) Cycling (8 mph) Table tennis Golf (carrying clubs) Dancing (foxtrot) Badminton (singles) Tennis (doubles) Many calisthenics
5–6 METs	Digging garden Shoveling light earth	Walking (4 mph) Cycling (10 mph) Canoeing (4 mph) Horseback riding ("posting" to trot) Stream fishing (walking in light current in waders) Ice or roller skating (9 mph)

TABLE 3.5 Continued

MET Value	*Occupational Activities*	*Recreational Activities*
6–7 METs	Shovelling 10 shovelfuls per min. (10 lbs.) Splitting wood Snow shovelling Hand lawn mowing	Walking (5 mph) Cycling (11 mph) Badminton (competitive) Tennis (singles) Folk or square dancing Light downhill skiing Ski touring (2½ mph) Water skiing
7–8 METs	Digging ditches Carrying 80 lbs. Sawing hardwood	Jogging (5 mph) Cycling (12 mph) Horseback riding (gallop) Vigorous downhill skiing Basketball Mountain climbing Ice hockey Canoeing (5 mph) Paddleball Touch football
8–9 METs	Shovelling 10 shovelfuls per min. (14 lbs.)	Running (5½ mph) Cycling (13 mph) Ski touring (4 mph—loose snow) Squash racquets (social) Basketball (vigorous) Handball (social) Fencing
10 or more METs	Shovelling 10 shovelfuls per min. (16 lbs.)	Running: 6 mph = 10 METs 7 mph = 11½ METs 8 mph = 13½ METs 9 mph = 15 METs 10 mph = 17 METs Squash (competitive) Handball (competitive) Ski touring (5+ mph—loose snow)

Adapted from Samuel M. Fox, et al. "Physical Activity and Cardiovascular Health." *Modern Concepts of Cardiovascular Disease.* American Heart Association, June 1972. Reprinted by permission of the American Heart Association, Inc.

As you work through your Activity Record, if you do not find your activity in the tables and you have to approximate, err to the *lower* side. If you err one-half MET on the higher side for several hours of activity per day, you may become convinced that you're a metabolic wreck and/or that the MET system is crazy. Just as in counting the calories you eat, you must honestly record what activity you have done or your feedback will be erroneous.

TABLE 3.6 Calorie Expenditure per Minute for Various Activities

Activity	*Body Weight in Pounds*																					
	90	*99*	*108*	*117*	*125*	*134*	*143*	*152*	*161*	*170*	*178*	*187*	*196*	*205*	*213*	*222*	*231*	*240*	*249*	*257*	*266*	*275*
Archery	3.1	3.4	3.7	4.0	4.5	4.6	4.9	5.2	5.5	5.8	6.1	6.4	6.7	7.0	7.3	7.6	7.9	8.2	8.5	8.8	9.1	9.4
Badminton (recreation)	3.4	3.8	4.1	4.4	4.8	5.1	5.4	5.6	6.1	6.4	6.8	7.1	7.4	7.8	8.1	8.3	8.8	9.1	9.4	9.8	10.1	10.4
Badminton (competition)	5.9	6.4	7.0	7.6	8.1	8.7	9.3	9.9	10.4	11.0	11.6	12.1	12.7	13.3	13.9	14.4	15.0	15.6	16.1	16.7	17.3	17.9
Baseball (player)	2.8	3.1	3.4	3.6	3.9	4.2	4.5	4.7	5.0	5.3	5.5	5.8	6.1	6.4	6.6	6.9	7.2	7.5	7.7	8.0	8.3	8.6
Baseball (pitcher)	3.5	3.9	4.3	4.6	5.0	5.3	5.7	6.0	6.4	6.7	7.1	7.4	7.8	8.1	8.5	8.8	9.2	9.5	9.9	10.2	10.6	10.9
Basketball (half-court)	2.5	3.3	3.5	3.8	4.1	4.4	4.7	4.9	5.3	5.6	5.9	6.2	6.4	6.7	7.0	7.3	7.5	7.6	8.2	8.5	8.8	9.0
Basketball (moderate)	4.2	4.6	5.0	5.5	5.9	6.3	6.7	7.1	7.5	7.9	8.3	8.8	9.2	9.6	10.0	10.4	10.8	11.2	11.6	12.1	12.5	12.9
Basketball (competition)	5.9	6.5	7.1	7.7	8.2	8.8	9.4	10.0	10.6	11.1	11.7	12.3	12.9	13.5	14.0	14.6	15.0	15.2	16.3	16.9	17.5	18.1
Bicycling (level) 5.5 mph	3.0	3.3	3.6	3.9	4.2	4.5	4.8	5.1	5.4	5.6	5.9	6.2	6.5	6.8	7.1	7.4	7.7	8.0	8.3	8.6	8.9	9.2
Bicycling (level) 13 mph	6.4	7.1	7.7	8.3	8.9	9.6	10.2	10.8	11.4	12.1	12.7	13.4	14.0	14.6	15.2	15.9	16.5	17.1	17.8	18.4	19.0	19.6
Bowling (nonstop)	4.0	4.4	4.8	5.2	5.6	5.9	6.3	6.7	7.1	7.5	7.9	8.3	8.7	9.1	9.5	9.8	10.2	10.6	11.0	11.4	11.8	12.2
Boxing (sparring)	3.0	3.3	3.6	3.9	4.2	4.5	4.8	5.1	5.4	5.6	5.9	6.2	6.5	6.8	7.1	7.4	7.7	8.0	8.3	8.6	8.9	9.2
Calisthenics	3.0	3.3	3.6	3.9	4.2	4.5	4.8	5.1	5.4	5.6	5.9	6.2	6.5	6.8	7.1	7.4	7.7	8.0	8.3	8.6	8.9	9.2
Canoeing, 2.5 mph	1.8	1.9	2.0	2.2	2.3	2.5	2.7	3.0	3.2	3.4	3.6	3.7	3.9	4.1	4.7	4.4	4.6	4.8	5.0	5.1	5.3	5.5
Canoeing, 4.0 mph	4.2	4.6	5.0	5.5	5.9	6.3	6.7	7.1	7.5	7.9	8.3	8.7	9.2	9.4	10.0	10.5	10.8	11.2	11.6	12.0	12.4	12.9
Dance, modern (moderate)	2.5	2.8	3.0	3.2	3.5	3.7	4.0	4.2	4.5	4.7	5.0	5.2	5.4	5.7	5.9	6.2	6.4	6.7	6.9	7.2	7.4	7.6
Dance, modern (vigorous)	3.4	3.7	4.1	4.4	4.7	5.1	5.4	5.7	6.1	6.4	6.7	7.1	7.4	7.7	8.1	8.4	8.7	9.1	9.4	9.7	10.1	10.4
Dance, fox-trot	2.7	2.9	3.2	3.4	3.7	4.0	4.2	4.5	4.7	5.0	5.3	5.5	5.8	6.0	6.3	6.6	6.8	7.1	7.3	7.6	7.9	8.1
Dance, rumba	4.2	4.6	5.0	5.4	5.8	6.2	6.6	7.0	7.4	7.8	8.2	8.6	9.0	9.4	9.8	10.2	10.6	11.0	11.5	11.9	12.3	12.6
Dance, square	4.1	4.5	4.9	5.3	5.7	6.1	6.5	6.9	7.3	7.8	8.1	8.5	8.9	9.3	9.7	10.1	10.5	10.9	11.3	11.7	12.1	12.4
Dance, waltz	3.1	3.4	3.7	4.0	4.3	4.6	4.9	5.2	5.5	5.8	6.1	6.4	6.7	7.0	7.3	7.6	7.9	8.2	8.5	8.8	9.1	9.4
Fencing (moderate)	3.0	3.3	3.6	3.9	4.2	4.5	4.8	5.1	5.4	5.6	6.0	6.2	6.5	6.8	7.1	7.4	7.7	8.0	8.3	8.6	8.9	9.2
Fencing (vigorous)	6.2	6.8	7.4	8.0	8.6	9.2	9.8	8.7	11.0	11.6	12.2	12.8	13.4	14.0	14.6	15.2	15.8	16.4	17.0	17.6	18.2	18.8
Football (moderate)	3.0	3.3	3.6	4.0	4.2	4.5	4.8	5.1	5.4	5.7	6.0	6.2	6.5	6.8	7.1	7.4	7.7	8.0	8.3	8.6	8.9	9.2
Football (vigorous)	5.0	5.5	6.0	6.4	6.9	7.4	7.9	8.4	8.9	9.4	9.8	10.3	10.8	11.3	11.8	12.3	12.8	13.2	13.7	14.2	14.7	15.2
Golf, twosome	3.3	3.6	3.9	4.2	4.5	4.8	5.2	5.5	5.8	6.1	6.4	6.7	7.1	7.4	7.7	8.0	8.3	8.6	9.0	9.3	9.6	10.0
Golf, foursome	2.4	2.7	2.9	3.2	3.4	3.6	3.9	4.1	4.3	4.6	4.8	5.1	5.3	5.5	5.8	6.0	6.2	6.5	6.7	7.0	7.2	7.4
Handball	5.9	6.4	7.0	7.6	8.1	8.7	9.3	9.9	10.4	11.0	11.6	12.1	12.7	13.3	13.9	14.4	15.0	15.6	16.1	16.7	17.3	17.9
Hiking, 40 lb. pack, 3.0 mph	4.1	4.5	4.9	5.3	5.7	6.1	6.5	6.9	7.3	7.7	8.1	8.5	8.9	9.3	9.7	10.1	10.5	10.9	11.3	11.7	12.1	12.5
Horseback riding (walk)	2.0	2.3	2.4	2.6	2.8	3.0	3.1	3.3	3.5	3.7	3.9	4.1	4.3	4.5	4.7	4.9	5.1	5.3	5.5	5.7	5.8	6.0
Horseback riding (trot)	4.1	4.4	4.8	5.2	5.6	6.0	6.4	6.8	7.2	7.6	8.0	8.4	8.8	9.2	9.6	10.0	10.4	10.8	11.2	11.6	12.0	12.4
Horseshoe pitching	2.1	2.3	2.5	2.7	3.0	3.3	3.4	3.6	3.8	4.0	4.2	4.4	4.6	4.8	5.0	5.2	5.4	5.6	5.8	6.0	6.3	6.5
Judo, Karate	7.7	8.5	9.2	10.0	10.7	11.5	12.2	13.0	13.7	14.5	15.2	16.0	16.7	17.5	18.2	19.0	19.7	20.5	21.2	22.0	22.7	23.5
Mountain climbing	6.0	6.5	7.2	7.8	8.4	9.0	9.6	10.1	10.7	11.3	11.9	12.5	13.1	13.7	14.3	14.8	15.4	16.0	16.6	17.2	17.8	18.4
Paddleball, Racquetball	5.9	6.4	7.0	7.6	8.1	8.7	9.3	9.9	10.4	11.0	11.6	12.1	12.7	13.3	13.9	14.4	15.0	15.6	16.1	16.7	17.3	17.9
Pool, Billiards	1.1	1.2	1.3	1.4	1.5	1.6	1.7	1.8	1.9	2.0	2.1	2.2	2.4	2.5	2.6	2.7	2.8	2.9	3.0	3.1	3.2	3.3
Rowing (recreation)	3.0	3.3	3.6	3.9	4.2	4.5	4.8	5.1	5.4	5.6	6.0	6.2	6.5	6.8	7.1	7.5	7.7	8.0	8.3	8.6	8.9	9.2
Rowing (machine)	8.2	9.0	9.8	10.6	11.4	12.2	13.0	13.8	14.6	15.4	16.2	17.0	17.8	18.6	19.4	20.2	21.0	21.8	22.6	23.4	24.2	25.0
Running, 11-min. mile (5.5 mph)	6.4	7.1	7.7	8.3	9.0	9.6	10.2	10.8	11.5	12.1	12.7	13.4	14.0	14.6	15.2	15.9	16.5	17.1	17.8	18.4	19.0	19.6
Running, 8.5-min. mile (7 mph)	8.4	9.2	10.0	10.8	11.7	12.5	13.3	14.1	14.9	15.7	16.6	17.4	18.2	19.0	19.8	20.7	21.5	22.3	23.1	23.9	24.8	25.6

TABLE 3.6 Continued

Activity	*Body Weight in Pounds*																				
	90	*99*	*108*	*117*	*125*	*134*	*143*	*152*	*161*	*170*	*178*	*187*	*196*	*205*	*213*	*222*	*231*	*240*	*249*	*257*	*266*	*275*
Running, 7-min. mile (9 mph)	9.3	10.2	11.1	12.9	13.1	13.9	14.8	15.7	16.6	17.5	18.9	19.3	20.2	21.1	22.1	23.0	23.9	24.8	25.7	26.6	27.5	28.4
Running, 5-min. mile (12 mph)	11.8	13.0	14.1	15.3	16.4	17.6	18.7	19.9	21.0	22.2	23.3	24.5	25.6	26.8	27.9	29.1	30.2	31.4	32.5	33.7	34.9	36.0
Stationary running (140 counts/min)	14.6	16.1	17.5	18.9	20.4	21.8	23.2	24.6	26.1	27.5	28.9	30.4	31.8	33.2	34.6	36.1	37.5	38.9	40.4	41.8	43.2	44.6
Sprinting	13.8	15.2	16.6	17.9	19.2	20.5	21.9	23.3	24.7	26.1	27.3	28.7	30.0	31.4	32.7	34.0	35.4	36.8	38.2	39.4	40.3	42.2
Sailing	1.8	2.0	2.1	2.3	2.4	2.7	2.8	3.0	3.2	3.4	3.6	3.8	3.9	4.1	4.3	4.4	4.6	4.8	5.0	5.1	5.3	5.5
Skating (moderate)	3.4	3.8	4.1	4.4	4.8	5.1	5.4	5.8	6.1	6.4	6.8	7.1	7.4	7.8	8.1	8.3	8.8	9.1	9.4	9.8	10.1	10.4
Skating (vigorous)	6.2	6.8	7.4	8.0	8.6	9.2	9.8	9.9	11.0	11.6	12.2	12.8	13.4	14.0	14.6	15.2	15.8	16.4	17.0	17.6	18.2	18.8
Skiing (downhill)	5.8	6.4	6.9	7.5	8.1	8.6	9.2	9.8	10.3	10.9	11.4	12.0	12.6	13.1	13.7	14.3	14.8	15.4	16.0	16.5	17.1	17.7
Skiing (level, 5 mph)	7.0	7.7	8.4	9.1	9.8	10.5	11.1	11.8	12.5	13.2	13.9	14.6	15.2	15.9	16.6	17.3	18.0	18.7	19.4	20.0	20.7	21.4
Skiing (racing downhill)	9.9	10.9	11.9	12.9	13.7	14.7	15.7	16.7	17.7	18.7	19.6	20.6	21.6	22.6	23.4	24.4	25.4	26.4	27.4	28.3	29.3	30.2
Snowshoeing (2.3 mph)	3.7	4.1	4.5	4.8	5.2	5.5	5.9	6.3	6.7	7.0	7.4	7.8	8.1	8.5	8.8	9.2	9.6	9.9	10.3	10.6	11.0	11.4
Snowshoeing (2.5 mph)	5.4	5.9	6.5	7.0	7.5	8.0	8.6	9.1	9.7	10.2	10.7	11.2	11.8	12.3	12.8	13.3	13.9	14.4	14.9	15.4	16.0	16.5
Soccer	5.4	5.9	6.4	6.9	7.5	8.0	8.5	9.0	9.6	10.1	10.6	11.1	11.6	12.2	12.7	13.2	13.4	14.3	14.8	15.3	15.8	16.9
Squash	6.2	6.8	7.5	8.1	8.7	9.3	9.9	10.5	11.1	11.7	12.3	12.9	13.5	14.2	14.8	15.4	16.0	16.6	17.2	17.8	18.4	19.0
Swimming, pleasure (25 yds./min.)	3.6	4.0	4.3	4.7	5.0	5.4	5.7	6.1	6.4	6.8	7.1	7.5	7.8	8.2	8.5	8.9	9.2	9.6	10.0	10.3	10.6	11.0
Swimming, back (20 yds./min.)	2.3	2.6	2.8	3.0	3.2	3.5	3.7	3.9	4.1	4.2	4.6	4.8	5.0	5.3	5.5	5.7	6.0	6.2	6.4	6.6	6.9	7.1
Swimming, back (30 yds./min.)	3.2	3.5	3.8	4.1	4.4	4.7	5.1	5.4	5.7	6.0	6.3	6.6	6.9	7.2	7.4	7.9	8.2	8.5	8.8	9.1	9.4	9.7
Swimming, back (40 yds./min.)	5.0	5.5	5.8	6.5	7.0	7.5	7.9	8.5	8.9	9.4	9.9	10.4	10.9	11.4	11.9	12.3	12.8	13.3	13.8	14.3	14.8	15.3
Swimming, breast (20 yds./min.)	2.9	3.2	3.4	3.8	4.0	4.3	4.6	4.9	5.1	5.4	5.7	6.0	6.3	6.5	6.8	7.1	7.4	7.7	7.9	8.2	8.5	8.8
Swimming, breast (30 yds./min.)	4.3	4.8	5.2	5.7	6.0	6.4	6.9	7.3	7.7	8.1	8.6	9.0	9.4	9.9	10.3	10.8	11.1	11.5	11.9	12.4	13.0	13.3
Swimming, breast (40 yds./min.)	5.8	6.3	6.9	7.5	8.0	8.6	9.2	9.7	10.3	10.8	11.4	12.0	12.5	13.1	13.7	14.2	14.8	15.4	15.9	16.5	17.0	17.6
Swimming, butterfly (50 yds./min.)	7.0	7.7	8.4	9.1	9.8	10.5	11.1	11.9	12.5	13.2	13.9	14.6	15.2	15.9	16.6	17.3	18.0	18.7	19.4	20.0	20.7	21.4
Swimming, crawl (20 yds./min.)	2.9	3.2	3.4	3.8	4.0	4.3	4.6	4.9	5.1	5.4	5.7	5.8	6.3	6.5	6.8	7.1	7.3	7.7	7.9	8.2	8.5	8.8
Swimming, crawl (45 yds./min.)	5.2	5.8	6.3	6.8	7.3	7.8	8.3	8.8	9.3	9.8	10.4	10.9	11.4	11.9	12.4	12.9	13.4	13.9	14.4	15.0	15.5	16.0
Swimming, crawl (50 yds./min.)	6.4	7.0	7.6	8.3	8.9	9.5	10.1	10.7	11.4	12.0	12.6	13.2	13.9	14.5	15.1	15.7	16.3	17.0	17.4	17.9	18.8	19.5
Table Tennis	2.3	2.6	2.8	3.0	3.2	3.5	3.7	3.9	4.1	4.2	4.6	4.8	5.0	5.3	5.5	5.7	6.0	6.2	6.4	6.6	6.9	7.1
Tennis (recreation)	4.2	4.6	5.0	5.4	5.8	6.2	6.6	7.0	7.4	7.8	8.2	8.6	9.0	9.4	9.8	10.2	10.6	11.0	11.5	11.9	12.3	12.6
Tennis (competition)	5.9	6.4	7.0	7.6	8.1	8.7	9.3	9.9	10.4	11.0	11.6	12.1	12.7	13.3	13.9	14.4	15.0	15.6	16.1	16.7	17.3	17.9
Timed calisthenics	8.8	9.6	10.5	11.4	12.2	13.1	13.9	14.8	15.6	16.5	17.4	18.2	19.1	19.9	20.8	21.5	22.5	23.9	24.2	25.1	25.9	26.8
Volleyball (moderate)	3.4	3.8	4.0	4.4	4.8	5.1	5.4	5.8	6.1	6.4	6.8	7.1	7.4	7.8	8.1	8.3	8.8	9.1	9.4	9.8	10.1	10.4
Volleyball (vigorous)	5.9	6.4	7.0	7.6	8.1	8.7	9.3	9.9	10.4	11.0	11.6	12.1	12.7	13.3	13.9	14.4	15.0	15.6	16.1	16.7	17.3	17.9
Walking (2.0 mph)	2.1	2.3	2.5	2.7	2.9	3.1	3.3	3.5	3.7	4.0	4.2	4.4	4.6	4.8	5.0	5.2	5.4	5.6	5.8	6.0	6.2	6.4
Walking (4.5 mph)	4.0	4.4	4.7	5.1	5.5	5.9	6.3	6.7	7.1	7.5	7.8	8.2	8.6	9.0	9.4	9.8	10.1	10.6	10.9	11.3	11.7	12.0
Walking 110–120 steps/min.	3.1	3.4	3.7	4.0	4.3	4.7	5.0	5.3	5.6	5.9	6.2	6.5	6.8	7.1	7.4	7.7	8.0	8.3	8.6	8.9	9.2	9.5
Waterskiing	4.7	5.1	5.6	6.1	6.5	7.0	7.4	7.9	8.3	8.8	9.3	9.7	10.2	10.6	11.1	11.5	12.0	12.5	12.9	13.4	13.8	14.3
Weight training	4.7	5.1	5.7	6.2	6.7	7.0	7.5	7.9	8.4	8.9	9.4	9.9	10.3	10.8	11.1	11.7	12.2	12.6	13.1	13.5	14.0	14.4
Wrestling	7.7	8.5	9.2	10.0	10.7	11.5	12.2	13.0	13.7	14.5	15.2	16.0	16.7	17.5	18.2	19.0	19.7	20.5	21.2	22.0	22.7	23.5

Adapted from Frank C. Consolazio, et al. *Physiological Measurements of Metabolic Functions in Man*. New York: McGraw-Hill, 1963. Reprinted by permission.

A.M.

6:00	Sleep	.85	6:15	Sleep	.85	6:30	Shower	1.5	6:45	Dress	1.5
7:00	B'fast	1.5	7:15	Read Paper	1	7:30	Drive	1.5	7:45	Fast Walk to class	3

FIGURE 3.3. Sample from Lisa's Activity Record

TOTAL CALORIE OUTPUT OF YOUR ACTIVITIES

When you have all the blocks filled in your Activity Record, add each line across and then add down that column to find the total METs for the day. Multiply that figure by your quarter-hour caloric expenditure, and the result will be the number of calories you expended that day. (See Figure 3.4 for an example.)

In the two hours of the sample Lisa had 11.7 METs of activity. Multiplying these METs by her quarter-hour calorie usage (15), you can see that she burned 175.5 calories over this period of time.

Compare Input to Output

Once you have determined your approximate caloric expenditure in a day, compare it with your caloric intake. Unless you don't vary much in your activity or diet, one day won't tell you anything about your weight trend. But at the end of a week, calculate your total output (for seven days) and compare it with your total input (for seven days). If you show a caloric deficit around 3,500 calories, the scale will probably reflect the loss of that pound.

Remember, however, that although the calorie concept is a basic principle in weight reduction, there are other considerations, such as water retention (especially for females), when you weigh yourself, whether you are starving yourself, what kinds of food you are eating, and so on. Give yourself some time to get used to your new lifestyle. If you follow the whole program, pounds will come off and stay off.

Don't throw out this system if it doesn't please you at the end of one week or seems too difficult to deal with in the beginning. As you learn to use the system, you will learn to simplify it just as you did in counting your caloric intake.

Other Calorie Counters

Table 3.6 shows another way to calculate the approximate calories burned for many popular sports and other activities such as walking

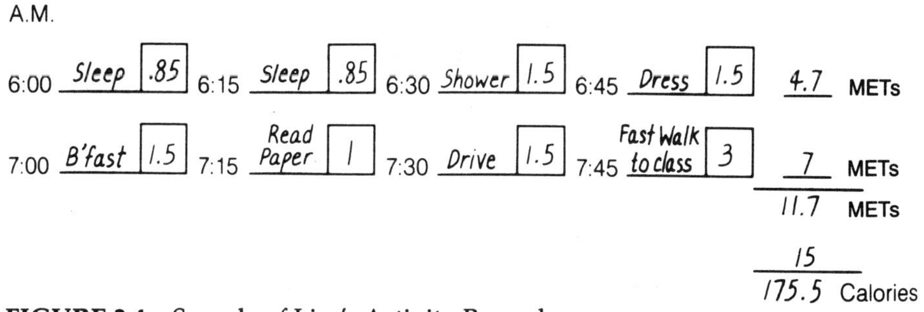

FIGURE 3.4 Sample of Lisa's Activity Record

and dancing. Find the column that represents your weight in pounds the closest and multiply the figure given for your activity by the number of minutes that you engage in it. I find that this is a good adjunct to the MET system because it does list more sports activities than the MET tables.

To use it with the MET system, just substitute the calories burned in this activitiy for 15, 30, or 45 minutes (and so on) for the MET calories you have approximated (or perhaps couldn't approximate).

Did It Surprise You?

As you look at your days' activities with the MET values filled in on your Activity Record, are you surprised to see so many time periods with a MET value of 1 or 2? If you don't have any activities worth more than 2 or 3 METs, this record is telling you what you will have to do in order to start your thinness lifestyle – find higher MET activities to engage in. Lisa solved her problem by adding a dance class three times per week that gave her an added output of 150 calories per class; she started running four times each week, worth about 180 calories per run; and she expended 100 calories per day in walking from the far end of the parking lot to her classes. She also cut 250 calories per day from her menu. So at the end of the week she was seeing on her record a deficit of 1,750 calories from eating and 450 calories added to her output from dancing, 500 from walking, and 720 from running. Her excess output over input averaged 3,520 calories per week, which was equal to one pound of fat.

Lisa's pound of fat per week came off almost perfectly, and she met her goal in 10 weeks. Lisa designed her program to lose 10 pounds in a very successful manner – she didn't try to reduce weight too quickly, she decreased her food intake only a little; she added some activities that were fun for her, fit her time schedule, and in which she had some group support. By understanding and using the calorie concept, Lisa is still (three years later) maintaining her desired weight successfully.

References

Consolazio, Frank C., et al., *Physiological Measurements of Metabolic Functions in Man*. New York: McGraw-Hill, 1963.

Fox, Samuel M., et al. "Physical Activity and Cardiovascular Health." *Modern Concepts of Cardiovascular Disease*. American Heart Association. June 1972, p. 27.

Van Itallie, T.B. "Some Determinants of Body Fat Content," in Conn, H. L., Jr., DeFelice, E. A. & Kuo P. (Eds). *Health and Obesity*. New York: Raven Press, 1983.

Suggested Readings

Drews, F., et al. *A Healthy Life*. New York: Benchmark Press, 1986.

Martin, D., et al. *Harper's Review of Biochemistry*. 20th Edition. Los Altos, CA: Lange, 1985.

Pollock, M., et al. *Exercise in Health and Disease*. Philadelphia: W. B. Saunders, 1984.

Reader's Digest. *The Complete Manual of Fitness and Well-Being*. Pleasantville, NY: Reader's Digest Association, 1984.

4 FAT: HOW THE HUMAN BODY STORES EXCESS FOOD

Storage Systems

Because humans do not constantly eat (in the way that horses or cows continually graze), nature has endowed humans with storage systems for the specific foodstuffs to be used when blood sugar, amino acids, or energy levels drop below a certain optimal level.

Actually, *proteins* (specifically, their components, amino acids) have no storehouse except that which maintains the delicate balance in the blood. However, nonessential amino acids can be synthesized by the body from other substances, and so one might say there is a limited reserve of protein building blocks in an individual who is fed.

Carbohydrates have a storage form—liver and muscle *glycogen*. The storage system cannot accommodate enough glucose (blood sugar) per se to sustain life for very long because the body would need too much water to balance out the number of particles of glucose that would supply sufficient energy until refeeding. So the body puts many glucose particles together in the crystallized form of glycogen, which needs little water to offset it when compared to the water needed by the individual glucose molecules. During starvation, glycogen stores can feed a person for about half a day.

Glycogen is made from glucose when blood sugar goes above starvation level. *Liver glycogen* stores are immediate suppliers of glucose when it is needed for energy or blood sugar, but *muscle glycogen* cannot be released from the muscle cell to assist blood glucose levels—it can be used only for energy demands of the muscle cell itself. Again, nature designed a storage system so that if an emergency arose, the body would have "instant energy."

With limited ability to store protein and carbohydrates, the human body uses *fat deposits* as its greatest energy reserve. In our modern affluence we tend to think of body fat as ugly, a stroke of bad luck, rather than as life-sustaining, stored energy. During starvation periods our fat stores are extremely important—they provide muscle and other organ tissues with energy while blood glucose is reserved for the brain and other specialized tissues, and proteins are reserved for structural purposes.

If you eat breakfast at 7:00 A.M., lunch at noon, and dinner at 6:00 P.M., you are using stored fat for energy before each meal, even though during each of these time periods you are not actually "starving" as the word is commonly meant.

Fat Cells and Adipose Tissue

When a sponge is dipped into water, the cells become engorged and will retain the water until it runs out, is squeezed out, or dries out. In dry form, the sponge cells are diminished in size but have the potential for swelling. Although not quite so simply, fat cells in the adipose (or fat) tissues of the body act in somewhat the same fashion. Each fat cell is a potential space to be filled with fat made from foods that are eaten but not utilized for energy. Unfortunately, you cannot just squeeze the fat out or wait for it to dry out, as in the case of the sponge. Instead, your body must break down the contents of the fat cell and utilize it by expending energy.

NUMBER AND LOCATION OF FAT CELLS

Each individual is endowed with a given number of fat cells that are distributed throughout the body (about half the body fat is subcutaneous—just under the skin; the other half surrounds the deep organs such as the heart and liver). Inheritance and gender determine which parts of the body will have more or less fat than others. Females characteristically have more potential for fat deposits around the hips, upper thighs, breasts, and back, while males generally have greater potential for deposits around the waist and abdomen.

Each individual who loses and gains weight may notice a pattern of loss or gain—for example, one may lose weight in the chest area first, then the waist, then the thighs, and finally in the hips and buttocks. Weight gain will generally occur in the reverse pattern. Most of those who continually seek a lower target weight have one area that seems loathe to give up its fat, but it generally has the most fat and thus is the last area to respond to a weight reduction program.

Genetic pattern decides where the individual will lose weight first or last, and no amount of cajoling, hip bumping against the wall, waist twisting, or body wrapping will induce the fat cells in a specific area to dissolve and remove the fatty acids from inside the cell. When energy demand becomes high enough, the body will tap various sources, and if this continues long enough, unsightly fat deposits will eventually be utilized as energy. Localized exercise is good for increasing muscle tone, and inches may be lost if the muscle is contracted with greater strength and more often than previously. But waist exercises, for example, will not unequivocally take fat off the waist. That is, the energy required to do a specific waist exercise will not necessarily come from the fatty acids stored in the adipose tissue around the waist.

THE FAT CELL

To further understand the concept of fat loss from adipose cells, you should understand fat cells themselves. The structure of a *fat cell* is seen in Figure 4.1. *Adipose tissue deposits* contain many fat cells that are held together with fascia-type (membranous connective) material. The number of fat cells you have is dependent upon heredity and perhaps upon early feeding.

Subcutaneous adipose tissue consists of about 3 percent protein (membranous tissue), 14 percent water in and around the fascia, and 83 percent concentrated fat. Fat deposits can also be found in muscle. The fat cell (or adipocyte) consists of a large proportion of fat, a membrane coat, and a small proportion of cytoplasm that houses organelles (nucleus, mitochondria, and so on) that can generally be found in all cells of the body.

In early growth and development fat cells have the ability to increase in number or multiply. Normally, this occurs during the first nine months of life, then there is a slight increment around age 7 and a final spurt during adolescence (Kannel, 1983). Research indicates that overnutrition, or overfeeding, in early life promotes fat cell multiplication (Wishon, et al., 1983), and so we are learning that a fat baby is not necessarily a healthy baby. For some years it was thought that adipose tissue cell multiplication occurred only during these critical periods before adulthood. More recent research shows that fat cell

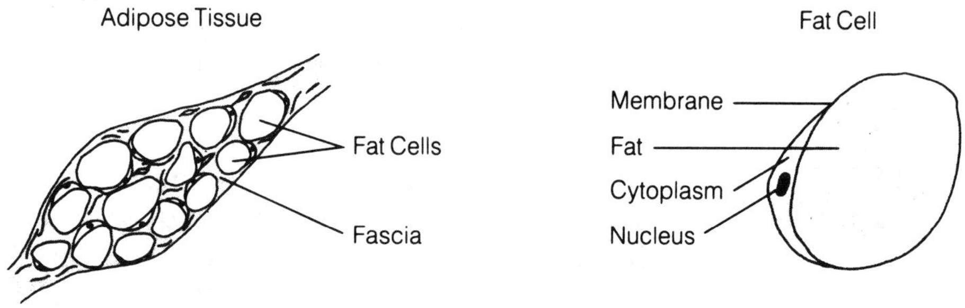

FIGURE 4.1 Adipose Tissue and Fat Cell

multiplication does occur in adulthood as a response to filling the fat cells to their maximal size (Bjorntorp, 1983).

Triglycerides—The Storage Form of Fat

The part of the fat cell of most interest to those who are weight conscious is the vacuole or potential space that can be filled with *fatty acids* that have been joined to a carbohydrate substance, *glycerol.* When three fatty acids are joined to glycerol, the substance is called a *triglyceride,* and in the majority of cases this is the form of stored fat.

The whole process of gaining weight centers on the synthesis and storage of triglycerides, while weight reduction occurs with the breakdown, removal, and utilization of this substance from the fat cell. The main factors in this process are the three basic foodstuffs—carbohydrates and simple sugars, fats, and protein. The manner in which these foodstuffs are eaten—how often, how much, exercise patterns, the presence of necessary vitamins and minerals, and even one's state of mind—will determine what happens to the lowly fat cell. Before examining each foodstuff as a contributor to fat stores, let's consider four general concepts about eating and whether our bodies store what we eat or not. These concepts are:

1. All foods can become fat—there are no "good guys" such as tuna and broccoli and no "bad guys" such as potatoes.
2. Blood glucose controls when the body will store fat and when it won't.
3. Calories are the currency of energy.
4. Energy is the final goal of eating for the human body.

ALL FOODS CAN BECOME FAT

All of the foods that we eat can be changed into fat if they contain calories. Perhaps our ability to make and store fat from all food sources is a protective mechanism, carried over from primitive times when the next meal was not just a few steps away in the cupboard or the refrigerator. A kill had to be eaten immediately as primitive people had no skills in preserving foods, and the time between kills might be lengthy. Only people with good fat storage survived. Thus, we arrive at well-documented fact: The longer the time is between meals, the greater is the body's efficiency in forming fat from whatever is eaten (Lukert, 1982). The next chapter discusses this fact more fully.

BLOOD GLUCOSE IS IN CONTROL

Blood glucose, or blood sugar, the final product of carbohydrate digestion, is absorbed in the small intestine into the blood vessels there, taken back via the blood to the heart, and pumped throughout the body. Carbohydrates are the first foodstuffs to be digested (by enzymes in the mouth rather than in the stomach or the intestines). Perhaps this was planned because, of all the foodstuffs, carbohydrates are the most immediate contributors to blood sugar supply, which is vital to minute-to-minute survival.

Maintaining a constant blood sugar level is vital because the central nervous system, the red blood cells, the retina of the eye, the germinal epithelium of the reproductive system, and a few other specific cells and/or tissues utilize glucose as their primary or only source of energy—they cannot use fats as an energy source. This is important information to remember as you read about blood sugar levels.

Blood glucose levels rise after a meal and fall between meals. If the system is quickly flooded with glucose (which happens when refined sugar is ingested), it has a protective mechanism—it stimulates insulin release, which allows the excess glucose to escape from the blood into the other tissues of the body that make up about three-quarters of the body mass. When the glucose levels become low between meals, the liver puts glucose back into the bloodstream and muscles are no longer allowed to use this precious food supply for energy (they must burn fats). The glucose is, of course, saved to be used by the special organs and tissues described above.

If insulin levels do not drop as blood sugar levels drop, the muscles and adipose tissue use up available glucose, and the central nervous system and other special tissues have nothing to use for energy. This is what happens in insulin shock or hypoglycemic shock. In these instances, if glucose levels are not immediately reestablished, the individual in shock could die. When there is an *excess* of blood sugar, however, insulin helps bring the level down to normal so that high glucose levels do not create pathogenic problems and so that glucose is not lost from the body through excretion in the urine.

Figure 4.2 shows what happens to blood glucose when its level is high and when it is low.

What then should supply the energy for most of the body if glucose is kept at a lower level? *Fat* is the answer—a high energy food that breaks down slowly, constantly supplying energy for the muscles and other tissues that can burn fat.

A good carbohydrate tolerance means that the body efficiently lowers blood sugar after a meal and keeps it in a healthy range. As the individual arises in the morning there are about 80 milligrams of glucose per every 100 milliliters of blood in the body (or, in kitchen terms, less than a quarter teaspoon of sugar per quart of blood). This "starvation" level of blood glucose varies from person to person, but unless diabetes (high blood sugar) or hypoglycemia (low blood sugar) is present, starvation level will be in the range of 75 to 90 milligrams per 100 milliliters of blood. After a meal, if blood sugar level does not rise higher than 120 milligrams, then normal blood sugar utilization in the body can be assumed. A higher peak level might signify diabetes mellitus, while a diminished curve might signify hypoglycemia (see Figure 4.3). The problems and progress of hypoglycemia and diabetes and how they are related to nutrition, exercise, and obesity are discussed in great depth in Chapter 9.

Under normal conditions (at least two to three mixed meals per day) ample glucose is supplied for maintenance of blood glucose level with

FIGURE 4.2
What Happens to Blood Glucose

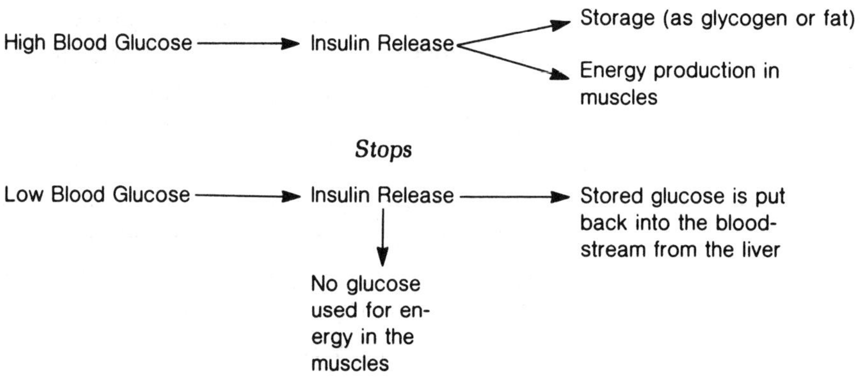

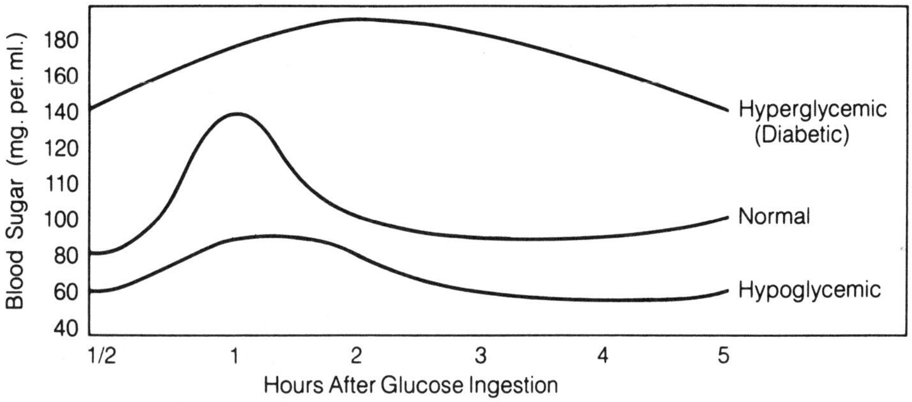

FIGURE 4.3 Normal and Abnormal Blood Sugar Curves as Seen in Glucose Tolerance Tests

some left over for energy production, for restoration of carbohydrate stores in the form of liver and muscle glycogen, and in many people, for synthesis of fatty acids that are stored in adipose tissue.

Whether weight will be lost or gained depends on the blood sugar level. If blood sugar level is low, the body will use an alternative source of energy—protein and/or fat. If blood sugar level is high, glucose will be used for energy and will also be stored as shown in Figure 4.2.

CALORIES ARE THE CURRENCY OF ENERGY

As discussed in Chapter 3, fat is measured in the calories it will produce when used by the body, and energy expenditure is based on calories burned. The system of energy exchange is fairly straightforward: If you *eat* 1,500 calories a day and you *burn* 1,500 calories in that same day, weight will remain the same. Usually the two processes balance over a long period of time such as a week or a month.

There are various factors that will unbalance this seesaw of calories, such as metabolic rate of food and water retention in the system. But over a period of time weight will be determined by "calories in" versus "calories expended" (Bray, 1983).

ENERGY IS THE FINAL GOAL

We must eat in order to provide ourselves with energy. Energy is stored in the body in the form of *adenosintriphosphate* (which, fortunately, is abbreviated to *ATP*)—an amino acid plus a sugar with, most importantly, three phosphates connected by "high energy" bonds that explode when broken (see Figure 4.4). When one of these high energy phosphate bonds is broken it gives off energy, some of which is used to perform work, the rest dissipating as heat. When energy is used, ATP is broken down; when energy is stored, ATP is put back together again. This is the story of our lives—eating food to create energy so that we may move, express ourselves, feel, experience, that is, *live.*

All cells of the body use ATP—for contraction in muscle cells, for enzyme synthesis in glandular cells, for transport of substances through membranes, and for all types of work in each cell. All cells also store a small amount of ATP, but when energy is spent, more foodstuff is necessary to reestablish ATP, bringing this discussion back full circle to the basic food sources (carbohydrates, proteins, and dietary fats) that supply the chemical products that form energy.

Let us now proceed to the three basic foodstuffs and see how they may contribute to weight control problems.

Carbohydrates

The simplest foods taken into and used by the body are the *carbohydrates* (see Figure 4.5 for the structure of a long-chain carbohydrate). This foodstuff derives its name from its basic components—carbon, hydrogen, and oxygen—and is often abbreviated CHO. A *starch* is a long-chain carbohydrate made up of simple sugar (*monosaccharide*) molecules attached to each other as seen in Figure 4.5. (Long-chain carbohydrates are found in such foods as bread, potatoes, spaghetti, beans, corn, peas.) Digestion breaks these down into maltose, a *disaccharide,* which in turn is broken down into two molecules of *glucose,* the most abundant simple sugar in the body (and thus called "blood sugar").

The simplest sugars that we usually consume are the disaccharides: *sucrose* (table sugar) and *lactose* (milk sugar). Sucrose breaks

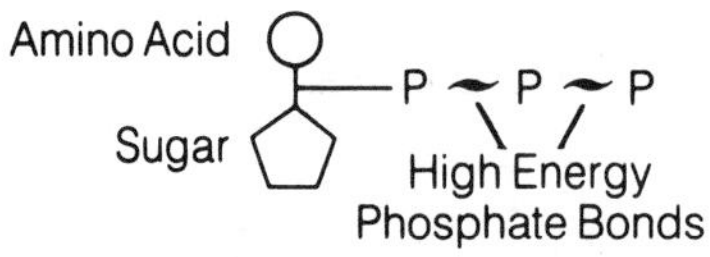

FIGURE 4.4 ATP—The Form of Energy in the Body

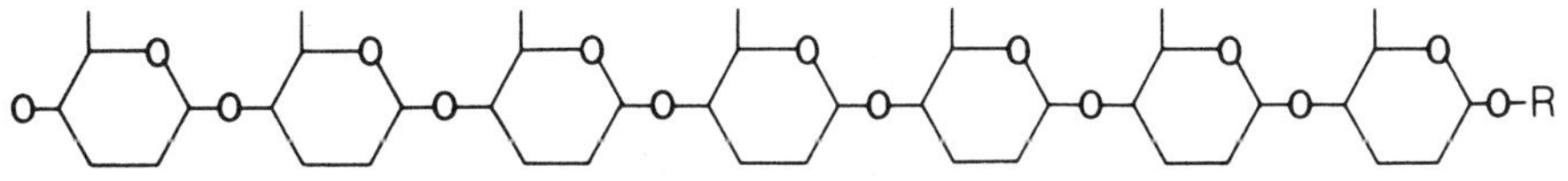

FIGURE 4.5 A Long-Chain Carbohydrate

down into one molecule of glucose and one molecule of fructose during digestion. Lactose is broken down by intestinal enzymes into one molecule of glucose and one molecule of galactose. A composite of carbohydrate digestion is shown in Figure 4.6 where you can see that most of the breakdown results in glucose, or blood sugar.

THE BREAKDOWN MIRACLE

The intricacies of glucose metabolism are small wonders of engineering. This tiny molecule of carbon, hydrogen, and oxygen is taken apart step by step to produce energy for the system. Instead of releasing all its energy at once (which would mean losing much in the way of heat production and reserving little for actual work of the cell), CHO slowly releases elements that become small sparks of energy as the original molecule is continually transfigured, until all that remains is water, carbon dioxide, and the energy that has been produced. Complete breakdown and use of one gram of glucose produces four calories of energy for the body.

1 gram of glucose = 4 calories of energy

ROUTES OF GLUCOSE USE

As carbohydrates are broken down and enter the bloodstream, the level of blood glucose rises and the body must do something to maintain a normal blood sugar level. The body apparently has three methods or routes whereby it can "detoxify" the blood of high sugar levels:

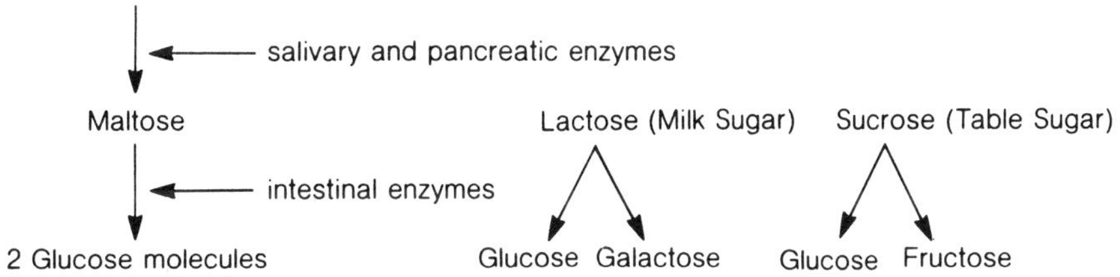

FIGURE 4.6 Carbohydrate Digestion

1. Energy production
2. Glycogen production (storage in liver and muscle tissue)
3. Fat production (storage in adipose tissue)

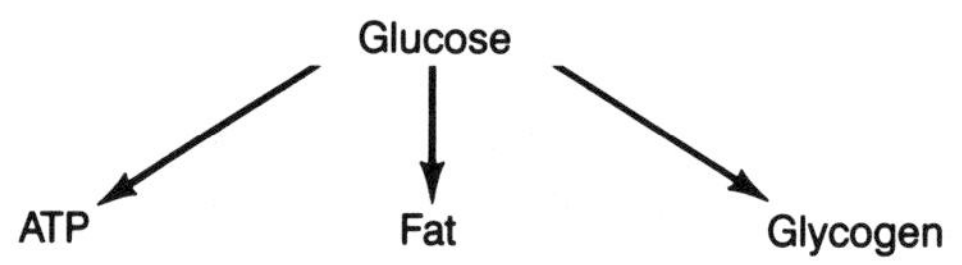

Route 1: Energy Production. If route 1 is taken, the glucose follows the energy metabolism path, breaking glucose down all the way to ATP (or energy) synthesis. This metabolic process of energy production occurs in the central nervous system and other special tissues without the necessity of having insulin present. However, high glucose levels stimulate the release of insulin so that muscle and adipose tissue can also take in the glucose and use it for energy or store it as glycogen or fat.

Route 2: Glycogen Production. Usually route 2 (*glycogenesis*, that is, making new glycogen) occurs at the same time as route 1 because the body lowers an excessive blood glucose level immediately in every way it can (perhaps so that this vital substance will not be lost from the body; perhaps also because high blood sugar levels create some of the degeneration that occurs in diabetes and the body is trying to protect itself).

As glucose enters muscle cells, some is used for regeneration of ATP (energy), if needed, and some is used to reestablish glycogen stores that have been spent since the last meal. Muscle glycogen stores consist of only about 2 to 3 percent of the muscle weight and last only a short time after blood sugar levels go back down to a low level.

Route 3: Fat Production. The third route shown—that of fat production—occurs concomitantly with the other two. As soon as insulin lets glucose into the fat cell, the glucose is metabolized partly and when the cell needs no more glucose for making glycogen or for energy production, the glucose molecules are shoved into the fat-making process.

Thus, the carbohydrates (broken down into glucose molecules) that are not used for energy are stored; a small amount is stored as glycogen and the rest is stored in the form of fat.

Proteins

Sugars and carbohydrates are our most immediate source of blood glucose and energy. Proteins contribute second most readily to our energy needs and are easily converted into blood glucose and fats. A protein has the same elements as carbohydrates (carbon, hydrogen, and oxygen) but also has nitrogen. Each of the building blocks of protein has one or more amino and acid groups, and thus are called "amino acids." Some complicated proteins may have many thousands of amino acids, so as one eats meat or eggs or dairy products, the intake of amino acids is high.

BREAKDOWN OF PROTEIN

The digestion of protein first occurs in the stomach, as this foodstuff touches off a reaction of hydrochloric acid and a basic protein proenzyme (a substance that stimulates enzyme production), *pepsinogen*, which in turn stimulates a strong proteolytic or "protein-eating" enzyme, *pepsin*, to break down the chemical linkages between amino acids so that each unit may be utilized. The amino acids can be used in several ways:

1. As building blocks for body tissues
2. In enzyme production
3. As an energy source
4. Converted into blood sugar
5. Converted into fat and stored

As three-quarters of the solid body parts are made of proteins, our obligatory protein intake is utilized in reproducing spent cells and enzymes. However, if a person eats more protein than the body needs for structural purposes or if the body is getting only small amounts of carbohydrates or fat (that is, a high protein, low carbohydrate diet), then amino acids will be converted into blood glucose for energy or changed into triglycerides and stored as fat.

There are 21 amino acids in significant quantity in the body and 10 of them must be ingested through the diet as they cannot be synthesized either sufficiently or at all by the body—thus they acquired the name, "essential" amino acids. All amino acids, however, can be converted into fat- or carbohydrate-building products, each requiring specific enzymes and other natural body chemicals to do so. Once these products are formed, they will be used as the body dictates: as fuel for energy, as blood sugar if blood sugar level is low, stored as fat if blood sugar is adequate and if carbohydrate stores are filled, or reconverted into nonessential amino acids for structural purposes. If used for energy, one gram of protein produces about four calories of energy in the body.

1 gram of protein = 4 calories of energy

Fats

Fats are the great energy producers of metabolism—more than twice the energy (nine calories) is derived from a gram of fat versus a gram of carbohydrate or protein. Similarly, twice the energy *output* is needed to use up a gram of stored fat as is needed to utilize a gram of stored carbohydrate (glycogen).

1 gram of fat = 9 calories of energy

FATTY ACIDS

Dietary fats are made up of two different kinds of fatty acids: saturated and unsaturated. Saturated fat (or saturated fatty acids) in the diet is usually in the form of triglycerides (for example, fat on a beef steak). Of all the fats, this triglyceride is the hardest—or at least takes the longest time—to digest. Because unsaturated and polyunsaturated fats (or fatty acids) have double bonds between their carbon elements, they are easier to break down into short carbon chains that yield to digestion and metabolism more readily than saturated fats do. A good example of rapid breakdown of polyunsaturated fats is the oil in fish—if allowed to sit too long, fish turns rancid and quickly smells because of fat breakdown. More detailed information on these fatty acids is in Chapter 9.

FAT BREAKDOWN AND CLEARANCE

Foodstuffs are available to the blood and body cells as they are digested: Initial breakdown of carbohydrates occurs in the mouth; proteins are acted upon in the stomach; and finally, fats are broken down in the small intestine. Virtually no fat metabolism (other than butter fat) occurs until fats leave the stomach and enter the small intestine where they cause bile (as an emulsifier) and digestive enzymes to be released.

After a high fat meal, the blood may become turbid and yellowish due to the high concentration of fat transport molecules. In a healthy person, the plasma is cleared of these new dietary fats within several hours. Exercisers, especially those who exercise regularly doing aerobic activity, have a shorter clearance time than sedentary individuals. And "Type A" (coronary-prone) individuals and persons suffering from heart attack have a longer fat clearance time. Present scientific thought regards shorter clearance times as healthier than longer clearance times (Matarazzo, et al 1984).

Fat is cleared from the blood by an enzyme, *lipoprotein lipase*, which is found in adipose tissue, heart muscle, skeletal muscle, and also, to a lesser extent, in the blood. Incidentally, all of these tissues can use fatty acids for energy. Lipoprotein lipase breaks triglycerides down into fatty acids that are then made into energy or stored again in the adipose tissue as triglycerides.

FAT STORAGE AND RECALL

Why a person loses or gains weight depends basically on that person's fat synthesis and deposition and on the breakdown and release of fat from the adipose tissue. As discussed earlier:

1. Adipose tissue consists mainly of triglycerides.
2. Fats can be made from all three basic foodstuffs, and if not used for energy, will be stored.
3. Stored fat will be removed from adipose cells and used *when it is needed by the body for energy purposes.* It can be removed from fat cells by a false stressor such as nicotine or caffeine, but if after removal, greater energy output does not occur, the fatty acids will only circulate in the blood until they are stored again in the adipose tissue.

With these basics in mind, let's examine the foundations of weight gain and weight loss, taking first the all-too-real example of overeating and weight gain. An adult man weighing 175 pounds eats his dinner at 7:00 P.M. The meal consists of:

A large platter of spaghetti with tomato sauce and three meatballs
Three slices of garlic-butter bread
Dinner salad with dressing
12 ounces of whole milk

This is followed by:

A large piece of chocolate cake
One scoop of ice cream
One cup of coffee with cream and sugar

This dinner consists of about 2,200 calories, most of which will be introduced into the bloodstream within a two- to three-hour period, with the sugars entering first (in one-half to one hour), then animal followed by vegetable proteins within an hour or so, then the long-chain carbohydrates (spaghetti, flour), and finally the fats from meatballs and oil from the dressing hitting the bloodstream more than three hours after the meal—up to six hours later.

A 175-pound man at rest burns approximately 80 calories per hour, and the man in this example sits down after dinner and watches three and one-half hours of television after which he retires for the night. So, in this evening he uses about 300 calories of the 2,200 calories he ate. Most of the energy he did expend came from utilization of blood sugar, the level of which was greatly increased by sugars and carbohydrates and perhaps some protein in his dinner.

Imagine now, if you will, this man's body cells that are trying to deal with a surplus of food. Instead of eliminating foodstuffs not necessary at any one time (such as the body does with water soluble vitamins, for instance), the excess food elements continue to circulate until some storage mechanism in the cells converts them into stored energy.

As soon as the blood sugar of this diner went above "starvation" level, his liver enzymes were stimulated, which caused glucose to be polymerized into its stored form, glycogen. Increased blood sugar levels also stimulated the release of insulin from the pancreas so that excess blood sugar would be moved into muscle and adipose tissue. In his muscles the glucose was used minimally for energy, and the rest was made into glycogen. In the adipose tissue a small amount of blood sugar may have been used for energy but most was converted into fatty acids that combined with glycerol and were stored as triglycerides.

This 175-pound man has suffered the common effects of affluent Western diners—the excess foodstuffs eaten were turned into fat.

Some of those fats will be used overnight while he sleeps to keep his cells alive, but eight hours of sleep will require only 500 calories for this individual (energy requirements in sleep are about 85 percent of awake, resting needs). So he will accumulate about one-third of a pound of fat due to his eating and exercise routine for this short period of time.

In review, any excess glucose (above starvation blood sugar level) can be metabolized and subsequently synthesized into fatty acids. Amino acids in excess of structural needs can become stored fat in the same manner. The schema of fat storage is shown in Figure 4.7. Dietary fats, starches, sugars, and proteins are broken down by digestion and changed biochemically to form fatty acids, which in turn are stored as triglycerides.

Figure 4.8 shows the interrelationships in the metabolism of foodstuffs: Glucose is used for energy or stored. Amino acids may be changed into glucose to supply blood sugar, metabolized for energy,

FIGURE 4.7
Fat Synthesis and Storage

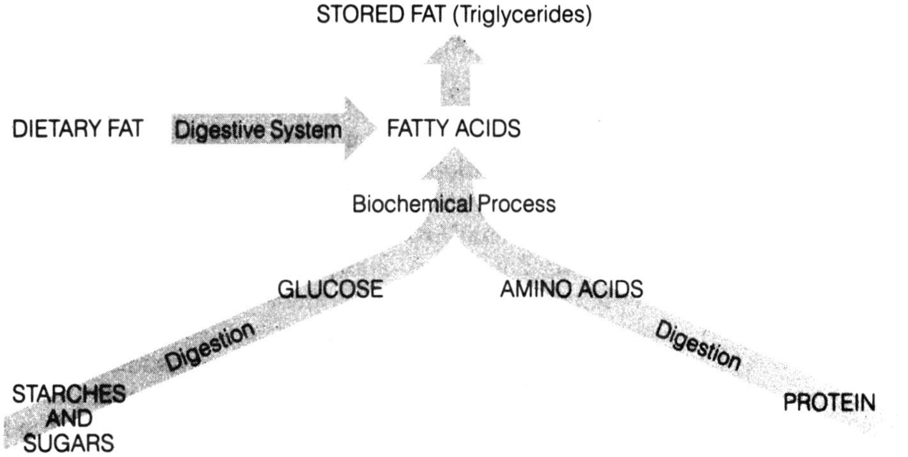

FIGURE 4.8 A Flowchart of Food Metabolism

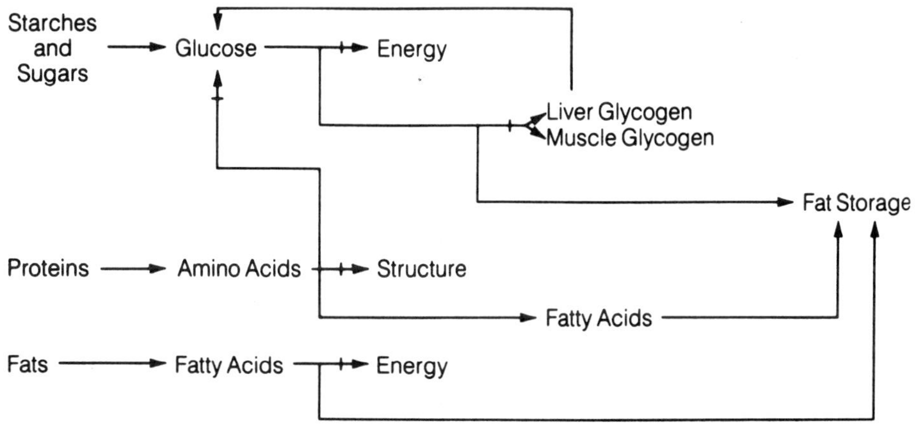

or made into fat or protein structures. The glycerol in triglycerides can be utilized to supply blood sugar, as it is a carbohydrate product. Liver glycogen can supply blood sugar. But fats can be used only as energy suppliers in those tissues that have specific enzymes to break the fatty acids down into their component parts. These parts are then used to make ATP or energy.

Perhaps this process offers an insight into nature's design—glucose may be meant mainly for supplying energy to those tissues that must have constant instant energy, especially the central nervous system (glucose is the easiest food to metabolize). These specialized tissues do not demand huge energy supplies for work production (neurons are never asked to physically swing a sledgehammer). So carbohydrates, proteins, and the glycerol portion of stored fat can all be changed into blood glucose to ensure a continuous necessary level of sugar. Unless large quantities of glucose are present at any one time in the bloodstream, glucose is not used for energy except by select tissues.

Summary

By now you must realize that weight loss and weight gain involve more than just fat. Fat removal and storage are dependent upon all the food sources, respond to blood sugar level, and also are highly dependent upon energy output. Therefore, eating patterns, nutrition and physical activity have central roles in the process of fat removal and fat storage. Stress and mental attitude also affect fat storage and fat utilization. The following chapters of this book deal with all of these aspects.

References

Bjorntorp, Per. "The Role of Adipose Tissue in Human Obesity," in Greenwood, H. (Ed.). *Obesity*. New York: Churchill Livingstone, 1983.

Bray, G. "Metabolic Response to Positive Energy Balance," in Hansen, B. *Controversies in Obesity*. New York: Praeger, 1983.

Kannel, W. B. "Health and Obesity," in Conn, H., et al. (Eds). *Health and Obesity*. New York: Raven Press, 1983.

LeVielle, G. and D. Romsos. "Meal Eating and Obesity," *Nutrition Today* (Nov.–Dec. 1974): 4–9.

Lukert, B. "Biology of Obesity," in Wolman, B. (Ed). *Psychological Aspects of Obesity*. New York: Van Nostrand Reinhold, 1982.

Matarazzo, J., et al (Eds). *Behavioral Health: A Handbook of Health Enhancement and Disease Prevention*. New York: Wiley, 1984.
Wishon, P., et al. "Childhood Obesity," *Young Children* 39 (1): 21–27, 1983.

Suggested Readings

Atrens, Dale. *Don't Diet*. New York: Morrow, 1988.
Curtis-Prior, P. (Ed). *Biochemical Pharmacology of Obesity*. New York: Elsevier, 1983.
Guyton, A. *Human Physiology and Mechanisms of Disease*. 3rd Edition. Philadelphia: W. B. Saunders, 1983.
Martin, D., et al. *Harper's Review of Biochemistry*. Los Altos, CA: Lange, 1985.

5 NEVER HUNGRY, NEVER STUFFED: THE 6-MEAL-A-DAY PLAN

THERE ARE A COUPLE of well-kept secrets about eating that should be shared by the research community—concepts that have been known in medical literature for some time but somehow have not been communicated very well to all of those who might benefit from this knowledge.

Don't Starve Yourself

One of these "secrets" is that starving yourself is really a self-defeating way to try to reduce your weight. As you decrease your energy input below an obligatory level, your body's metabolic rate decreases, so it becomes harder to utilize the foods you *do* allow yourself. This is the basic conservation of energy law designed by nature for your survival.

If you decrease your intake to, say, fewer than 1,000 calories per day, that severe denial of food will cause your body to "shut down" because it wants to survive. The body seems to know it isn't being fed much so it reduces the amount of energy that it would normally produce. Also, when you "starve" yourself, you lose muscle mass, so there is less lean tissue to metabolize the fat you're trying to get rid of.

MORE IS BETTER

I knew a woman who, wanting to lose about ten pounds, drastically decreased her intake—to 500 calories per day. Her meals consisted of instant oatmeal with a token amount of milk in it for breakfast, an apple and carrot sticks for lunch, and three fishsticks, a cup of green beans, and a glass of milk for dinner—week after week after week. Even with regular physical activity (running, badminton, or tennis) she was not losing weight as she felt she should. When she related this to her friends who were sophisticated in the knowledge of caloric balance, they accused her of cheating—she must be hiding in the bathroom, eating chocolate chip cookies. They thought that anyone eating only 500 calories per day and engaging in the kind of activities this woman was would surely be losing a great deal of weight.

Christmas arrived and the woman gave up her 500-calorie diet in favor of a prudent and controlled combination of turkey, salads, vegetables, and even a few Christmas cookies. She was astonished that she began to lose weight after a short while. Through her experience she discovered the secret—don't starve yourself when you want to lose weight. Starvation (1) decreases metabolic rate; (2) seriously limits the intake of vital nutrients, especially protein, vitamins, and minerals, all of which can be vital to weight loss; and (3) promotes self-defeat, which makes you rather cranky about life in general.

The woman in this example, by increasing her caloric intake, lost weight, and she has successfully maintained her weight over the last ten years through good nutrition and exercise.

Many clients I have worked with, especially young, college-age females, take this same starvation route. Thinking it noble and stoic to stay on a 500- to 800-calorie daily intake, they find it difficult to understand that eating *more* than their few hundred calories can help them lose weight. But most of them grudgingly increase to 1000 calories or so, add some activity, and break through the starvation plateau. It is one time that they find that more is better, and they are rewarded both physically and mentally.

Generally adults should keep caloric intake above 1,000 calories (or more) per day, depending on how much they weigh. According to the facts, you don't have to literally starve yourself in order to lose weight.

MORE REASON NOT TO STARVE YOURSELF

A serious effect of starvation is the loss of lean body mass, that is, muscle. When food intake is too low for the demands of the body, the body uses up available amino acids to keep the blood glucose level stable. It is well recognized in research concerning starvation that *initial* weight loss is about two-thirds lean vital tissue, and only one-third fat loss (Kraus and Mahan, 1984). It is also recognized that if a dieter is replenishing the body periodically with food, *fat* loss is greater than it is during starvation (if all other variables are held equal).

In other words, *weight* loss may be greater in starvation, but much of that reduction in weight is from use of body protein and the water related to it rather than from fat loss. This principle also applies to semistarvation when the body slows its metabolism, begins to store fat efficiently, and then must use protein to maintain blood glucose. As lean body tissue mass diminishes, there is proportionally less of the body to oxidize or burn up fat.

Don't Gorge Yourself

The second "secret" that must be passed along is that it is important not to eat all of your calories, or a large portion of them, *at one time.* Such gorging creates two problems. One is that when many calories are introduced into the bloodstream at once, the body must store the excess. When you gorge repeatedly, your body becomes very efficient at changing your food into fat and storing it. A second problem of gorging at one or two meals is that between these meals, the body thinks it's being starved (which, in fact, it is because it usually takes no longer than five to six hours to process an entire meal into an energy-producing or a fat-producing form). When this occurs, the starvation syndrome previously described comes into play and the body preserves its energy.

NIBBLERS VERSUS GORGERS

Research on the frequency of meals has shown that "nibblers" are better off than "gorgers" (Edwards, 1988; LaVielle and Romsos, 1974; Leiter and Marliss, 1982). Those who eat 4–6 small meals a day are less efficient at storing fat and have the health benefits of lower cholesterol and better carbohydrate tolerance as well! In contrast, those who gorge (eat all of their calories in three or fewer meals per day) are just the opposite. They become very efficient at making fat from all foods, exhibit higher cholesterol levels, and generally have a poorer carbohydrate tolerance. They have what Bray (1972) calls "adaptive hyperlipogenesis," a sophisticated way of saying that they adapt to the high surge of calories by making fat very efficiently.

Two professors at Michigan State University found that 440 elderly men who spread their caloric intake over five or more "meals" each day were healthier in the categories mentioned above than those who ate fewer meals per day (LaVielle and Romsos, 1974). These researchers also pointed out the typical cycle that American dieters fall into—the "yoyo syndrome."

To illustrate the yoyo syndrome, let's suppose your neighbor wants to lose 10 pounds in a few weeks to appear slim at a wedding. Typically, that person will start cutting out breakfast and/or lunch (perhaps will drink coffee or diet soda) and will eat a modest dinner—no snacks all day, just dinner. This caloric intake is less than usual and so the dieter does in fact lose weight. But as weight is being lost, much of it may be lean body mass, and in a week's time the body responds to the 18- to 20-hour starvation period (the hours that food is not entering the metabolic process) by storing more of what food it does get. The body is also being bombarded by far too many calories at once. If this person eats 1,000 calories per dinner, then that amount will be too much energy to expend in the several hours after the meal when the blood sugar level is high.

Suppose your neighbor loses the weight (because of a caloric deficit), looks slim at the wedding, and then wishes to resume a maintenance diet. So breakfast and lunch are added again (also increasing calories to a maintenance level) and what happens? The body has become so efficient at making and storing fat that the scale starts to groan again. The yoyo syndrome is solidly based in this "adaptive hyperlipogenesis" process—weight increases again after the diet because the dieter's body has become skilled at making and storing fat.

The 6-Meal-A-Day (MAD) Plan

The 6-meal-a-day plan and the contrasting 3-meal-a-day plan might look like the illustration in Figure 5.1. With the same amount of calories consumed, the lower figure—six meals per day—makes more sense as an eating plan. Just by looking at it you can see that it is a plan whereby you'd never be stuffed and you'd never be hungry. It is apparent in the top figure that each of three meals exceeds the energy needs for the next period of time. That excess (above the dotted line) will be stored as fat.

A 6-MAD MENU

To put into operation the 6-meal-a-day plan shown in Figure 5.1, let's plan a 1,500-calorie per day intake. A good, wholesome breakfast can be 300 calories; for example, two slices of whole wheat toast at 65 calories apiece; one egg at 75 calories; one-half tablespoon of margarine at 50 calories; and eight ounces of tomato juice for 50 calories—all

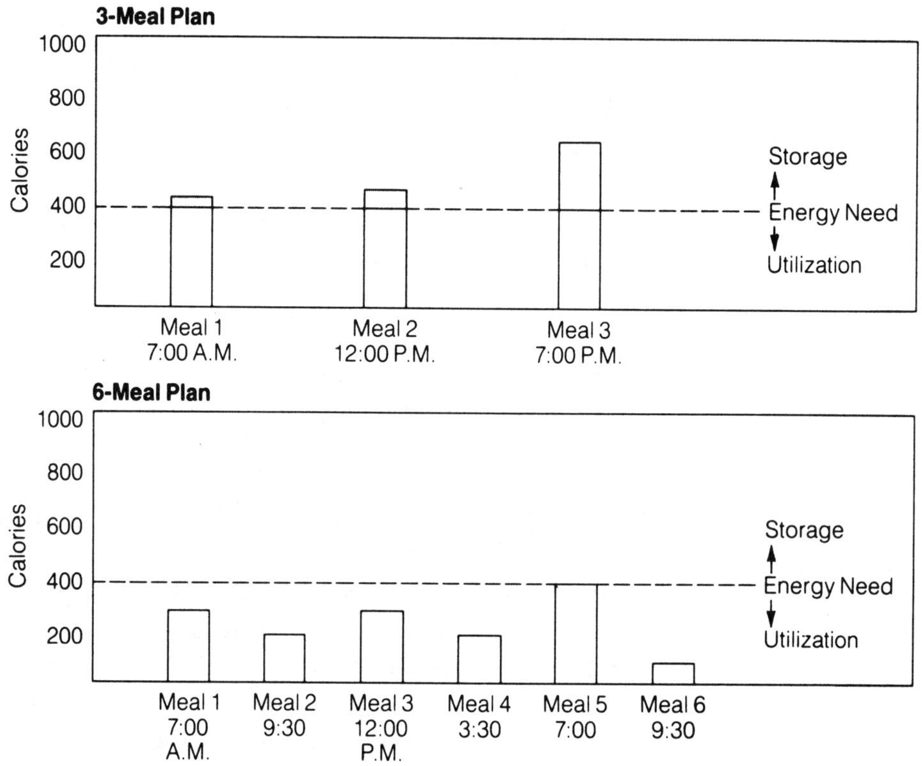

FIGURE 5.1 3-Meal-a-Day Plan versus 6-Meal-a-Day Plan (1,500 calories per day)

total 305 calories. You can drink all the black coffee or tea you should allow yourself. (Caffeine is not recommended by experts on health.) Breakfast is important—eat it early every day to decrease the length of the starvation period.

After breakfast, then, 1,200 calories are eaten in meals that might be broken down something like this: 200 calories in the midmorning snack, 300 in the noon meal, 200 in the midafternoon snack, 400 in the evening meal, and 100 in the bedtime snack. (Specific suggestions for each meal are given later in the chapter.)

You'll note that the traditionally large evening meal is still somewhat larger than the other meals so that the plan fits into cultural traditions. This evening meal might contain some of the higher calorie protein sources such as ham, beef, or other meats, but poultry and/or fish are good protein sources at lower calorie levels. These entrees (if you use meat rather than follow a vegetarian diet) can be supported by many delicious, low-calorie vegetables to round out the meal.

The snacks of 100 to 200 calories might be fruit, raw vegetables, nuts, cheese, or other favorite, creative munchies. One of my students who was "addicted" to potato chips for years as a midafternoon snack satisfied her desire for something to munch by measuring in a small plastic bag one ounce of Rice Chex or Wheat Chex (any nonsugar cereal would do) to crunch. Then her boyfriend began demanding his bag of cereal in the afternoon, too!

Many students generally appreciate the theory of the 6-MAD plan but explain that they can't put it into practice for different reasons: "I'm in class all day"; "I have to feed five people on five different schedules"; "I eat in the dorm"; "I work the swing shift." When someone says to me, "I can't," what I hear them saying is, "I won't—it's too much trouble, it isn't important enough to me, I'd have to do a lot of preplanning," and so on.

Planning to eat your calories in six or more "meals" a day requires nothing more than a little math skill and an urge to do it. Probably you will have to modify the traditionally large evening meal, but not too much more. Planning and carrying two snacks with you for the day if you are away from home can be as simple as buying some fruit, vegetables, crackers, and so forth, putting them in your purse or pack, and eating them when it's time! And if the family rebels, modify your *own* caloric intake and enjoy the benefits. Give the rest of the family the chance to make the choice (because this plan has health benefits for them, too), but don't think you can or must eat like the five-year-old or your spouse.

SUMMARY OF THE 6-MAD PLAN

The rules of healthy fat reduction in the 6-MAD plan are:

1. Don't starve yourself.
2. Spread your caloric intake throughout the day.

Some of the benefits of the 6-MAD plan are:

1. You're never hungry.
2. You're never stuffed.
3. Fat storage becomes less efficient.
4. Your carbohydrate tolerance and cholesterol level may be improved.

Designing Your 6-MAD Plan

When you have decided how many calories you must eat and how many calories you are going to expend through exercise to trim your body down to your target weight and size, take some time to plan how to eat your calories. To do this, follow the steps given here. Examples are given at the end of this worksheet for a 1,500-calorie 6-MAD plan. If any of the food choices given there appeal to you, add them to your plan. However, the choices given in the examples are some of my own and I know that I can stay on this plan because it has foods that *I* like in it. You must do the same for yourself if you want the best chance for this plan to work for you. After the examples there is another worksheet that you will want to fill out after you have progressed through all the chapters in this book. You may find that, after reading about good nutrition, the benefits of exercise, foods that may contribute to stress, and so on, you want to modify your food and calorie choices.

STEPS IN YOUR 6-MAD PLAN

1. Split your caloric intake into six meals. Be creative but be realistic.
2. What foods do you (or would you) like to eat for breakfast? List as many as you can think of.
3. Now write down the calories contained in each food. Books that might help if you cannot find the caloric content of foods are: Barbara Kraus's *Dictionary of Calories and Carbohydrates* (New York: Grosset and Dunlap), and Corinne T. Netzer's *Brand-Name Calorie Counter* (New York: Dell).
4. Design five different combinations that total the number of calories you plan to eat for breakfast. Designing menus for a five-day period will get you started. After this, plan your menu for a week at a time.
5. What kind of snacks do you like to eat? List some examples.
6. Write down the calories contained in each snack food.
7. Choose five different snack combinations for midmorning, five for midafternoon, and five for bedtime that correspond with the number of calories you allotted yourself for each.
8. What would satisfy you for lunch? List your favorites.
9. Write down the calories contained in each food.
10. Choose five different combinations that total the number of calories you have allowed yourself for lunch.

11. What foods do you like for dinner (other than what you have listed for breakfast and lunch)? List them.
12. Assign calories to these new foods.
13. Choose five different combinations that total the number of calories you think you should have at dinner.
14. Now put your choices together for a five-day plan: Choose one breakfast, one midmorning snack, one lunch, one midafternoon snack, one dinner, and one bedtime snack for each of five days. (You can identify them by the number on this worksheet, for example: breakfast 3.2; midmorning snack 5a5; lunch 7.3; afternoon snack 5b2; dinner 9.5; and bedtime snack, 5cl.

	Breakfast	*Snack*	*Lunch*	*Snack*	*Dinner*	*Snack*
Day 1						
Day 2						
Day 3						
Day 4						
Day 5						

EXAMPLE OF A 6-MAD PLAN

1. Calories allotted per meal on a 1,500 calories per day plan

Breakfast: 300 calories

Midmorning snack: 200 calories

Lunch: 300 calories

Midafternoon snack: 200 calories

Dinner: 400 calories

Bedtime snack: 100 calories

All the black coffee, black tea, diet soda, and water allowed myself throughout the day

2. Foods I like for breakfast:

FRUIT

2″ wedge honeydew melon	50
½ medium cantaloupe	50
½ cup grapefruit sections	50
2 small nectarines	50
½ cup orange juice	50
1 large tangerine	50
8 oz. tomato juice	50
1 apple	75
1 cup strawberries	50
1 banana	100
2 medium figs	100
½ cup prune juice	100

BREAD/CEREAL

1 slice whole wheat bread	65
1 biscuit	50
1 muffin	125
½–¾ cup dry cereal	75
1 cup puffed	50
1 biscuit shredded	100
¼ cup grapenuts	100
1 cup oatmeal	130
1 bagel	165
3 graham crackers	100

MEAT/EGGS

2 links sausage	125
2 slices bacon (crisp)	90
1 egg (boiled or poached)	75

MILK

1 cup whole	165
1 cup 2%	145
1 cup skim	85
8 oz. plain yogurt	150

3. Some combinations of these foods for breakfast (about 300 calories):

1.

1 egg	75
2 bacon slices	50
4 oz. tomato juice	25
1 bran muffin	125
1 pat butter	35
	310

2.

1 cup strawberries	50
1 cup puffed rice	50
½ glass whole milk	80
½ sliced banana	50
1 poached egg	75
	305

3.

4 oz. orange juice	50
2 sausage links	125
1 poached egg	75
1 biscuit	50
	300

4.

1″ wedge honeydew melon	25
8 oz. whole milk	165
3 graham crackers	100
	290

5.

½ banana	50
½ cup strawberries	25
¼ cantaloupe	25
1 small nectarine	25
½ tangerine	25
4 oz. yogurt	75
1 slice whole wheat toast	65
	290

4. Snacks I like (same fruit suggestions as breakfast):

1 boiled egg	75	1 Fig Newton	50
1 piece Ry Krisp	25	1 T. peanut butter	90
1 Ritz cracker	15	2 oz. peanuts	210
1 stalk celery	5	3 oz. creamed cheese	320
1 carrot	20	2 cups popcorn with oil/salt	80
1 tomato	40	2 twists or 25 sticks pretzels	50
1 oz. cheese	110	1 cup ice cream	255
2 oz. cottage cheese	60		

5. Some combinations for snacks:

a. Midmorning (about 200 calories)

1. 1 boiled egg	75	2. 2 oz. peanuts	210
1 Ry Krisp	25		
1 banana	100		
	200		
3. 1 carrot	20	4. carrot and celery sticks	25
2 celery stalks	10	1 Fig Newton	50
2 T. peanut butter	180	4 oz. yogurt	75
	210	½ cup strawberries	25
			175
5. 1 deviled egg	100		
1 sliced tomato	40		
2 Ry Krisp crackers	50		
	190		

b. Midafternoon (about 200 calories)

1. 4 oz. grapefruit juice	50	2. ½ cantaloupe	50
¼ cup cottage cheese	65	1 Ry Krisp	25
1 tomato	40	2 celery stalks	10
1 Fig Newton	50	1 oz. cream cheese	110
	205		195
3. 4 Ritz crackers	60	4. 1 oz. cheddar cheese	110
1 T. peanut butter	90	4 Ry Krisp crackers	100
1 peach	50		210
	200		
5. 4 oz. 2% milk	75		
1 blueberry muffin	125		
	200		

c. Bedtime (about 100 calories)

1. 1 cup popcorn	40	2. 1 cup strawberries	50
6 oz. tomato juice	40	½ oz. cheese	55
1 nectarine	25		105
	105		
3. 25 pretzel sticks	50	4. ⅓ cup ice cream	85
6 oz. tomato juice	40	¼ cup strawberries	15
	90		100
5. ½ cup puffed wheat	50		
½ cup skim milk	40		
1 tsp. honey	20		
	110		

6. I like for lunch (also, same fruit, bread and cereal, and milk products as listed for breakfast and snacks):

½ cup greens	25	2 oz. crab	50
½ cup green beans	25	2 oz. shrimp	50
1 cup cauliflower	25	1 oz. pickled herring	75
½ cup spinach	25	1 oz. very lean beef	75
¼ cup broccoli	25	1 oz. very lean ham	75
1 medium potato	100	1 oz. tuna in oil	75
1 small sweet potato	100	1 oz. brook trout	75
1 oz. chicken	50	1 oz. lake trout	100
1 oz. fish	50	1 oz. liver	50
		½ cup pickles	12½

7. Some combinations for lunch (about 300 calories each):

1. 4 oz. cottage cheese	120	2. 1½ oz. cheese	165
1 tomato	40	sprouts	15
2 Ritz crackers	30	1 slice whole wheat toast	65
1 apple	75	1 large tangerine	50
	265		295
3. tomato stuffed with	40	4. 2 slices whole wheat	
tuna (2 oz.)	150	bread	130
1 Ry Krisp	50	2 oz. ham	150
¼ cantaloupe	25	1 dill pickle	10
	265	lettuce	10
			300

5. 3 oz. chicken salad	150
1 T. salad dressing	65
1 celery stalk	5
pickles	5
lettuce	10
1 tomato	40
1 carrot	20
	295

8. Foods I like for dinner (same selections as already listed):

1 oz. spaghetti	40
1 oz. spagetti sauce	30
1 oz. lean ground beef	65
1 cheese enchilada	130
3 oz. red wine	70
12 oz. lite beer	97
green salad:	
1 carrot	20
1 tomato	40
1 cup lettuce	25
½ zucchini	12½
1 celery stalk	5
1 boiled egg	75
1 strip crisp bacon	45
sprouts	12½
	235
1 bean burrito	250
1 corn tortilla	42
1 oz. hot sauce	10
3 T. lowfat blue cheese dressing	35

9. Some combinations for dinner (about 400 calories):

1. green salad	235
salad dressing	35
2 oz. fish	100
½ cantaloupe	50
	420

2. 2 oz. spaghetti	80
tomato sauce	60
½ green salad	120
dressing	20
8 oz. skim milk	85
1 nectarine	25
	390

3. 1 tortilla	42
hot sauce	10
1 bean burrito	250
1 lite beer	97
	399

4. 4 oz. barbecue chicken	200
1 cup green beans	50
lettuce	13
1 sliced tomato	40
8 oz. skim milk	85
	388

5. 1 oz. pickled herring	75
raw cauliflower and broccoli pieces	50
2 oz. lean beef	150
½ cup spinach	25
½ baked potato	50
3 oz. red wine	70
	420

10. Menu Plan for Five Days:

	Breakfast	*Snack*	*Lunch*	*Snack*	*Dinner*	*Snack*
Day 1	3.4	5a5	7.4	5b1	9.1	5c4
Day 2	3.5	5a1	7.1	5b2	9.4	5c5
Day 3	3.1	5a4	7.3	5b3	9.2	5c1
Day 4	3.3	5a2	7.5	5b4	9.3	5c3
Day 5	3.2	5a3	7.2	5b5	9.5	5c2

ADDITIONAL SUGGESTIONS

Some ideas that might work for you are:

1. Use scissors to cut out your meal and snack combinations and then work with them as you would a deck of cards, laying them out into a satisfying day's worth of food for yourself.
2. Don't feel that you can't have the same snack two or three times (or more often) in a week if there is something that you especially like and is good for you. This is true of all meals and snacks, but many people like variety in their menus.
3. Keep adding new foods to your deck of cards.
4. Sit down at the beginning of the week and deal yourself the week's menu. Then do your grocery shopping with that menu.
5. Always be conscious of good nutritional balance, especially with nutrients you cannot store in your body such as the B vitamins, vitamin C, and protein. You need to have them every day in appropriate amounts. Calcium and iron should also be noticeable in your diet each day.

STEPS IN YOUR 6-MAD PLAN (FIRST REVISION)

1. Split your caloric intake into six meals. Be creative but be realistic.
2. What foods do you (or would you) like to eat for breakfast? Name as many new foods as you can and repeat the old ones that worked for you.
3. Now write down the calories for the foods.
4. Design five different combinatations that total the number of calories you plan to eat for breakfast.
5. Snacks: List old ones you liked and new ones you have found.
6. Write down the calories contained in each snack food.
7. Choose five different snack combinations for midmorning, five for midafternoon, and five for bedtime that correspond with the number of calories you allotted yourself for each.
8. List those foods you have found that will satisfy you for lunch.
9. Write down the calories contained in each food.
10. Choose five different combinations that total the number of calories you have allowed yourself for lunch.
11. List those foods you have found that are good for dinner.
12. Assign calories to each food.
13. Choose five different combinations that total the number of calories you think you should have at dinner.
14. Now put your choices together for a five-day plan.

	Breakfast	*Snack*	*Lunch*	*Snack*	*Dinner*	*Snack*
Day 1						
Day 2						
Day 3						
Day 4						
Day 5						

References

Bray, George. "Lipogenesis in Human Adipose Tissue: Some Effects of Nibbling and Gorging," *Journal of Clinical Investigation* 51 (1972): 537–547.

Edwards, T. *Weight Loss to Super Wellness*, 2nd Edition. Champaign, IL: Life Enhancement, 1988.

LaVielle, G., and D. Romsos. "Meal Eating and Obesity." *Nutrition Today* (Nov.–Dec. 1974): 4–9.

Leiter, L., and E. Marliss. "Survival during Fasting." *JAMA* 248 (1983): 2306.

Sassoon, H. "Time Factors in Obesity." *American Journal of Clinical Nutrition* 26 (1973): 776–783.

Suggested Readings

Carper, J. *The Brand Name Nutrition Counter*. New York: Bantam, 1985.

Kraus, Barbara. *Calorie Guide to Brand Names and Basic Foods*. New York: Signet, 1988.

Kraus, Barbara. *Carbohydrate Guide to Brand Names and Basic Foods*. New York: Signet, 1988.

Netzer, Corinne. *The Complete Book of Food Counts*. New York: Dell, 1988.

Powers, P. *Obesity: The Regulation of Weight*. Baltimore: William and Wilkins, 1981.

6 WHY DID YOU EAT THAT?

DO YOU EVER STOP to wonder why you eat, what motivates your food choices, why you accept food when you don't want to eat it? Let's take a look at some possible answers through a hypothetical interview. The interviewee begins the day with a breakfast of one egg, two slices of whole wheat toast with margarine and strawberry jam, one-half a glass of orange juice, and a cup of Morning Thunder tea with honey.

This breakfast eater tells us that breakfast always starts with orange juice. But why orange juice? we ask. Why not tomato or grapefruit or prune juice? And why drink it before eating the eggs and toast? Just half a glass, not a whole glass of O.J.? What kind is it? Frozen concentrate, fresh, canned? What was the choice based on? All these questions about one little glass of orange juice!

On to the main course. One egg? Why not two? Why two pieces of toast? Why whole wheat, and of what particular brand? Why not butter instead of margarine? Strawberry jam? Isn't that full of sugar? And why tea that has a strong shot of caffeine? Why not coffee? Why use honey?

And then the big question, "Why did you eat breakfast at all?"

You didn't know breakfast could be such a struggle, did you? To clarify a bit of the struggle, let's look at some possible answers the interviewee could give for why certain foods are eaten. You will probably identify with some of the answers yourself.

WHY DID YOU EAT BREAKFAST?

I was hungry when I woke up.

I *always* eat breakfast.

I'm usually not hungry, but I know I should eat breakfast.

Someone cooks it for me, so I eat it.

WHY ORANGE JUICE?

It's cheaper than tomato juice.

It has my RDA of vitamin C.

I like the taste.

I'm thirsty when I get up.

I want something cold to drink in the morning.

WHY HALF A GLASS OF ORANGE JUICE?

I can't drink a whole glassful.

I always drink half a glass.

It lasts longer that way.

My breakfast partner drinks the other half and it's fun to share.

WHY THAT PARTICULAR BRAND?

They have a cute jingle.

It's cheap.

It's the brand they have at the closest store.

It tastes sweeter than the other brands.

My mother always bought that kind.

WHY DID YOU DRINK IT FIRST?

I always drink my juice first.

It freshens my "overnight mouth."

I don't like cold drinks with hot eggs and toast.

It's something to do while I wait for the rest of breakfast.

WHY EGGS AND TOAST?

They keep me going all morning.

They're good for you.

They're cooked for me.

They're easy to cook.

WHY ONLY ONE EGG?

I'm cholesterol conscious.

I'm not a big eater.

That's what I always eat.

Eggs last twice as long in the refrigerator.

WHY WHOLE WHEAT TOAST?

It tastes better than white.

It's more nutritious than white.

It fills me up.

It smells great as it toasts.

WHY TWO SLICES?

It fills me up.

I eat one with my egg and the other is a kind of dessert—I put jam on it.

I need two slices to fulfill half my grain needs for the day—you know, the Basic Four.

WHY THE STRAWBERRY JAM?

It has more fruit and less sugar than other jams and jellies.

I love strawberries.

I have to have something sweet for breakfast.

My mom used to make the best strawberry jam.

WHY TEA?

I like the taste.

I can drink it after it cools off, but I have to drink coffee hot.

It's better for you than coffee.

Dr. Frank always drinks it.

WHY HONEY?

Somebody gave it to me and I couldn't throw away good honey.

I like the taste.

It's more wholesome than sugar or artificial sweetener.

I have to have something sweet in my tea; I grew up that way.

Through this hypothetical interview, you can see that people eat what they eat and when they eat for a multitude of reasons. For every question here, all of the answers proposed could be true for any individual, and each person could add more reasons.

The reasons given here can be separated into several categories: *habit* ("I always eat one egg"); *memories* of mom ("Mom used to make the best strawberry jam"); *respect* for someone who uses the product ("Dr. Frank always drinks it"); *advertising* ("They have a cute jingle"); *finances* ("It's cheap"); *hunger or thirst* ("I'm hungry and thirsty when I get up"); *smell* ("It smells great as it toasts"); *taste* ("It tastes sweeter than the other brands"); *necessity* ("That's my only choice"); *intellect* ("They're good for you"); *energy* ("They keep me going all morning"); *health* ("I'm cholesterol conscious"); or *social* interaction ("it's fun to share").

Take a minute to reflect on why you ate breakfast. And if you didn't eat breakfast, why did you eat lunch or dinner or that granola bar this afternoon on your way to work?

Eating is a very complex behavior. All the realms of human motivation come into play. Apart from the physical need for food, people are social beings with their own individual childhood learning and development, current finances, moods, desires, and appetites. Psychology has overriden the basic physiological response to hunger and satiety. People are constantly bombarded with psychological messages to "eat, child, eat." I call this phenomenon of mind over physiology "cerebral override" or the "telencephalization of eating."

I have had numerous clients in my weight management groups who have never felt a hunger pang! Their reasons for eating were mainly psychological. One of my most exciting moments in this business was when a 52-year-old woman I was working with came into the group session one day very excited and declared that yesterday she had experienced hunger for the first time in her life! The group cheered!

In working with people in weight management, I ask them to spend several days writing down what and when they eat, whom they are with, where they are, and how they feel at the time (what their moods are and how they're feeling about themselves and their relationships with others). This is no novelty as a weight reduction technique—behavior modification therapists have used it for years. I also ask my clients to analyze their motivation for starting to eat each particular food and then the motivation for cessation of eating that food. Table 6.1 shows this exercise in chart form. Fill it in for a day or two and discover what your eating behavior is really like.

The responses of my clients have ranged from hunger to anger, from finances to tradition. Some examples are given below. You will undoubtedly have some elements in common with these responses, which clearly divide into categories that will be embellished in this chapter.

RESPONSES TO "WHY I ATE IT"

It looked so good	To be social	Tradition
Availability	It's good for me	Frustrated
Lonely	Angry	Worried
It was a reward	Love the taste	Sad
Special occasion	Depressed	It smelled good
Time to eat	Hungry	Upset
I paid for it	Couldn't throw it away ($$)	For energy
Bored	Habit	Love the texture

RESPONSES TO "WHY I STOPPED"

It was gone!	I was bloated
I was full	It wasn't worth the calories
I allow myself just so much	It didn't taste good
Angry	The table was cleared
Will power	I was upset
Too sweet	I just wasn't hungry

TABLE 6.1. Your Eating Chart

Food	*How Much*	*When*	*Where*	*With Whom*	*Mood*	*Why Started*	*Why Stopped*

In analyzing the responses to "Why I Ate It," you can see that they fall into four general categories: (1) positive affect—there's something rewarding about eating a particular food, or about eating a food at a particular time; (2) physiological; (3) negative affect—food is consumed as the result of a negative mood or emotional state; and (4) physical environment, relating to the situation that precedes and promotes eating. The responses can be redistributed into these categories:

POSITIVE AFFECT	*PHYSIO-LOGICAL*	*NEGATIVE AFFECT*	*PHYSICAL ENVIRONMENT*
Looked good	Hungry	Bored	Availability
To be social	Good for me	Worried	Financial
Smelled good	Energy	Sad	Habit
Reward		Lonely	Time to eat
Special occasion		Angry	
		Upset	
Taste		Depressed	
Tradition		Frustrated	
Texture			

You may be able to identify your own reasons in one of these categories. If your motivation to eat is mainly physiological or physical, you will have less trouble in reducing your weight and maintaining it than someone whose main motivation is affect—positive *or* negative.

Rarely will a person's reasons fit into just one category. Eating is a complex behavior. But the physiological category may not be represented in the motivation patterns of some overweight persons. Early in obesity research Dr. Albert Stunkard (1976) discovered that obese individuals did not perceive hunger pangs when, in fact, their stomach muscles were contracting—a physiological signal that nonobese patients recognized and reported as hunger. Subsequent research has shown that the obese tend to respond more to external cues, and that they are less aware of their physiological state of being than the nonobese. What is this physiological mechanism that can tell a person to eat or to stop eating? How can some recognize it better than others? Does everybody have it?

The Physiological Basis of Hunger and Satiety

GENETICS

The earliest "research" on what makes one person fat and another person (perhaps with the same biological background) skinny dealt mainly with genetics. The hypothalamic feeding centers hadn't been discovered yet, but body build could be observed.

It was noted by Mayer (1968) that in the 1920s Davenport's research showed that in the matings of two slender parents, only slender offspring were produced (very seldom were there "fleshy" offspring); two fleshy parents produced predominantly fleshy offspring; and when one parent was fleshy and one slender, the majority of the offspring were still fleshy. It was concluded that there were several genes that controlled body build, and one of them was dominant because out of the possible pairings, the "fleshies" predominated.

It is known that there are definite strains of mice that are obese. For example, the New Zealand obese mice have an abnormal glucose tolerance that is genetically transmitted, and hereditary obese-hyperglycemic mice are thought to become obese because of the absence of an enzyme-depressor (also genetically determined). The study of humans is not so clear-cut because they cannot be experimentally manipulated like mice, and the human cerebral override can make just about anybody an obese person!

Even though research at this time cannot say there definitely are a fat gene and a skinny gene (or perhaps just the absence of a fat gene), a person may have an innate tendency to become overweight. An abnormal carbohydrate mechanism, an abnormally efficient fat storing mechanism, or any number of physiological traits that are passed on genetically could "tip the scale" toward obesity. But even if a person has the genetic tendency to become overweight, the cerebral override can prevent obesity. If such a person wants to be a healthy weight, he or she can fight the extra measure needed to keep the extra pounds off. In laboratory testing I worked with one woman who had half the oxygen utilization of what was considered normal. This meant that she had to eat half as much or exercise *twice* as much as others of her weight in order to have the same caloric deficit to lose or maintain weight. And so she did a little of each and did indeed control her weight at 115 to 120 pounds, just what she wanted it to be. A picture of her with her four sisters lined up with their backs to the camera provided evidence for the genetic theory. Although they were all different heights and weights, they all carried the same "double hip" problem of one fat pad at the buttocks and one at the top of the thigh!

If you think you are genetically "cursed" and can never lose weight even though you really want to, consider it a genetic challenge and get started on the program.

PHYSIOLOGICAL HUNGER AND SATIETY

Before we look at the elaborate mechanism of the most inner parts of the brain that govern eating behavior, we should define what hunger, satiety, and appetite are.

Hunger is the physiological drive to hunt for food and ingest it. It is manifested by stomach contractions and a complexity of nervous system impulses that involve smelling, tasting, and seeing food.

Appetite is the desire to eat when you are not necessarily hungry. Something may look good, smell good, strike a pleasant memory, or just be available when there's nothing else to do; so the appetite says, "Eat it." Appetite and hunger work in a seesaw relationship: The hungrier you are, the less appetizing or attractive the food has to be. The less hungry you are, the more you have to have an appetite for something specific or for some specific reason.

How many times after a huge Thanksgiving dinner have you accepted a piece of pumpkin pie with whipped cream? Were you *hungry* for it? Probably not. It was your anticipation, force of habit, memory of Mom's pumpkin pie, or some other cerebral stimulation that made you want to eat that pie.

Knowing the difference between hunger and appetite, you might want to analyze your eating behavior more precisely. When you confront yourself with food, ask yourself if you need it (hunger) or want it (appetite). Let yourself satisfy both, but let your choices lean toward hunger and you have a better chance of getting rid of that extra weight and then maintaining your lower weight. It's not impossible for a weight loser to have an incredible appetite for only low-calorie foods that are loaded with vitamins and minerals.

Satiety is the feeling of fullness that comes after eating—a feeling that you don't really *need* anything else to eat. Lethargy, sleepiness, and a satisfied feeling may accompany satiety.

All of these terms—*hunger, appetite,* and *satiety*—indicate quite subjective feelings in humans (and also in domesticated animals—obesity in the house dog is nearing the proportions of obesity in the owners). And so they are not easy terms to deal with. If a light came on when the body was hungry and went off when satiety occurred, and if appetite could be satisfied only when the light was on, then people would not have to learn how to recognize when they are actually hungry and when they are sated.

HUNGER AND SATIETY REGULATION

Some of the early experiments to find out why animals eat were done by Jean Mayer, famed nutritionist. In looking into the question, Mayer and his colleagues evaluated existing theories—the thermostatic theory that the body increased its fat storage in the cold and expended it in hot temperatures, and the gastric theory that hunger was caused by stomach contraction, and satiety occurred when the stomach was distended. These theories could not withstand close scrutiny because they did not answer some basic questions. The first question was, of course, are there controlling processes or body regulations for the intake of calories? Then the researchers asked, what is regulated, how well does the regulator work, and in what way does it work?

Short-Term Regulation. Early study by numerous investigators showed that under normal conditions mice, fish, rats, and other animals generally ate each day what they needed for energy purposes and no more. If more energy was expended on one or two days of the week, food intake would increase at some time so that the extra energy drain was compensated for over a period of time, usually within a day or two. People tend to respond in the same manner. You probably find that if you have a day or two of strenuous activity, you spend the next day or so inadvertently eating a little more than usual. Or if you've overeaten at one meal, you may find that you are not as hungry the next day. Your biologic nature will keep you in balance if you don't try to outwit it.

From experimental study it is suspected that there is, in fact, some sort of short-term regulatory mechanism that keeps the human body in balance from day to day—*if you don't override it*! So the answer to the first question—are there controlling processes—is "yes," there does seem to be some sort of regulatory mechanism.

What Is Regulated? It appears that the answer to this question is *intake*. If you expend more than normal energy, you respond by taking in more food. If you eat too much, you respond by subsequently taking in less food (rather than spontaneously exercising more) to put your body back into caloric balance.

To understand the precision of this mechanism, researchers looked to the animal kingdom (especially nondomesticated animals) to see how well it *can* work. However, research on humans shows that humans tend to maintain the same weight from day to day under normal circumstances. This short-term mechanism seems to be more precise than any long-term mechanism, as "creeping obesity" can be seen throughout society. Long-term regulation will be discussed later in this chapter.

What Is the Mechanism? In looking for the biologic regulating mechanism, early researchers knew that many biologic factors were involved, such as metabolism (how fast the body burns its fuel), metabolic defects (for example, carbohydrate intolerance), the feelings of hunger (especially hunger pangs or stomach muscle contractions), the biologic mechanism itself (wherever it may be), and the feelings of satiety. Any substantial theory of regulation had to show all these factors in a cause-and-effect relationship.

The gastric theory was popular as early as the late eighteenth century, as everyone knew that when you were hungry your stomach growled, and when you ate and the stomach became distended, you *felt* full and could *see* it looking full. In the early 1900s research substantiated the subjective data. Subjects were asked to swallow balloons and then these were inflated and connected to an outside pressure gauge. And, sure enough, as the subjects became hungrier, their stomach contractions became stronger. But further investigation showed that when the splanchnic nerves (those that carry the message of stomach contraction to the brain) were cut, hunger still occurred and food intake was still regulated! Also, vagotomy (cutting the vagus nerve between the brain and the stomach) eliminated stomach contractions, but hunger and eating regulation still occurred. So, back to the drawing board!

The Satiety Centers. In the 1930s researchers developed a new theory, as it was found in autopsies that some very obese people had portions of the hypothalamus that appeared to have lesions.

The hypothalamus (see Figure 6.1) normally regulates the automatic functions of the body, such as heart rate, breathing, water balance, temperature control, and so on. So it was thought that perhaps the hypothalamus controls metabolism, too. Soon researchers found that there are, in fact, two tiny nerve depots in the hypothalamus that must have something to do with food regulation, because when they were destroyed in experimental animals, the animals ate excessively and became obese. Experiments were carried out with mice, rats, chickens, and goats, and the same response occurred—overeating and obesity.

These tiny nerve centers were recognized as the *ventromedial nuclei* (VMN), and they became very popular targets of research. The next page in this story was the finding that when lesions were introduced in the VMN, animals showed a lack of satiety rather than an increase in hunger. That is, they did not work as hard for their food (by pressing a lever), and their satiety periods were shorter than animals' without such lesions. And so, it became increasingly apparent that the VMN are more concerned with satiety than with hunger. The VMN normally put a stop to eating and thereby control intake of calories somehow; and when they are not stimulated, hunger occurs.

The Hunger Centers. Then it was found that animals *would* stop eating if hypothalamic areas lateral to the VMN had lesions induced, and the entire hypothalamic theory was put together: The *lateral hypothalamic* (LH) *areas* govern hunger, and the VMN govern satiety (see Figure 6.2). It was assumed that since the LH and the VMN are

FIGURE 6.1
The Brain and the Brainstem

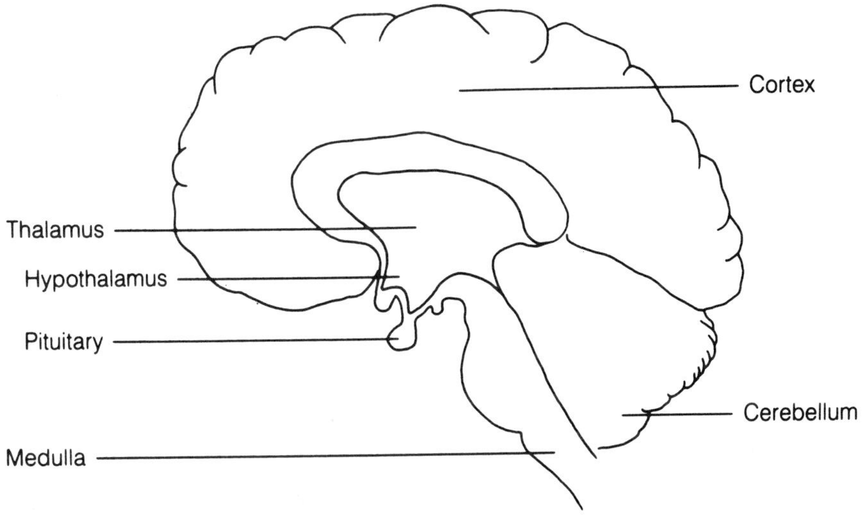

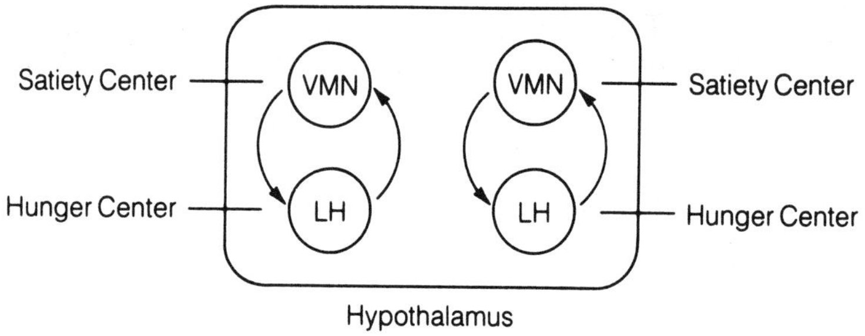

FIGURE 6.2 Hypothalamic Hunger and Satiety Centers

intimate neighbors they therefore might have a close communication system. This was in fact the case, as research continued to expose nature's plan of controlling hunger and satiety.

Glucose Receptors. In 1967 Mayer and his colleagues traced nerve fibers from the satiety centers to the hunger centers. Having discovered the anatomical basis, they proceeded to ask, what do these centers respond to? What stimulates them to tell the body, "eat," or "stop eating"?

It is known that blood passes through the hypothalamus unfiltered by the blood-brain barrier that protects the cortex. As the blood passes through the hypothalamus, special cells test how thick or thin the blood is so the body can maintain water balance by saving or getting rid of water. The hypothalamus also measures the temperature of the blood so that body temperature is maintained by sweating, shivering, and other devices.

So, based on early speculation, researchers suspected that the hunger and satiety centers respond to the level of blood sugar, and the theory was tested. Again, Mayer did some insightful research on the hypothesis that glucoreceptors (sensors of glucose in the blood) exist in the satiety centers (the VMN). He biochemically attached gold to glucose (creating a structure called goldthioglucose, GTG), knowing that if the VMN were in fact glucose receptive, the gold attached to the glucose would damage the receptor. If the receptors were poisoned by the gold, they would no longer work, the animal would begin to overeat, and become obese (see Figure 6.3).

When other sugars such as galactose or other substances whose structures are close to that of glucose were used, there was no effect on the VMN. Another convincing aspect of this glucostatic theory is that diabetic animals showed no lesions from the glucose-gold combination—because without insulin, glucose cannot enter the VMN.

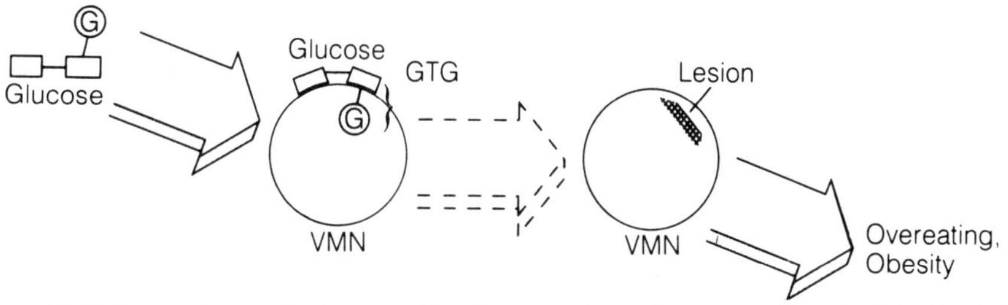

FIGURE 6.3 Mayer's Process for Discovering Glucoreceptors in VMN: Goldthioglucose is induced into bloodstream; gold is received by glucoreceptors; gold poisons receptors, causing lesions in VMN. Overeating and obesity follow.

More proof of the existence of glucose receptors in the satiety centers was added when the activity of single neurons in the VMN was shown to correspond with glucose utilization. When glucose levels are high, the VMN electrical activity is high, and when blood glucose levels are low, so is the electrical activity of these centers (see Figure 6.4).

So it appeared that the VMN control the process: When blood sugar is low, the satiety center allows the hunger centers to take over and food-seeking behavior begins. After eating, when the blood sugar levels rise again, the VMN starts increasing its activity again to shut off the feeding centers.

The Final Common Pathway. A refined model of hunger and satiety regulation was advanced by Balagura (1972) who noted that the lateral hypothalamus is also receptive to glucose, that is, it also has glucoreceptors. This newer finding somewhat contradicted the older

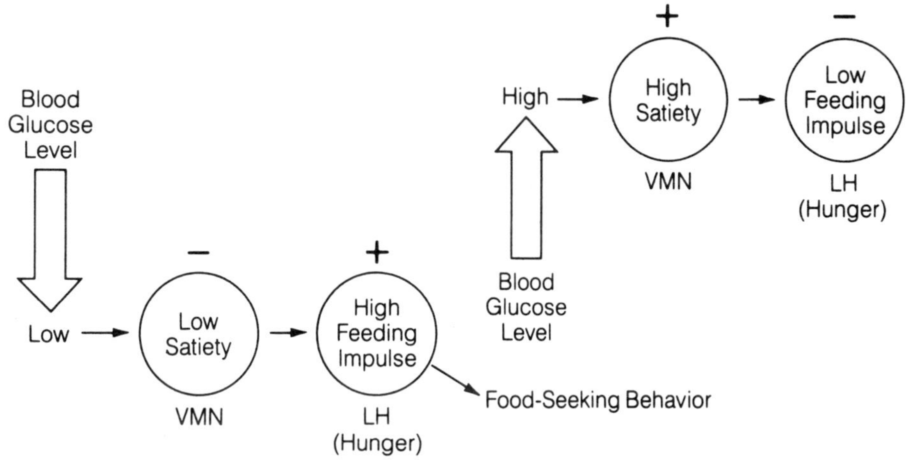

FIGURE 6.4 Electrical Response of Glucoreceptors to Blood Glucose Levels

theory that stated that the satiety center controls everything with an on-off switch. (In other words, while the VMN is stimulated by satiety, it turns off the hunger center and no eating occurs; then when satiety wanes, the hunger center is allowed by the VMN to take over.)

In finding glucoreceptors in the lateral hypothalamus, researchers discovered its autonomy. Low glucose is the stimulus for the animal to start moving its feet to find food and whatever other kind of feeding movement is needed. When this stimulus (low glucose level) occurs, a motor pathway originating in the lateral hypothalamus and continuing out the hypothalamus and down the brainstem carries the impulses to the parts of the anatomy responsible for getting and eating food. Balagura called this the "final common pathway of eating" (see Figure 6.5). The reciprocity of the satiety and hunger centers is still apparent as satiety and hunger do not occur at the same time; when one is turned on, the other is turned off. Each is responsive to blood sugar and the presence of insulin (Rodin, 1984).

Peripheral Helpers The hypothalamic control centers appear to be the bases of human feeding behavior, but you know you cannot ignore the fact that your stomach growls when you're hungry or that your mouth waters when you smell or see something delicious being served. These factors, too, are physiological but are representatives of *peripheral* regulatory mechanisms that aid the central controls in the hypothalamus.

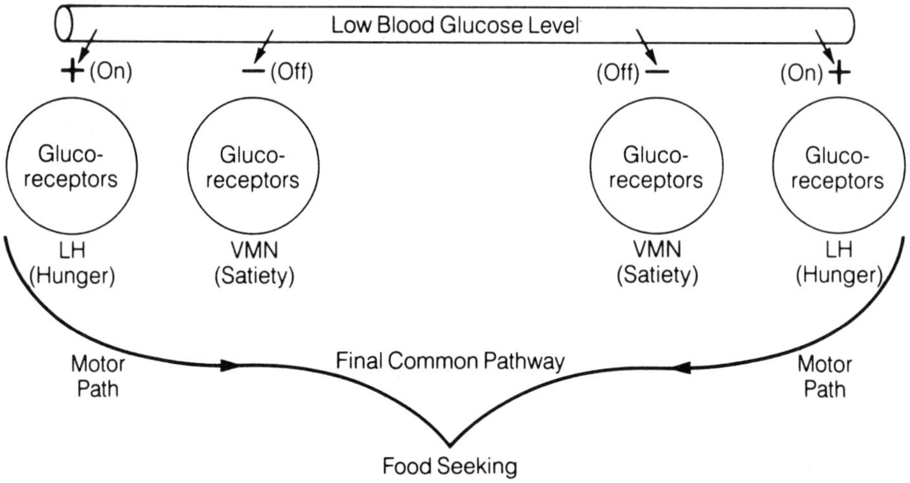

FIGURE 6.5 Balagura's Model of the Final Common Pathway of Eating

The Stomach. There are some tiny nerve fibers (the Bundles of Schutz) between the VMN and the vagus nerve that carry feedback to and from the gastrointestinal (GI) tract, especially the stomach. Apparently when the body is low on blood sugar, messages are sent to the stomach for it to start "growling" about not being fed lately. How often have you been engrossed in your work and then it suddenly occurred to you that it's time to eat because you hear this gurgling noise inside your stomach? Sometimes it's an embarrassment, but perhaps it's just another precaution against starvation. It usually gets your attention!

The Nose. What happens when you smell your favorite food cooking? Your mouth waters, and you have a great desire to eat that food. This response is also a physiological reminder to eat. There is a neurological pathway from the nose to a portion of the inner brain that appears to facilitate eating. Again, it seems that nature has taken precautionary measures to make sure you don't starve.

There is also an olfactory pathway that inhibits eating, perhaps to protect the body from rotten food. When something rancid turns your stomach, your natural senses are at work. These senses also keep you from stuffing yourself. Think back to past Thanksgivings or Christmas Days when the morning started smelling like baked turkey. The delicious aroma drifted through the house and you couldn't wait to eat the turkey. But what reaction did you have to that same smell after the dinner was over? It was probably a feeling of not needing to smell turkey again for a while. With this olfactory turnoff, you didn't want to eat any more turkey, either.

The olfactory sense (smell) is one of the strongest feeding senses. Even though humans have learned to rely on modes other than the nose to find food, this sense is still very strong in "lower" animals who rely on their noses for food seeking. However, even in humans, an accompanying terrible stench can extinguish unwanted eating behavior faster than any another mode of punishment (such as electric shock) can.

Taste. Taste is a facilitator to eating if the taste is pleasant, and an inhibitor to eating if the taste is bitter, sour, too salty, or too sweet. When you eat something that tastes good, it is an immediate reward that encourages you to have more. I have seen the "taste good" phenomenon in many of my clients; it drives them to eat more than they need. If you have ever seen the TV commercial where someone insists to another, "I'll bet you can't eat just one," you know what this phenomenon is. I worked with one student who was a doughnut "junkie." Every morning on her way to school she passed a doughnut shop. If she drove right by the shop, there was no problem. But if she stopped, she could never have just one doughnut. She would eat three at the shop and buy a half dozen to go. And she would eat all six on the way to school.

Taste can also be remembered from another time that a particular food was eaten, but remembered taste is not such a strong reinforcer as good-tasting food in your mouth this very minute. If you have a "bet you can't eat just one" problem, a good way of handling it is to program how many (much) you can have before you start eating. Freeze the rest, or give it to a neighbor, or don't buy any more than you can have, or lock your refrigerator or cupboard door if you have the weakness for more (some of my clients have bought locks for such a purpose—and have used them).

Sight. The sight of food is also a peripheral mechanism that helps determine when and how much you eat. Subliminal commercials (such as showing during a theater movie one frame of film that depicts a food item, for example, popcorn) have been outlawed. But the fact that the use of such commercials was researched and that they were successfully used does indicate that the sight of a particular food can arouse interest in that food. Grocery stores take advantage of visual stimuli—they have prime space for certain products and that prime space is at eye level. This is one reason why many people should not shop when they're hungry. Visual input will fill the grocery basket with many unwanted or unusual items.

Think of the times you see food commercials on TV—breakfast food ads in the morning, candy bars ads predominantly in the afternoon and evening, dinner suggestions in the afternoon, and junk food snacks in the afternoon and evening. And what do you do during the commercials? Go find something to snack on!

Chewing and Swallowing. Chewing and swallowing appear to have some satiety value; that is, as food is "monitored" by the mouth and swallowed, it provides some satisfaction. Research has shown that when food is chewed and swallowed, but then is diverted from the throat through a surgical opening (called a fistula), animals will show satiety.

Appetite. Whether food is appetizing or not is an important psychological regulator of what and how much is eaten. Sight, smell, and taste are all related to appetite as they trigger some psychological memory about certain foods. As mentioned before, as hunger diminishes, appetite must increase in order for a person to keep eating.

Whether these peripheral aspects have a physiological basis or whether they are psychological in nature, they do come into play in the regulation of food intake.

LONG-TERM REGULATION OF EATING

Through animal research it has been shown that there is a physiological basis for regulating food intake. Some of these regulatory mechanisms are buried deep in the inner brain and some are more peripheral, such as signals from the stomach. It is apparent that humans—so-called "highly evolved beings"—have learned to ignore the physical signals and override them with thoughts and feelings. For this reason, humans have a greater problem with maintaining their weight than do animals (those who have not been spoiled by humans, that is). In spite of the human appetite, however, most people seem to balance their weight from day to day. Usually it is a crisis that causes weight change. Then the new weight is maintained from day to day after the crisis is over. Perhaps animals have some kind of long-term regulatory mechanism that seems to be lacking in affluent human populations where overweight and obesity are the rule rather than the exceptions.

The Dual Lipostatic Theory. Through extensive research with animals with VMN- and LH-induced lesions, a theory of long-term weight maintenance has emerged. This theory states that humans have a lower weight threshold or set point that is governed by hunger and an upper weight threshold that is governed by appetite. Body weight is maintained between the upper and lower set points according to the dual lipostatic theory of Sclafani and Kluge (1974). Researchers testing this theory induced lesions in the satiety centers of experimental animals and found that the body weights of these animals increased greatly at first, but then leveled off at a new, higher set point (see Figure 6.6). After the new appetite body weight threshold was set, weight was again maintained.

When this theory is applied to humans, some trauma other than the cutting or a lesion of the satiety center may cause a new set point—perhaps worry, anxiety, depression, anger, or any of the ego emotions.

My Pet Theory. I have a pet theory of my own regarding a long-term weight regulation mechanism for weight. Part of the reason people keep their weight down year after year just may be the size of their clothes! Most people don't continually buy clothes at a rate to fit their size—they buy something that fits and then try to stay the same size as the garment. Then they try to buy the same size replacement clothes, not wanting to buy larger sizes. With the thinking and emotional components inherent in human eating behavior, this theory could be more than just a little humor aimed at the scientific community.

SO, IS THERE A PHYSIOLOGICAL CONTROL?

It does appear scientifically correct to believe there is some sort of biological control of human eating behavior. Logically, it seems unthinkable that nature would *not* supply all animals with some kind of eating regulator that would prevent starvation. Animals that are not domesticated (and some that are) use their biological mechanisms quite effectively to maintain their adult weight over a period of many years. Human beings, however, tend to fill their heads with ego emotions that can obliterate physiological feelings of hunger and satiety unless these physical feelings are extreme (or in some cases, aren't felt at all). The next section explains some of the psychological aspects involved in becoming overweight and staying there, or trying to become thin and staying there.

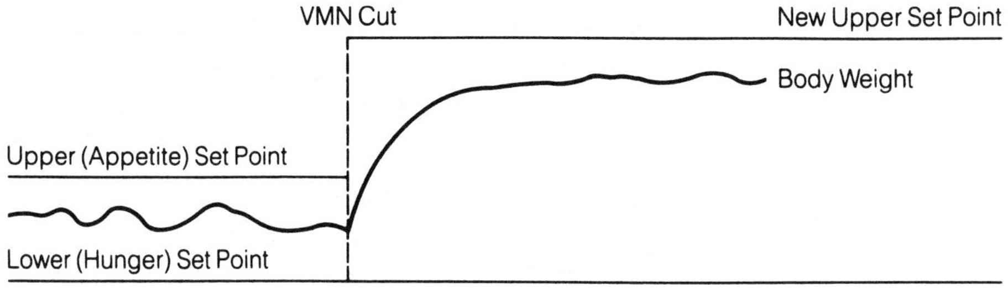

FIGURE 6.6 Dual Lipostatic Theory: Weight increases after VMN is cut but then levels off at a new set point.

The Psychological Aspects of Eating

If people could be aware of and respond to only their physiological need for food, everyone would be in great shape. Unfortunately, weight and body composition reflect to a large extent what people think about themselves and their body images. A large body size can be used for power, to hide behind, to scare away suitors, or for many other psychological purposes. And those who are overweight or obese and stay at such an enlarged size experience some kind of reward for staying large.

PSYCHOLOGICAL MODEL FOR EATING

Hilde Bruch, famed psychiatrist who works with individuals with eating disorders, especially children, explained a model for the psychological basis of eating that has great merit (1969). Going beyond the physiological basis of hunger, Bruch defined hunger in terms of the psychological factors as well. *Psychological hunger* is an unpleasant drive that you feel when you're deprived of food. This results in searching for, and perhaps even fighting for, food to relieve the torment.

Bruch's hypothesis is that hunger awareness is not innate biological knowledge but rather a learned response. Learning is necessary for hunger and satiety to become organized into a recognizable pattern. For proper learning of hunger awareness to take place an infant must repeatedly experience a defined sequence:

1. Feel discomfort
2. Express discomfort
3. Have signal recognized by feeder
4. Feed
5. Feel relief

Current knowledge of neurophysiology, child development, and communication theory is compatible with Bruch's theory.

In a graduate obesity theory class one of my students had recently become a father, so I asked him how he knew when to feed his new daughter. He replied, "When she cries, we check her temperature, her diaper, her position, and her clothing. If they're all okay, we feed her."

Eating disorders start very early when an infant does not properly learn the hunger-satiety pattern. Learning an improper pattern is the fault of the responder or feeder (usually the mother, but can be the father or some other responsible adult). Incorrect and confusing patterns result in an infant's not being able to differentiate between hunger and other bodily discomforts. Let's look at some inappropriate responses that my graduate student could have made when his daughter cried about various body discomforts.

If the infant was crying from pain, an inappropriate response would be to feed her, bringing her no relief. Feeding an infant who is crying because of wet diapers or an uncomfortable position would also be inappropriate. (In the latter case, the child may stop crying simply because she is being held.) The parents must respond appropriately to the cause of the child's crying—feed her because she is hungry, not because she is in pain, lonely, wet, or uncomfortable.

A nonresponsive parent or other family member may easily confuse the learning infant. Some parents, annoyed by the baby's crying, will automatically stick a bottle in the baby's mouth so that they can get some peace. Have you seen this happen?

A child growing up is often bribed with food (especially sweet treats) to be quiet, to do what the parents wish, as a reward for being a good boy or girl, to occupy the child while the parents are busy, and so on. Think of your early years: "If you're a good girl, I'll take you for an ice cream cone." "If you're a good boy and eat your meal, I'll give you some dessert." "I brought you a candy bar because you've been so good lately." "I bought you this lollipop just as a reminder that I love you." You probably still do this with the persons you like or love—you bake their favorite cake or give them a box of candy to show them that you care for them. It would be better to use a nonnutritive reward, especially with children. But adults may also fall into the trap.

It is no wonder that some people eat when they are sad, lonely, or bored. The early feeding that was a response to pain or discomfort easily connected those feelings with eating, especially when the factors of being held close by a warm, loving parent are included.

It is difficult as a parent not to use food as a pacifier, but each time it is done, the learning pattern of the child deviates further and further from a proper hunger-satiety response. And the improper responses learned early in childhood stay to haunt the grown person until they are relearned. Most people fail even to recognize that they are acting in the old pattern; therefore, they don't attempt to learn a new one.

Bruch, in her extensive psychiatric practice with obese patients, reported that many of her patients do not or cannot recognize the feeling of satiety, of having had enough. Many also cannot feel hunger. How, then, can they exert willpower over a function or need that they cannot even recognize? If the response was improperly learned at one time, it can be unlearned, and a new pattern can be learned. Behavior modification techniques may help in the relearning of this behavior.

SECONDARY GAIN

Whenever a person has little or no success in any kind of change program (whether it is a weight, fitness, stress or other kind of management program), the psychologist would have to guess that the person is getting what is called "secondary gain," or rewards, from the old behavior. Secondary gains are usually at a subconscious level, so they are not easily identified by the individual who is not having a successful program. The emotional ties that people (especially women) have with food are often at the core of the problem, as are other psychological/emotional issues. Four of the common secondary gains from emotional blocks found in weight management clients are:

1. *The issue of nurturing.* Many female clients spend a large proportion of their lives nurturing others with little vocal complaint that no one is nurturing them in return. Food becomes a nurturer for them. Whenever the "dieter" rewards herself with forbidden sweets she is nurturing herself. Many use alcohol for the same purpose. Successful weight management clients realize that they need and want to be nurtured, and make a plan whereby they get nurturing without rewarding themselves with food.
2. *Protection.* One's fat may act as a buffer zone between him or her and the outside world, not only as a physical barrier, but also as added bulk to scare off others. When this is an issue, weight reduction often brings with it the "phantom body size" phenomenon because the person has so completely identified himself or herself as a formidable person. Very often the underlying issue in the use of fat for protection is low self-concept, low level of self-empowerment, and the resultant fear of the outside world in general and of close personal relationships in particular. Learning to be assertive in telling others of needs and feelings is especially helpful for these individuals.

3. *Being stuck, or waiting.* Gawain (1986) attributes excess weight problems to blockage of energy. Psychosomatic research goes even further in pointing out that individuals carry their weight quite obviously in the location(s) where energy is being trapped. Learning to release pent-up thoughts and actions overcomes the inertia and depression that often accompany excess weight and unsuccessful weight reduction.
4. *Eating as a release for negative emotions such as anger, fear, and anxiety.* In the buildup and release of stressful situations there are normally four stages: conflict, tension, release, and relaxation. However, the last stage, relaxation, is not reached unless there is release. A healthy release comes from resolving the situation, but individuals often substitute behaviors that are not appropriate for release of the emotion. Food may appease them and it becomes their tranquilizer. Becoming familiar with emotions and ways to truly release them is a healthy endeavor for those who use this kind of secondary gain.

CLASSIFICATIONS OF OBESITY

Although classifications tend to be limited in describing the personality of an overweight or obese person, they also may illuminate a particular problem by naming it. So the following classifications are offered to give greater understanding of problems related to being overweight or obese.

Bruch's Classification. The first classification given here defines the relationships between psychological reaction patterns and obesity, as identified by Hilde Bruch (1969).

1. *Absence of psychopathology.* These individuals are overweight or obese without emotional difficulty. They are well adjusted to a larger size and feel no compulsion to change it. They may, though, use their size as a rationalization for their problems of everyday life: "I can't do that because I weigh too much."

2. *Developmental obesity.* Obesity plays a significant role in the growth and development of these individuals. They become obese in childhood and are quite preoccupied with their size and weight. Generally, they do not tolerate frustration well or delay gratification well. As was explained earlier in Bruch's hunger-satiety theory, these people recognize internal stimuli poorly because of inappropriate early learning.

Fat children are constantly reminded of being fat—by childhood playmates and schoolmates, by adults, and by family. In school they usually acquire a fat-related nickname such as "Chubby," "Fatty," "Tubby," "Piggy," and so forth. They become accustomed to being the last ones chosen for teams and realize early that their size is a negative factor. As these children grow up many find it is difficult to buy clothes, be comfortable in a swim suit, or fit into a theater seat.

Another name given to this class of obesity is *childhood onset* obesity. The prognosis for weight loss is not as good for this group of obese individuals as it is for individuals in the other classes.

3. *Reactive obesity*. This group of individuals has become overweight or obese usually as a response to a psychological trauma. Eating is used to reduce feelings of psychological discomfort such as anxiety, fear, depression, tension. There may also be an underlying fear of starvation that is rekindled with any kind of disappointment.

You may recognize the person who has this underlying fear of starvation. For instance, when sharing an order of french fries to accompany your separate orders of sandwiches, this person will gobble down french fries from the common dish before eating his or her own sandwich. This phenomenon is not limited to obese individuals.

Reactive obesity is also called *adult onset* obesity. The prognosis for weight loss is much better for these individuals, as they do not have a lifetime psychology, sociology, and biology of obesity.

A classic case of adult onset or reactive obesity was characterized by Donna, a 25-year-old student. She had been a thin child and all the way through high school she had an attractive figure. Her first year in college was active and rewarding; she found her true love and together they were the "perfect couple." Donna became pregnant and wanted the child, but her boyfriend insisted that she have an abortion. So she did. Their relationship broke up. She started eating excessively and stopped all of her activities except going to class and studying. In a three-month period she gained 45 pounds and none of her casual friends recognized her. Her family was astounded and quite disgusted.

Donna's problem in weight loss was recovering from this emotional reaction. By the end of the weight control program, she was feeling better about herself and had lost 15 pounds.

4. *Thin-fat people*. This group consists of those who have successfully lost weight and no longer look fat, but still feel fat. They are preoccupied with their body size and weight and constantly focus

on food and eating. Some become real fanatics about what they can eat and what they cannot eat, and their most prized possessions are their scales.

One of the most outstanding examples of this "phantom body size" syndrome that I have seen is one of my former students, Liz, who had a surgical bypass operation. She went from 225 to 140 pounds in the nine months prior to entering my program. She shared pictures that showed her as a 225-pound bathing beauty, and it was hard for the group to believe that this was the same person. It was even harder for her to believe it! One of her greatest concerns was that she would never think of herself as "thin" (although she ended the program at a thin 125 pounds).

When you live inside a fat person for 20 years or more, it takes a while to get rid of the fat-person image, fears, and emotions. Constant positive feedback from those around you helps tremendously, but in some instances those who are used to the former fat person will discourage the new thin person by complaining: "You look emaciated." "A big wind is going to come along and blow you away." "God, you look awful!" They are accustomed to the way you used to look.

If the newly thinned person lives with fat people (especially family members), he or she will likely be discouraged because becoming thin is a constant reminder that the others are fat. Just as someone successful in Alcoholics Anonymous moves away from old alcoholic friends, so should the newly thinned person move away from the environment of negative reinforcement or punishment from fat persons nearby.

Hamburger's Classification. Hamburger (1956) in summarizing the obesity of his patients classified them according to type of overeating. This classification of four types may provide a little more enlightenment regarding obesity (and especially eating behavior).

1. *Overeating in response to dysphoric feelings*; that is, eating beyond normal satiety due to depression, anger, boredom, and so on. Most people do this to some extent, but Hamburger's patients reacted by extreme overeating.
2. *Overeating due to reactive situations*. Much like Bruch's reactive obese people, patients in this category respond to stressful life situations by overeating. These situations might be intolerable stress at

work, divorce-qualifying arguments at home, or any unpleasant or frustrating situation in their lives.

3. *Overeating as symptomology of emotional illness.* This group of patients overate to keep themselves from falling into deep depression or breaking into hysteria.

4. *Overeating as a food addiction.* This group used food to produce sedation—if they were eating, the situation was under control; but if deprived of food, they experienced a "withdrawal" reaction. With food restriction these patients would show behavioral changes that supported the concept of psychological dependence on food. In this category might be seen the eaters who have food hidden in various places around the house (usually carbohydrates such as cookies, doughnuts, and so on) so they will always have a food supply.

Stunkard's Classification. One other way to classify obesity types is by patterns of eating. Albert Stunkard (1976), in his extensive study and practice, discovered and identified two main types of eating patterns in the obese.

1. *The binge eater.* This person usually goes on a food binge in response to stress. Some of Stunkard's patients tell of binges that are hard to believe. One person ate full dinners at two different restaurants, then went to a grocery store and bought two large bags of cookies, cakes, doughnuts, pretzels, popcorn, and so on that he devoured as he drove around the city.

A binge eater at home might attack a whole frozen pumpkin pie or two, a can of whipped cream, several dozen cookies, a box of cake mix, a gallon of hot chocolate, three cans of fruit cocktail, a pound of peanuts, and various refrigerator leftovers in one binge. Having begun eating, a binge eater just cannot seem to get enough.

After the binge, the person is usually filled with self-condemnation and is bewildered about how he or she could have done this massive eating.

2. *The night eater.* Much like binge eating, the night eating syndrome involves eating a great amount of food, but only at night. The night eater is anorexic (has no hunger or desire for food) in the morning and may not eat until lunch or dinner of the following day, and these meals are likely to be normal.

Self-condemnation was not found by Stunkard to be a reaction to this kind of overeating.

Classification Summary. These classifications may give insight into the psychological profile of obese persons as we look at the behavioral characteristics that tend to differ between obese and normal weight people. The classifications have been given here for general observation and not as a basis to "psychoanalyze" yourself or your friends. If you see yourself in some of the classifications, you may be alerting yourself that you do have a behavior that happens to have been observed in others. Recognizing an area of problem behavior is the first step in correcting it—when you are ready.

THE EATING DISORDERS: BULIMIA AND ANOREXIA NERVOSA

There is widespread concern about the growing number of bulimics and anorectics in this country, especially in the teenage female population and in activities where it is important to meet weight requirements or otherwise be thin (activities such as gymnastics, high school and college wrestling, and ballet).

Bulimia. Bulimia is characterized by first gorging or binging and then vomiting, using laxatives or even exercise to purge or cleanse the body of the food or its caloric effects. The prevalence of bulimia among college students is estimated to be about 10 percent of the student body, overall. However, it is estimated that more than 90 percent of bulimics are women and that more than 1 out of 10 women between the ages of 16 and 24 may be bulimic. Most bulimics are white and belong to the middle or upper-middle class.

The medical complications of bulimia include tooth decay from vomited stomach acids, enlargement of the parotid (salivary) glands at the base of the jaw, disturbances of the sodium-potassium balance, kidney problems, and hemorrhages in the conjunctiva of the eye. Bulimics may even die from their disorder from gastric rupture, heart attack, liver damage, susceptibility to infection, or suicide (Gross, 1984). The symptoms of bulimia include skin rash, swelling, pain, and tenderness of the salivary glands; water retention and subsequent swelling of the ankles and feet; swelling over the abdominal area; and frequent dental caries and erosion of tooth enamel. These symptoms occur due to dehydration, electrolyte imbalances, and nutrient losses that occur from constant purging.

The bulimic, when on a binge, may eat tremendous amounts of food. One binge-purger told of taking food out of the garbage can and eating it. Patients suffering from this syndrome are unable to control their eating; they feel they must eat everything in sight. Many realize that they are trying to heal some psychological hurt (such as rejection or grief) or to prevent one. They may also enjoy the sense of self-control that vomiting gives them.

A former client, Sarah, was a 21-year-old college student with bulimia. She frequently went on eating binges that might have included a half gallon of ice cream with a pint of chocolate syrup poured over it, a package of cookies, a dozen donuts, and a box of chocolate-cream candies. Sarah knew that she was consuming an astronomical number of calories and was terrified of becoming fat, so she learned to make herself vomit after a binge. She also took laxatives and diuretics to further purge her body.

Sarah's binges produced an emotional numbness that helped her ward off feelings of depression, loneliness, boredom, and anxiety. The binging, however, was followed by guilt and self-condemnation, together with a fear of becoming fat. This led her to vomiting and other compensatory behaviors, such as taking laxatives, diet pills, and diuretics; fasting; or bouts of excessive exercise.

Sarah's bulimia was medically linked to depression (nearly 80 percent of clinical patients have experienced a major depression or a manic-depressive episode sometime in their lives). Treatment for Sarah's depression and attending syndromes was a long process that called for clinical intervention and family support.

Anorexia Nervosa. Anorexia nervosa is an eating disorder in which dramatic weight loss occurs due to continuous self-starvation or from severe self-imposed dieting in an attempt to attain the perfect thin body. Current figures suggest that the incidence of anorexia is on the rise, with about 1 out of every 250 U.S. females between ages 12 and 18 years old (Levenkron, 1982). These cases are only the serious clinical cases. There may be countless Kathy Rigbys (the U.S. women's Olympic gymnastic medal winner) who are performing well, even with their eating disorder, and are not identified as anorectics. A recent Gallup Poll projected that about two million American women between 19 and 39 and one million teenagers are affected by some symptoms of anorexia nervosa or bulimia nervosa, with males accounting for 5 to 10 percent of these cases.

The anorectic fears gaining weight and goes to dangerous lengths to become thinner and thinner. Even though she may become very thin and unhealthy, she still sees herself as being heavy. Anorectics often binge-purge and take laxatives to keep food cleared out of their systems. They may also take diet pills. Both diet pills and laxatives cause the body to build up a tolerance, and anorectics are forced to take more and more of them to get any effect.

The symptoms of bulimia also occur in anorectics, but in anorexia the electrolyte (sodium-potassium) balance may be even worse because of the habitual taking of laxatives. Severe electrolyte imbalances may cause muscle spasms, kidney problems, or cardiac arrest. Other symptoms include dryness of the skin, falling hair, constipation from insufficient fluid and food and from dulled intestinal nerves, abdominal pain, and the stopping of menstruation.

This illness can be deadly and leaves its scars on the victim and the family. Because it is poorly understood and has caused much fear, pain, and suffering, early detection and treatment are important. If you know and care for someone who is obsessed with being thin, who secretly binges on large amounts of food, who purchases large quantities of laxatives or diet pills, and who exhibits the other symptoms listed here, you should consider the possibility of anorexia-bulimia and suggest help for that person (Girdano, Everly, and Dusek, 1985).

Anorexia and Athletics. Nearly all high school and college students who are serious athletes are concerned at some time or another about their performance weight. In some sports, such as wrestling, athletes must "make their weight," while lighter bodies in other sports may make a difference in speed or the ability to be lifted or carried. Still other activities, such as dance, may encourage thinness for appearance's sake. All of these reasons put extra pressure on individuals to lose weight in an unwise way, and may put such a focus on being thin that it becomes an obsession that may stay with them even after their performance days are over. This pressure seems to have an even greater affect on the athlete who has considered him/herself overweight in the past. With high energy output sports, it is difficult to determine the effects of the sport and the effects of an eating disorder, so many young athletes who are anorectic may go unnoticed and undiagnosed.

It is important that athletes (and coaches) use the basic guidelines as given in this book to change body composition. Athletes can reach their fitness and weight goals by following good eating guidelines, being cognizant of their mental and emotional health, and performing some kinds of stress management techniques while they are involved in a demanding athletic program.

IS THERE A PSYCHOLOGICAL PROFILE OF FAT PEOPLE?

Extensive research has been done to find a psychological profile of the overweight and obese, but very few concrete factors continue to appear. *Distorted body image* and *irregular eating behavior* are two characteristics that do keep appearing, and a number of others are continually suggested, but with contradictory research.

When studying the obese, remember there is much difference between those who have been obese from childhood and those who become obese in adulthood. Remember also the difference between clinical obesity and being varying degrees of overweight. One other cautionary aspect here is that some of the research done on the obese is limited to those who are having psychological or psychiatric problems with their obesity; therefore, the nonclinical cases are not represented in that research. My own research has been done mainly on overweight college-age students, with a small percentage that qualify as clinically obese. These differences, where pertinent, will be pointed out in the following text.

Body Image. Research shows that obese individuals may have distorted body images (Leon, 1982). They cannot see themselves as they appear to others as accurately as normal weight individuals can see themselves. The obese may be overly self-conscious about their body size and feel that everything bad that happens to them is due to their largeness.

In years of practice with college students and private clients, I have found that when overweight individuals come into my program, they have, on the average, lower body image scores than do students in other health education classes in the same university or locale. What has been particularly rewarding is the fact that the average body image score in the weight control program always improves over the period of the program (usually about 15 weeks), and the postprogram scores are then similar to the average scores of students not seeking help in weight control.

If you would like to examine what you think of your body, complete the following Abbreviated Body Cathexis Scale (Dusek et al., 1987).

*ABBREVIATED BODY CATHEXIS SCALE**

Directions: Below are listed 16 body features. For each feature, indicate which ones you are satisfied with exactly as they are, which ones you worry about, and which ones you would really like to change. Use the following scale:

1 = I strongly dislike this feature and wish I could change it.
2 = I don't like this feature but can put up with it.
3 = I really don't give this feature much thought.
4 = I am satisfied with this feature.
5 = I consider myself fortunate to have such a fine feature.

For each of the items below fill in the number that *best* represents how you feel about that feature.

____ 1. Weight	____ 9. Energy level
____ 2. Hips	____ 10. Profile
____ 3. Appetite	____ 11. Arms
____ 4. Body build	____ 12. Back
____ 5. Trunk	____ 13. Posture
____ 6. Waist	____ 14. Knees
____ 7. Legs	____ 15. Neck
____ 8. Exercise level	____ 16. Chest

Add your score and write the total here: ____

The average score of three separate groups of 25 individuals who recently experienced the holistic program was 37.5, 41, and 35.6 as they began the program. If your score is between 35 and 40, you might consider that you have no poorer or greater image of your body than most others starting a weight control program. If your score is less than 30, you have a fairly poor image of your body, and if your score is 45 or greater, you would appear to be well pleased with your body overall.

The mean scores for the three groups mentioned here at the end of the program were 44, 47, and 41.5, a six-point increase in each group (see Table 6.2). The postprogram scores were similar to the average scores in several health information classes. So if your body

*This is an abbreviated form of the Secord-Jourard Body Cathexis Scale (Secord and Jourard, 1953), factor analyzed and reduced from 46 items to 16. The correlation between the 46-item and the 16-item form was found to be r = .88 and r = .93 with two large groups of university students (Dusek et al., 1987).

image score is low, there is a good chance that by improving your exercise habits, nutrition pattern, coping behavior, and/or your attitude toward yourself and thereby losing weight, you will improve your body image score, too.

TABLE 6.2 Increase in Average Body Image Scores After a 15-Week Program

Before Program	*After Program*	*Increase in Score*
37.5	44	6.5
41	47	6
35.6	41.5	5.9

Eating Disturbances. Some of the eating disturbances seen in many overweight and obese individuals have been mentioned in the classifications and other information already presented. A few of them are the absence of feelings of hunger, experiencing overwhelming appetite, going on a binge, and the absence of feelings of satiety.

Internality and Externality. Related to eating disturbances are the research suggestions that fat people are more externally controlled than internally controlled. In the 1960s Stanley Schacter (Schacter and Rodin, 1974) did a great deal of ingenious research on the effect of time on eating, the effect of fear from shock, the effect of eating prior to experimentation that involved eating various kinds of food, and the effect of having to work to get food. Schacter found that overweight subjects appear to be more keyed into external events such as time, sight of food, availability of food, and ease in obtaining food than normal weight individuals are.

From his research findings, Schacter summarized that overweight persons are more highly controlled by external influences than normal or underweight individuals. For a few years Schacter's theory was embellished to state generally that obese individuals are aberrant in their psychological or internal responses to hunger and satiety and so base their eating behavior on external events.

This theory was partially rejected as other researchers began looking at some different aspects of eating behavior. They accepted that overweight people may indeed respond to external events, but argued that the valence (high or low palatability) of food and the anxiety level of the overweight individuals are also strong governing forces. Internality and externality were not discarded as differing aspects between over- and normal weight individuals, but the simplicity of its dichotomy was no longer exacting enough to explain the psychodynamics of eating behavior in overweight people.

M-M-M Good. When the valence of food was considered in the research laboratory as a variable in eating behavior, it was found that overweight individuals do, in fact, respond to the palatability of food. They are likely to eat more highly palatable food than normal weight people do. Overweight subjects also have shown less selectivity in judging food to be good tasting than normal weight subjects.

It is important to link the palatability of food to the physiological satiety center, the VMN. When the satiety centers of experimental animals were cut or lesions caused, it was found that the animals responded with overeating and obesity *if food was available* and *if it was palatable* (Mayer, 1968). Animals with lesions would not work harder for their food, thus showing that they were not driven by hunger but rather had lost their normal control over satiety and would eat far beyond it in a supportive environment. Overweight persons may have reset the upper body weight set point, governed by appetite, a psychological function. So the overweight individual will overeat highly palatable foods, govern eating by social events (such as time), and respond to appealing, *available* foods; but the same individual will not exert a lot of effort to overeat or eat foods with little appeal.

With the research evidence available now, it might indeed be expected that the valence of food makes a significant contribution to eating behavior, especially in the overeating by overweight individuals when the food is highly appealing and available.

Stress. In addition to the valence of food, one other aspect that consistently appears with overeating is psychological stress. Experimenters have shown that animals that are mildly stressed respond by overeating. Hans Selye (1976), father of the modern stress concept, noted early in his stress research that a common response to acute stress is anorexia, but the general response to chronic stress is weight gain.

It has been noted that eating past satiety is usually due to the overriding aspects of one's psyche (Wolman, 1982). Very early in life children learn to associate eating with warmth, love, and closeness in an accepting, caring mother, and to associate hunger with feelings of dysphoria, and feelings of insecurity, anxiety, or anger with a non-accepting mother. Then they learn to accept food for nonnutritive reasons, usually as a pacifier for bad feelings (loneliness, boredom, stubbornness, depression, despair, pain, and so on) or as a reward for being good. It is not difficult to see how, then, sooner or later such feelings as anxiety, tension, depression, and so forth become connected with eating.

Psychiatrists in the study of obesity (notably Bruch and Stunkard, two leaders in the field) contend that obese children have a higher incidence of psychiatric disturbances than do normal weight children. Obese children also tend to have antagonistic relationships with domineering mothers, be eventually rejected in the home, and have problems with interpersonal relationships outside the home. The thoughts and emotions of these children are often highly negatively charged, and this starts the chain reaction of gaining more and more weight. They are anxious so they overeat and become fatter, which makes them more anxious, so they continue to overeat. It's a vicious cycle.

For those not overweight as children, a similar link between food and emotions develops. Mothers learn to give food to their children for nonnutritive reasons and children accept the lesson. Then at a high emotional stress time, early behavior is reenacted.

In a study done at the University of Maryland, a researcher of psychosomatic obesity found that being overweight was significantly related to the number of stressful events in the lives of college students. Normal weight individuals had a significantly lower number of stressful life events than did the overweight students (Mann, 1979).

The facts are becoming apparent that stress is an integral component in weight gain, loss, and maintenance. Therefore, a separate chapter in this book is dedicated to stress management.

A Composite Model

Earlier in the chapter, the physiological controls of hunger and satiety, both central and peripheral, on short- and long-term bases, were reviewed. The model of physiological control showed body weight maintained between the appetite set point and the hunger set point. Normally you stay between these two set points. When your body weight falls too far, hunger drives you to eat, and when you overeat, your appetite is lost and you quit eating.

So what goes wrong? It is known that by tampering with the satiety center (rendering it inoperable) the appetite set point loses control, overeating occurs because satiety doesn't have the normal control, and this results in weight gain. In experimental animals, a new set point is eventually established, perhaps depending upon a period of healing time or another part of the brain to help as a control.

Enter the psyche. In humans, the resetting may occur from stress, tension, anxiety, depression, and so on, or an accumulation. A new set point may not be reached until the stress is over or handled properly. Once the weight is gained, it is difficult to lose it because of the new, higher set point of the appetite. Have you ever been bored or depressed and just wandered around the kitchen looking for something "good to eat"? You weren't really hungry, but you had to have something in the form of food. And it had to appeal to your appetite. This is appetitive eating—see the model in Figure 6.7. In this model you can see smaller stressful events coinciding with minor weight gain. Then a large stressful event or an *accumulation* of smaller events over a period of time is the trigger that resets the top threshold (the appetite set point). If overeating is not restrained at this time, body weight increases as the appetite soars. The valence of food and its availability are highly important at this point.

At the other end of the picture, as stress is alleviated and appetite returns to normal, so does body weight. It seems that the sooner the stress is managed and weight is lost, the more successful the individual is in keeping weight down. The longer the time a person has to get used to the new weight, the more likely he or she is to stay there. And the more often the higher set point is visited, the easier it becomes to go back or even beyond it.

This model helps explain how innate controls are overridden by psychological needs. You can learn how to lose weight, then, examining

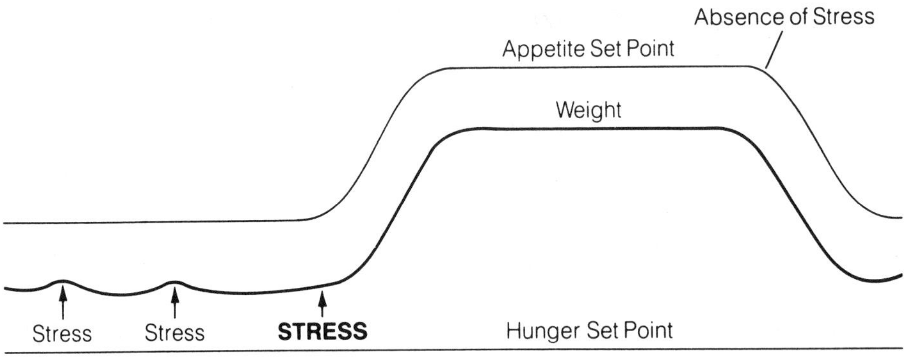

FIGURE 6.7 A Psychosomatic Stress Model of Weight Gain and Loss

how to loosen the hold of the psychological grip. The perfect prevention or cure is learning to manage stress, to eat the foods that you need in order to slim down and stay there, to exercise your body with the right activities, and to take control of your life with greater responsibility.

References

Balagura, S. "Neurophysiological Aspects: Hypothalamic Factors in the Control of Eating Behavior," In F. Reichsman (ed.), *Advances in Psychosomatic Medicine, Volume 7*. Basel, Switzerland: S. Karger, 1972.

Bruch, Hilde. "Hunger and Instinct." *Journal of Nervous and Mental Diseases* 149 (1969): 91–114.

Dusek, Dorothy, et al. *An Abbreviated Body Cathexis Scale*. Winter Park, CO: Paradox Publishing, 1987.

Gawain, S. *Living in the Light*. Mill Valley, CA: Whatever Publishing, Inc., 1986.

Girdano, D., and D. Dusek. *Changing Health Behavior*. Scottsdale, AZ: Gorsuch and Scarisbrick, 1988.

Girdano, D., G. Everly, Jr., and D. Dusek. *Experiencing Health*. Englewood Cliffs, NJ: Prentice-Hall, 1985.

Gross, M. "Medical Aspects of Bulimia," *Cleveland Clinical Quarterly*, 50 (1983): 19–24.

Leon, Gloria. "Personality and Behavioral Correlates of Obesity." In Wolman, B. (ed.). *Psychological Aspects of Obesity*. New York: Van Nostrand Reinhold, 1982.

Levenkron, S. *Treating and Overcoming Anorexia Nervosa*. New York: Charles Scribner's Sons, 1982.

Mann, Patricia. "Assessment of Personality Traits in the Overweight." Unpublished master's thesis, University of Maryland, 1979.

Mayer, Jean. *Overweight: Causes, Cost, and Control*. Englewood Cliffs, NJ: Prentice-Hall, 1968.

Mayer, Jean, and D. W. Thomas. "Regulation of Food Intake and Obesity," *Science* 156 (1967): 328.

Rodin, Judith. "Taming the Hunger Hormone." *American Health* (Jan.–Feb., 1984) 43–47.

Schacter, S., and Judith Rodin. *Obese Humans and Rats*. Potomac, MD: Earbaum, 1974.

Sclafani, Anthony, and Lawrence Kluge. "Food Motivation and Body Weight Levels in Hypothalamic Hyperphagic Rats: A Dual Lipostatic Model of Hunger and Appetite." *Journal of Comparative and Physiological Psychology* 86 (1974): 28–46.

Secord, P. F., and S. M. Jourard. "The Appraisal of Body Cathexis: Body Cathexis and the Self." *Journal of Consulting Psychology* 17 (1953): 343–347.

Selye, Hans. *Stress in Health and Disease*. Montreal: Butterworth, 1976.

Wolman, B. (Ed). *Psychological Aspects of Obesity*. New York: Van Nostrand Reinhold, 1982.

Suggested Readings

Arenson, Gloria. *Binge Eating*. New York: Rawson, 1984.

Bryan, Nancy. *Thin Is A State of Mind*. Minneapolis: CompCare, 1980.

Burckes-Miller, M., and D. Black. "Eating Disorders: A Problem in Athletics?" *Health Education* (Feb.–Mar., 1988): 22–25.

Byrne, K. *A Parent's Guide to Anorexia and Bulimia*. New York: Schocken Books, 1987.

Chapian, M., and N. Coyle. *Free To Be Thin*. Minneapolis: Bethany, 1979.

Chernin, Kim. *The Hungry Self*. New York: Times Books, 1985.

Ericksen, Ann. *Anorexia Nervosa The Broken Circle*. Boston: Faber and Faber, 1985.

Garner, D., and D. Garfinkel (Eds.). *Anorexia Nervosa and Bulimia*. New York: Guilford Press, 1985.

Grant, C., and I. Fodor. "Adolescent Attitudes Toward Body Image and Anorectic Behavior." *Adolescence* 21 (1986): 82, 269–280.

Griffin, S. "Eating Issues and Fat Issues." *T. A. Journal* 15 (1985)1: 30–33.

Hollis, J. *Fat is a Family Affair*. New York: Harper/Hazelden, 1985.

Orbach, Susie. *Hunger Strike*. New York: W. W. Norton, 1986.

Roth, Ganeen. *Breaking Free From Compulsive Eating*. New York: Signet, 1984.

Rowland, C. *The Monster Within: Overcoming Bulimia*. Grand Rapids, MI: Baker, 1984.

Stuart, M., and L. Orr. *Otherwise Perfect*. Pompano Beach, FL: Health Communications, 1987.

7 STRESS PROTECTION PROGRAM

STRESS IS a physiological reactive pattern that responds to perceived danger. In 1956, Hans Selye, the father of stress research, suggested that obesity may be a response to stress, and if so, it was the obese person's maladaptive response to some kind of stressor(s). It has been noted that laboratory animals respond to a stressor (pinching their tails) by becoming hyperphagic, that is, they overeat (Rowland and Antelman, 1976). Also, through your experiences you probably know people who react to stress by eating—they eat when they're angry or depressed or sad or fearful and many times even when they're happy. Yes, even happy events can be stressful. Vacations, birthdays, weddings, holidays, visits from relatives—any event that calls for a change from daily routine can be stressful. Not all stress is bad; in fact, you would not grow without some stress in your life. The "good" stress that motivates and energizes has been named *eustress* by Selye (1956), while the stress that debilitates and can eventually cause mental and physical harm is *distress*. This chapter is concerned with how you can protect yourself against *distress* and *distress-related eating*.

Appendix D consists of a four-part general stress test. Take a few minutes to answer the items on each test and place your scores for the 4 tests here:

Your score, Test 1 ______

Your score, Test 2 ______

Your score, Test 3 ______

Your score, Test 4 ______

Did your scores for any of the first three tests exceed 25, and is your score on test 4 less than 50? If so, this is an indication that the factual material and the exercises given in this chapter could be very important to your health, whether or not your stress is related to eating.

In Chapter 6 the discussion of why people eat pointed out that students and clients in weight control frequently eat because they are bored, worried, anxious, pressured by others, sad, lonely, angry, upset, depressed, or frustrated. These reasons bring about distress-related eating behavior. Although everyone engages in some distress-related eating behaviors, those individuals who can prevent or handle potentially distressful situations will engage in distress-related eating less often than those individuals who are more *stress-reactive* (that is, those who react more often, more inappropriately, and/or more intensely to stress). For example, a successful student of stress prevention and management would prevent boredom or would manage to respond to temporary boredom appropriately by finding someone interesting to be with and/or something exciting to do. Eating would be an inappropriate response to boredom.

The Distress-Related Eating Profile

Do you respond to stressful situations in your life by eating? Answer the following questions with a "yes" or "no" to see how distress may be related to your eating behavior. Total the number of "yes" answers at the bottom.

	YES/NO
1. I know that my mother/father/significant other gave me food "treats" when I fussed or cried as a child.	______
2. When I am angry at someone or about a situation or event, I respond by eating.	______
3. Many times I find myself eating because there is nothing else interesting to do.	______
4. When I'm worried about my health, I respond by eating.	______
5. Many times I eat because I am lonely.	______
6. I usually can't refuse something to eat or drink when I visit friends.	______
7. When I feel depressed or want to take my mind off my worries, I eat.	______

8. When I gain a lot of weight (for me, ______ pounds), I can usually remember a stress-related incident that "set me off." ______
9. When I get nervous or fatigued, I crave sweets or other special foods. ______
10. I usually drink three or more cups of coffee with breakfast, lunch, and/or dinner. ______

TOTAL ______

If your score was 5 or more, you may be eating as a psychological response to stress or discomfort such as boredom, loneliness, or anger. This is what I call "negative affect" eating. Although food may help at times to tranquilize you, it is not an answer to your discomfort. Sooner or later you will find that the answer lies in solving the problem, not taking a symptom to dinner. In addition, if you are gaining weight or maintaining an unhealthy high weight because of negative affect eating, you are increasing your stress and decreasing your capabilities of handling stressful situations of all kinds.

Also, if your score was high (over 5), the stress of social pressure may be encouraging you to eat or drink when you really don't want to. Pleasant or happy times are occasions when there is an abundance of good food that is difficult to refuse because of others' expectations.

You can be sure you are caught in the stress cycle when you crave sweets, caffeine, nicotine, chocolate, or alcohol. You may feel that if you don't have your "fix," you don't feel right. A common culprit in this situation is low blood sugar—a condition that may have been caused or exacerbated by stress. Remember—eating is an appropriate response to physiological hunger, not psychological "hunger."

Whether your signs of distress are *feelings* (conscious or subconscious) or *visible physical symptoms* such as muscle tremors, crying, or sweaty palms, it is important to recognize them and what reaction you have to them. Recognition is the first step in solving the problem.

Listed in Table 7.1 are some signs of distress. Go through the list and see if you have any of these symptoms now, or if you have had them in response to stressful situations in the past. If you have one or more of these symptoms and are responding to it (them) by eating more than usual, you can use one or more of the techniques in this chapter to help you (1) get rid of the cause of the symptom, (2) get rid of the symptom, and/or (3) get rid of the overeating response to the symptom.

TABLE 7.1 Some Physical and Emotional Signs of Distress

Bodily Complaints	*Muscular Tension*	*Conscious Feelings*
Cardiovascular	Jittery, easily startled	Fearful
Heart palpitations	Tremors, tics	Apprehensive
Rapid/erratic pulse	Clumsiness	Feeling of loss of control
Increased blood pressure	Hyperactivity	Mental disorientation and confusion
Faintness	Forehead wrinkles, scowls	Crying, tearful
Gastrointestinal	Frequent headaches	Trouble concentrating
Nausea	Easily fatigued	Obsessional or phobic fears
Hunger	Hands tremble	Overly shy, timid, fearful of offending an authority figure
Vomiting	Pacing the floor	Preoccupied
Diarrhea	Nervous mannerisms (nail biting, hair pulling, foot tapping, etc.)	
Constipation	*Other*	
Loss of appetite	Excessive perspiration	
Stomach, intestinal pain	Frequent urination	
Respiratory	Sleeplessness	
Breathlessness	Sweaty palms	
Frequent sighing		
Rapid, shallow breathing		
Inability to breathe deeply		

A Case of Distress-Related Eating

Most likely you will be able to relate to Julie, who came in for counseling when her scale read 175 pounds. Julie explained that she just really loved food and she had to do something about it. "Can't you hypnotize me or something?" was her plea. Instead of hypnosis, we encouraged her to talk about her parents, the rest of her family, her grades at school, her friends, and we soon uncovered a very unhappy and distressed Julie.

As she sat there on the verge of tears, she explained, "My parents expect all A's from me, just like Emily, my older sister, got when she was in school. So I have to stay home and study six nights a week. One way I can stall off my study hours is eating—I clean up every bowl at the dinner table. And then I'm nauseated all evening . . . and so I eat anything to get rid of the nausea. I'm tired when I go to bed, but I don't sleep well at all. I worry about tests and school, and whether my friends like me or not.

"When I go out with my friends after school or spend the one evening a week out with them, I usually end up treating them to pizza or hamburgers or whatever they want. I'm beginning to think that's the only reason they want me around . . . they laugh at how fat I am, especially in gym class. I just want to go home from school every day and eat!"

Julie responded to the psychological stress of parent expectations, perceived response from her classmates, self-doubt, and other negative feelings about herself by inappropriate eating. It was the only way she knew how to deal with her distress. Her case is not at all uncommon. In fact, in every instance of overeating or being overweight that I have encountered personally in counseling, there is a stress element. The problem is deeper than simple overeating. The answer is in the *reason* behind the eating response, and that reason is usually psychological stress of some nature.

After Julie's first visit, she soon realized that she was distressing herself about her parents and her friends, and she began caring more about how she felt about herself. She knew that if she carried her distress with her over a prolonged period of time she might start showing physical signs of disease such as gastritis leading to an ulcer. She gradually realized that her weight problem was linked to her distress because as she practiced her stress prevention and alleviation techniques, her weight began to normalize. As she became happier with herself, she grew thinner—almost as though her weight were taking care of itself. As she liked herself more, she treated herself to healthier foods and eating behavior, and she exercised more. All of these new habits created a healthier and happier Julie.

The stress protection program that Julie successfully used is explained in the rest of this chapter. Generally, it follows this outline:

1. Increase readiness and self-responsibility.
   a. Review Chapter 1.
   b. Recognize other social stressors (such as overload, frustration, diet, deprivation, and noise).
2. Exercise.
   a. Understand the benefits of exercise (Chapter 10).
   b. Engage in an aerobic exercise program (Chapter 13).
   c. Get benefits out of play.
3. Utilize relaxation techniques.
   a. Breathing
   b. Meditation
   c. Autogenic relaxation

Whether or not you respond to stress by eating, it is important to reduce the stress in your life. However, if you have determined that you are definitely *not* a distress-related eater, you may want to skip Chapter 8 and come back to the information in this chapter when you need it.

Increasing Readiness and Self-Responsibility

REVIEW OF PSYCHOSOCIAL STRESSORS

Your stress protection program started when you read Chapter 1 and determined your readiness to begin a health behavior change program and the self-responsibility that you would donate to the cause. You may already have won some of the battle against psychosocial stressors by following the prescriptions for changing behaviors in order to allow yourself to:

Be assertive.
Expect a little less from others.
Be in charge of your emotions.
Free yourself from guilt and worry.
Show your emotions.
Be independent.
Label yourself with positive characteristics rather than negative ones.

If you need to work more on the areas given in Chapter 1, go back now and review your answers to the Readiness Profile. *Psychosocial* and *personality engineering*—that is, guiding your experiences so as to avoid setting yourself up for stressful situations—are stress reducing (Girdano and Everly, 1987) and many suggestions for doing just that were given in Chapter 1.

OTHER SOCIAL STRESSORS

There are other social stressors not specifically mentioned in Chapter 1 that may be triggering your stress response—for example, overload, frustration, diet, deprivation, and noise. The stress from these can also be reduced with social engineering. Some suggestions for psychosocial engineering and responding appropriately to these stressors are given here.

Overload (or Overstimulation). If your job, schoolwork, family, and/or friends continually expect too much from you, you can:

1. Set up a time management schedule to fit in all the important people (those *you* think are important).
2. Eliminate unimportant items from your life. Assertiveness will help you limit the unreasonable expectations from your boss, family, friends, and maybe even from professors!

Frustration. Frustration occurs when you are thwarted or inhibited from doing what you want or attaining goals that you desire. Some of today's thwarting elements are overcrowding, finances, and prejudice. To socially engineer against *overcrowding*:

1. Give yourself extra time to reach where you are going so that a crowded freeway or impossible inner-city traffic won't interfere with your plans.
2. Do everything a little early – the crowd never gets there until the middle or the end! For example, on the day that license plates expire, the Department of Motor Vehicles usually has a line a mile long. Go get your plates the very first day that you can. You can think of a hundred instances when you can beat the crowd so they don't hold you back.

To engineer your *finances*, devise a budget for yourself. This requires discipline on your part, but you will find that your finances balance at the end of the month, which is better than worrying that you won't have enough money to pay bills at the end of the month.

Engineering against the stress of *prejudice* involves giving up prejudice yourself. Prejudice stems from fear – fear of unknown customs and people, fear of an outsider taking your job, fear that you won't get your share because of someone else. If you can realize what prejudice consists of, you will be more likely to give it up. You will also be more tolerant of those who still don't realize how stressful prejudice is.

Diet. Are these stressors part of your diet – caffeine, sugar, white flour, salt? *Caffeine* occurs in three common foods:

1. Coffee and tea – one cup contains about 100 milligrams of caffeine.
2. Colas – one 12-ounce can of cola (or "Pepper") beverage contains 50 to 60 milligrams of caffeine.

3. Chocolate—there are about 20 milligrams of caffeine in one ounce of chocolate.

Caffeine stimulates the sympathetic nervous system stress response. It gets the body ready to fight or run and if the stress products are not used up by fighting, running, or some other physical response, they circulate in the body where they can cause eventual trouble. If you have ever experienced a "coffee buzz," you know the effects of caffeine. To engineer caffeine out of your diet:

1. Substitute decaffeinated coffee or herbal tea for regular coffee or tea. Decaffeinated coffee still contains about half as much caffeine as regular coffee, however. When you see a label that says the decaffeinated coffee is only 3 percent caffeine, keep in mind that regular coffee is only 6 to 7 percent caffeine. *Herbal tea* is the best bet!
2. For cola beverages, substitute clear sodas such as ginger ale, or better yet, club soda—it has no calories. A much healthier substitute is *juice*—apple, cranberry, citric (orange, grapefruit), tomato, and so on. They are not made of sugar or carbonated water, and they contain vitamins and minerals you don't get in soda pop.
3. A good substitute for chocolate is *carob.* If you haven't tried it, don't discount it. In my household when I first suggested we try carob chips, I was drummed out of the house. Then when the local market manager, who happens to be a great cook, suggested that carob chips were better than chocolate chips in taste and price, I was granted permission to bring them into our diet. They're great.

   Carob is used by many people who are allergic to chocolate or who want to avoid caffeine. This substitute contains some sugar and fat, however, along with some protein, calcium, and phosphorus.

Most of the dangers of white or any refined *sugar* are discussed in Chapter 9. There are two specific stress involvements, though, that should be emphasized here. The first is that sugar consumption deregulates blood sugar, resulting in hypoglycemia (acute and/or chronic low blood sugar). The body responds to hypoglycemia with the stress response. The second is that the vitamins that are needed to break down sugar happen to be those that are also used to fight stress. Sugar has absolutely no vitamins or minerals, so to break it down the body must use vitamins that are already depleted by the stress response to sugar! It is a harmful, depleting process. If you respond to stress by eating sugar (or drinking it in colas or other sodas), recognize that such behavior may be a symptom of hypoglycemia.

The substitutes for sugar in the average American's diet are *honey* (about three times sweeter than sugar) and *artificial sweetener.* Although there are warnings of possible dangers involved in eating or drinking large amounts of artificially sweetened substances, some people may be better off using them rather than sugar or honey. Ideally, people should rely on natural fruit sugars to satisfy their taste for sweetness.

The nutritional dangers of *white flour* are about the same as those of refined sugar. The processing of white flour strips it of all vitamins and minerals; it is refortified with only three or four of them. But the body needs all the original nutrients to metabolize the flour—so the body is again robbed of vitamins essential to fighting stress.

The substitute here, of course, is *whole grain flour.* It is wise to put corn meal, rye, rice, and other whole grain foods into the family diet rather than just relying on whole wheat flour as a staple.

When excessive *salt* is consumed, the body will retain excessive water. Excessive fluid retention can cause increased nervous tension and increased blood pressure. While salt needs are low—less than one gram per day—Americans consume between four and eight grams per day! A popular salt substitute is *potassium chloride.*

Deprivational Stress. This stress occurs in the form of *boredom* and *loneliness,* two of the leading causes of distress-related eating in overweight people. Social and personality engineering can help you respond appropriately:

1. Join social groups that will present you with new people and/or interesting things to do.
2. Take classes in self-improvement, hobbies, and so on. These help you occupy time that you may have spent eating in the past.
3. Feel happier and more tranquil when you do spend time alone. If you enjoy the company of yourself, you're never bored or lonely.

Noise. Noise can elicit the stress response in you without your knowing it. It slips right into your brain whether you are awake or asleep. Sound that is 80 decibels or more is known to raise blood pressure, increase heart rate, and generally turn on the body's stress response.

Have you ever been outside sunbathing or sitting in a classroom when a lawn mower or other motor was in use within earshot? Your brain became used to it as you snoozed, or listened to the teacher, or read. But do you recall your sigh of relief when the motor was turned off? That sigh of relief told you that your body was becoming rather irritated with the noise. If you're eating because of irritation, but you don't know why you're irritated, check the noise level around you. If noise is a stress factor in your life:

1. Be assertive about the noise source, if possible—ask that the sound level be lowered.
2. Buy and wear ear plugs when you need them. A friend of mine always carries a pair of ear plugs in her purse, and I first saw her slip them in her ears when we went to a noisy disco in Houston. She told me that noise was never a problem for her—when she wanted to tune out somebody or something, she simply put in her ear plugs! They are a cheap, reliable way to obtain peace and quiet.

Exercise as a Stress Fighter

Exercise works in several different ways as a stress reducer. It tunes your body so that you can physically recover more quickly from stress; it aids in building self-assurance; and exercise is often the vehicle for fun, play, and laughter, which are all stress fighters. If your weight problem is distressful to you, a good exercise program also helps you become thinner and thus helps remove that problem.

Jacobson (1976), the creator of a well-known neuromuscular relaxation technique, remarked early in his study of relaxation that you cannot laugh and be stressed at the same time. Norman Cousins, in *Anatomy of an Illness* (1977), described how he fought off what had been diagnosed as a terminal illness with laughter and megavitamin therapy. Play is also a stress reducer when it is free, spontaneous play, void of ego. Probably all adults have stifled the child at play within them. Relearning how to play can be a relaxation technique.

Aerobic exercise can also be used as a treatment for stress. When you respond to any kind of stress, your body pours hormones and foodstuffs into your blood to help you handle the stress. If these biochemicals circulate in your system over a long period of time, they keep you "up" long after the stressful situation is over. However, if you exercise your total body (by running, swimming, and so on), the byproducts of stress will be burned up, your system will recover more quickly from the stress, and you will have received another bonus of exercise.

Thus, exercise is both a treatment after the fact (stress) and a preventive measure. In Chapters 10 through 13 you will discover the magic of exercise, the natural stress reducer.

Relaxation Techniques

The connection between health and stress is apparent. Thus, it seems obvious that any program for a change in lifestyle would include some information on stress management, alleviation, and prevention and how to protect yourself against stress in general and stress-related eating.

Before the specific relaxation techniques of breathing, meditation, and autogenic relaxation are presented step by step, let's look at the rationale behind the use of relaxation techniques.

RATIONALE

Important in learning to relax is the knowledge that the body is governed by two parts of the central nervous system (see Figure 7.1). One part is the *voluntary* system that controls the movements that you wish to make, such as raising your hand in class when you have a question. Your arm does not automatically pop up into the air; you put it there of your own volition. The other part of the system is the *autonomic* (or *automatic*) part that takes care of all the minute details of life in the body so you don't have to think about doing them. These duties include keeping the heart beating, the lungs breathing, the pupils of the eyes responding to varying amounts of light, your organs producing products that they should, the gastrointestinal tract

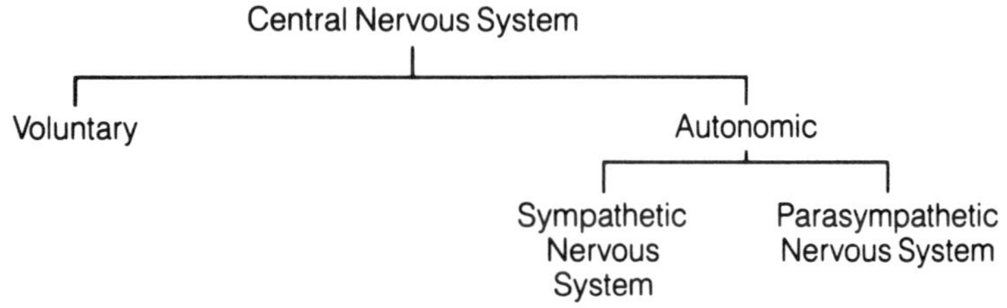

FIGURE 7.1 Parts of the Central Nervous System

moving, and so on. You can learn to control these functions voluntarily with the aid of biofeedback and other relaxation techniques. But rest assured that whether you can voluntarily control them or not, the autonomic nervous system is always there tending to all the life-sustaining functions (unless there has been some damage to the system).

The autonomic nervous system also has two divisions, and they are always vying for control of the organs. One part is the *sympathetic* nervous system that is responsible for the life-sustaining stress response. You may recognize the sympathetic nervous system as your "fight or flight" response. Most of the characteristics of the stress response pattern are due to stimulation of the sympathetic nervous system.

The other part of the autonomic nervous system is the *parasympathetic* nervous system. It is responsible for slowing down the heart rate and the respiratory rate and generally putting things back in order after they have been upset by stress.

Each of these two parts of your autonomic nervous system can be trained to respond to your will by practice. People who always become excited and respond emotionally to situations train the sympathetic nervous system to be dominant. They might not even recognize that they are in a vicious cycle, getting themselves ever more excited. They become "overreactors" to potential stress situations.

In contrast, some people practice allowing the parasympathetic nervous system to dominate. Their emotional reactivity level is lower and they calm down more quickly after a stressful bout than those with a dominant sympathetic nervous system. In order to train the parasympathetic nervous system, these people engage in one or more relaxation techniques regularly and/or do aerobic exercise regularly.

Another way to understand the need for the function of relaxation is to explore the different duties that each side of the brain performs. In Figure 7.2 you can see that the left hemisphere is the logic and business-oriented side of the brain. It is also considered the "ego" side. The right hemisphere of the brain is responsible for time-space orientation such as in art, music, and dance.

When you are protecting your ego, you are using mainly the left hemisphere, and when you go into "altered states of consciousness," such as daydreaming, your right hemisphere is in control. The egoless states of meditation, play, dance, fantasy, and so on are right-brain functions. Apparently if you can use natural means to exercise

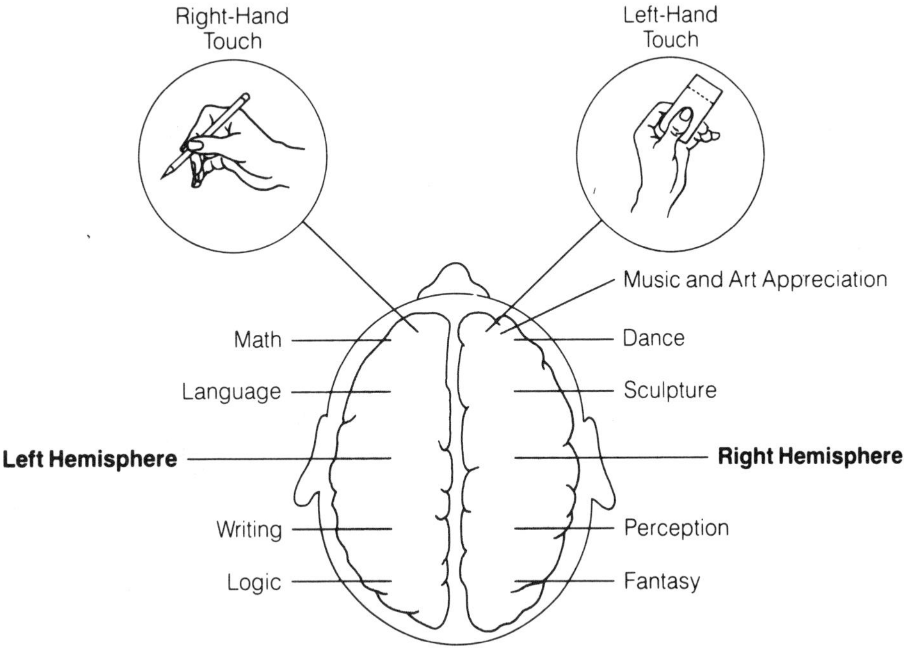

FIGURE 7.2 Hemispheres of the Brain and Their Functions

the right brain for a while, you will have better control over stress (Houston, 1982; Ornstein, 1977; Edwards, 1986). The relaxation techniques given in this chapter help you learn to use your parasympathetic system and explore your right brain in order to become less emotionally reactive and to calm down faster after you have reacted to stress.

You may be asking, "Do I want to dampen my stress reaction? Isn't it a healthy, necessary part of life?" The fact is that no matter how much relaxation training you do, the intensity of your stress response will *not* be dampened. What will happen is you will become better able to respond realistically and appropriately to stress and not let the harmful effects of the stress reaction linger to cause you harm.

Let's look at the difference in emotional reactivity between a person who does practice stress prevention and treatment techniques and one who does not. We will call them Reactor A and Reactor B, respectively. Their stress reaction profiles over a day would look like those shown in Figure 7.3. Each star in the figure is a stress incident of the same intensity and the linear movements indicate the stress reactivity throughout the day.

Reactor A, who trained his parasympathetic nervous system to take care of him, ended the day with little more emotional reactivity

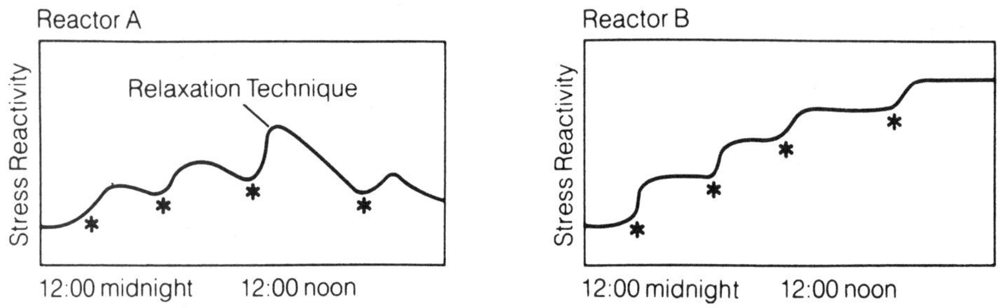

FIGURE 7.3 Stress Reaction Patterns

than he started with. It was especially helpful for him to use a relaxation technique when he needed it around noon. Poor Reactor B, however, had no resources to diminish his stress level during the day and probably went to bed with his head still buzzing, his heart rate above normal, and on an "adrenalin high." His sleep undoubtedly suffered and his stress level was probably still somewhat elevated the next morning.

Some of the techniques that Reactor A might have learned to fight stress successfully are social, psychological, and personality engineering; a stress-free diet; a regular aerobic exercise program; and specific relaxation techniques. All of these aspects have been covered in this chapter except the relaxation techniques. These special exercises in relaxation now round out the chapter.

The following are specific techniques that you can use to train your parasympathetic nervous system to protect you from the dangers of stress. They can be valuable at any time of the day, but you may find them especially useful when the urge to eat is stimulated by distress (such as boredom, loneliness, or fear).

BREATHING

Before you read on, place your hands on your chest and feel yourself breathe. Do you feel a rise and fall in your chest? If so, you are a typical Western breather. Western world residents, in general, breathe high and shallow. The chest rises and falls. This method of breathing wastes the lungs and the opportunity to use the surrounding air in a natural, tranquilizing manner. It doesn't matter *why* Westerners have not learned to use the entire lung capacity; the fact is that they haven't!

Ancient Eastern religion and philosophy revered deep breathing and knew that concentrated, deep, rhythmic breathing could control the mind and cause the whole body to relax. To gain these benefits from breathing, learn the following breathing technique.

Sit comfortably in a chair with your feet on the floor or sit on the floor with your legs crossed, in a half lotus position, or in a full lotus position – whatever is comfortable for you (see Figure 7.4 for these postures). Keep your back straight, but not stiff, to give your lungs a chance to expand fully.

When you are first learning, place your hands immediately over your belly so you can feel what is going on. Later you can place your hands on your thighs or knees if you find it more comfortable.

Breathe in slowly through your nose and let that air fill up the *bottom* of your lungs first. You will feel your belly expand under your hands as you do this. Continue to breathe in, but keep the air flowing to the bottom of your lungs until that part can hold no more air. Then slowly fill up the lungs from the bottom to the top as you would fill up a vase with water. You will feel your rib cage expanding outward as you fill up your lungs. The whole process of taking in air should take three seconds.

Now hold all the air in your lungs for three seconds and assure yourself, "My body is calm, relaxed, tranquil." This affirmation will help the breath to relax your body.

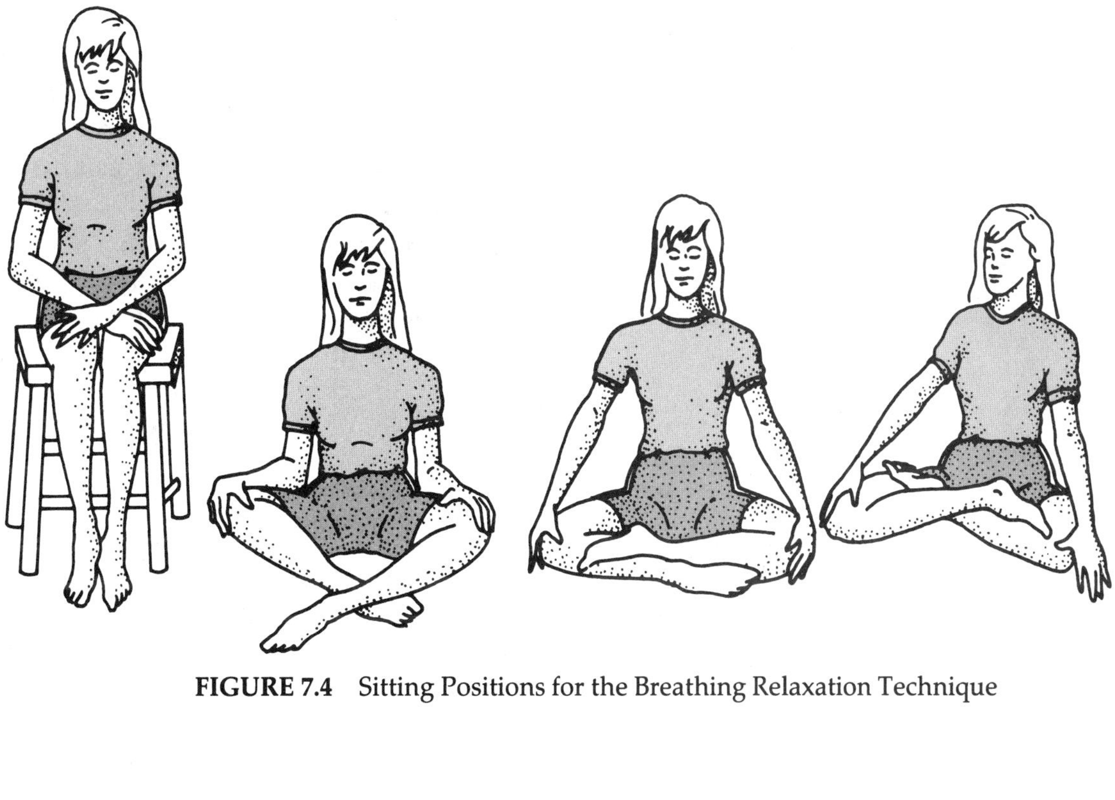

FIGURE 7.4 Sitting Positions for the Breathing Relaxation Technique

Next, take three seconds to exhale slowly through your nose. Let the air out of the *top* of your lungs first and work your way to the bottom of your lungs. Feel your chest wall recede and your belly go back in. When you have let all the air out, try to let out a little more and hold for three seconds while you tell your body that it is quiet and serene.

Repeat this procedure six times whenever you can, 10 to 15 times a day. Sit on the edge of your bed each morning and start the day this way. Do it before each meal and at bedtime. It is also a very helpful procedure when you become upset, anxious, angry, or out of sorts in any way during the day. As you can see, this procedure, like exercise, can be used as a treatment or it can be used to prevent stress reactivity. You may also realize that any physical exercise that makes you breathe hard is a form of this deep breathing exercise.

After the three-second intervals become comfortable for you, increase the time of inhalation, exhalation, and the hold that you do after each to four seconds each. Progress one second at a time and set your own limit.

MEDITATION

Millions of Americans have become meditators in the last two decades—some are practitioners of transcendental meditation (T.M.); some practice specific yoga meditations; some never learn a specific pattern, they do what feels good to them. In all forms of meditation, the main principle is to clear the mind (specifically, the left hemisphere of the brain where logic, ego, and social skills are housed), and in so doing, train the tranquil parasympathetic nervous system to dominate over the excited sympathetic system.

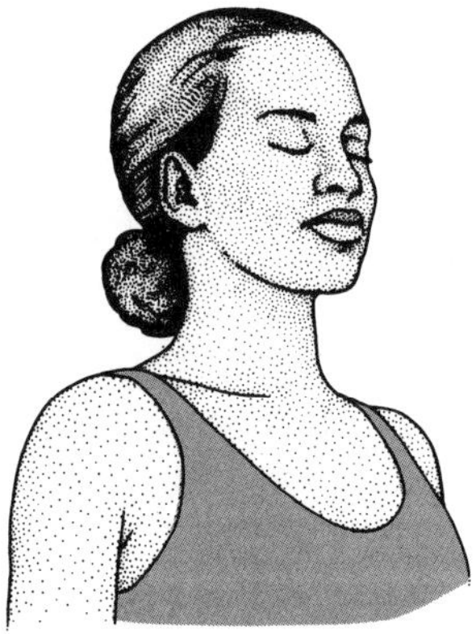

According to Zen Buddhism, the Eastern philosophy-religion, to become enlightened one must "let go of the mind." This philosophy contends that suffering comes from trying to hang on to power, possessions, and things the way they are rather than letting things change and grow—these are functions of the left hemisphere of the brain. So in Zen, meditation is a natural, necessary part of training the mind (Suzuki, 1964).

In the Western world, researchers tend to explain meditation in terms of psychophysiology: The left side of the brain houses the ego, and the ego causes or encourages stress problems. So to alleviate the basic problem, you have to learn not to let your left brain dominate. You can probably think of a time when you have allowed the left brain free rein. You may have been thinking about how unpleasant some meeting was going to be, and you mentally had a furious argument with someone. By the time of the meeting, you had worked yourself into a frenzy, causing a great deal of self-induced stress. And then perhaps the expected confrontation didn't even occur—the other person was pleasant and agreeable. All that stress for nothing—except to protect an ego that wasn't even attacked!

The way to train the right brain to take over is to stop any mind stories that involve the ego. To make it easier to drown out the left side of the brain meditators use words, numbers, music, or other soothing sounds. Then whenever they catch themselves thinking about not getting that pay raise, being turned down for a date, and so on, they merely turn their thoughts back to counting, repeating a word (sometimes called a *mantra*), or getting involved in the music again. There are many methods to use in order to meditate effectively, but here is one that you'll find relaxing and helpful.

First of all, choose a place where you will be comfortable and undisturbed for 10 to 20 minutes. Muzzle the telephone if you can (many home phones can be unhooked at the base of the phone); put out the cat and the dog; ask others in your household to refrain from disturbing you. Some of my students use a hot bath as their medium.

Close your eyes and/or turn out the lights to eliminate the stimulation that comes to you visually; you want to reduce the amount of outside stimulation as much as you can, especially when you are learning the technique.

Sit in an upright position with your hands resting on your thighs or knees. Ask your subconscious mind to awaken you in 10, 15, or 20 minutes (whatever time period you wish). You will be surprised the first time your subconscious does, in fact, alert you when the time is up. After that you will know that you can rely on it if you ask it to serve you.

Be aware of your breathing. Count 10 breaths, then as you breathe in, begin saying to yourself, "I am . . . ," and as you breathe out, say "relaxed" (or "at peace" or "tranquil"). Let your mind wander where it will, but every time it strays to a situation where you are defending your ego, go back to counting your breaths.

An alternative to counting breaths is to concentrate on a word. It should be a word that has no particular meaning to you, such as the Sanskrit *mantras* used in T.M. You might use the word *one* to recite each time you exhale. *Om* is also used as a mantra and when uttered aloud, it has great resonance. As you breathe out slowly, say, "aaaaaoooommmmm."

You can perform an activity of taking yourself mentally to a special place where you are comfortable, safe, warm, and cozy. For some it is the beach, for others it is up on a fluffy cloud, in a favorite room, floating on water, lying in a meadow, swinging in a hammock. As you go to that favorite place, really put yourself there—see and hear what's around you, feel the comfort and the warmth, smell the fresh air and the flowers. This is a fantasy trip that takes you into your right hemisphere. Stay there and let your mind wander.

You may feel your body floating, slowly descending, tingling, or many other pleasant sensations while you are meditating. Your mind may flash on creative ways of doing things, psychic occurrences, remembered experiences, and so on. Your mind is the only limitation to the experiences you can have during meditation.

Still another concentration technique is to begin counting backward from 100 or 10 (depending on your internal scale) or slowly descending a tall building in an elevator, counting the floors as you descend. Tell your body that with the passage of each number, your body will become more relaxed. When you reach zero (or the basement), you are in a most calm, relaxed, tranquil state. Stay there until your subconscious alarm clock goes off. It really will take care of you if you ask it to.

As you learn to relax and enjoy your meditation you will be able to blank out the environment around you and get into a relaxed, calm posture any time or anywhere you need it. It is a skill that you will master as you practice it.

Higher forms and/or specific forms of meditation can be learned from yoga, T.M., or other Eastern philosophies and/or religions. Zen Buddhists reach their highest enlightenment through meditation, and so the literature on that philosophy can take you beyond the beginning lessons given here. The suggested readings at the end of this chapter will give you some sources for further lessons in meditation.

AUTOGENIC RELAXATION

Autogenic refers to something that is produced by yourself. In autogenic relaxation, you tell your body what you want it to do, and it will learn to respond if you will let it do so. If you have practiced meditation as suggested in the previous section, you have already experienced some autogenic relaxation. When you told your body that you were relaxed, you probably felt more relaxed, especially at the end of the session. One of the keys to autogenics is using words that the body knows and then using the right words to cause relaxation.

Close your eyes now and think of a time when you were very relaxed. Get into that posture now and really let yourself relive that experience. If you cannot think of a particular time when your body was limp with relaxation, search in your mind for a person you have seen in a very relaxed posture. Then try to assume that posture. How would it feel to be that relaxed?

Once you reproduce the relaxed posture, describe how it felt then. Your arms and legs probably felt heavy and perhaps tingly. Your feet and hands were warm, your breathing slow and deep. Your heart rate slowed down.

Now that you have some descriptors, you can use them to relive the relaxed posture any time you want . . . your body knows the words *heavy, tingly, warm, relaxed, peaceful, tranquil,* and many more that you can add.

Start your autogenic training just as you would learn how to meditate—find a quiet place where you can sit comfortably. Close your eyes and concentrate on your breathing. Feel the energy surge into your body as you breathe in, then feel the tension drop away as you breathe out. In just reading this, you are probably letting your body relax.

After five breaths, *place your hands on your thighs* and say to yourself slowly, taking time to feel the reaction:

"My *right thigh* feels heavy."
"My right thigh feels heavy and warm."
"My right thigh is relaxed."
"My right thigh is relaxed, heavy and warm."
"My *right foot and leg* feel heavy and warm."
"My right foot and leg are relaxed."
"I am calm and relaxed."
"I am at peace."

Repeat with your *left thigh*, then your *left foot and leg*. Take about five to six minutes to complete this. See Figure 7.5 for the position you will assume for the technique.

Follow the same sequence with your *left* and *right shoulders* (where you said "thigh" before); and *arms and hands* (where you said "foot and leg" before).

After you have done this (which should take about five or six minutes), move on to your power center (or *chakra,* as it is called in yoga), your *solar plexus,* which lies just behind your navel. *Place a hand lightly on your navel,* over the solar plexus and slowly, quietly say to yourself:

"I am at peace."
"I am calm."
"I am relaxed."
"My solar plexus is warm."
"Heat radiates from my solar plexus."
"I feel the heat throughout my body."
"My whole body is relaxed and warm."
"My body is heavy and warm."
"I am relaxed."
"I am calm."
"I am at peace."

You will easily and quickly learn the sequence that helps you the most and you will find it easy to use anywhere you go. It is important to place your hands on your body parts that are involved in your conversation with yourself. They are *physical anchors* that, even when used in silence after you have practiced this technique, will elicit the autogenic relaxation response (Girdano and Dusek, 1988).

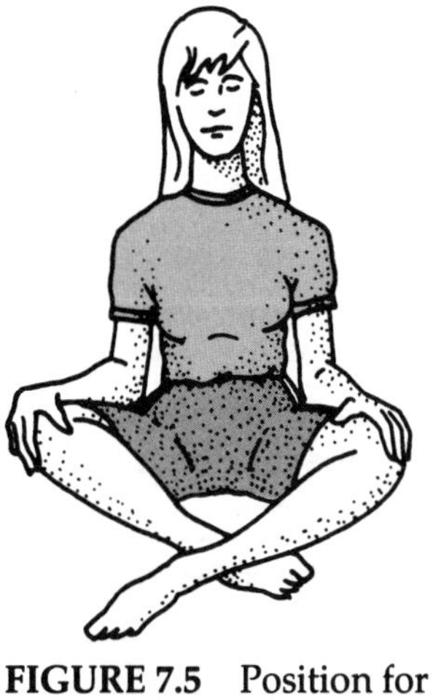

FIGURE 7.5 Position for Autogenic Relaxation of Shoulders, Arms, and Hands

A Summary

You now have learned many ways to combat stress and many techniques to put into your stress protection program. Enjoy the relaxation techniques when you get up in the morning, when you go to bed at night, before each meal (especially during the "empty" hours at the end of the afternoon when it seems that dinner time will never arrive), and especially when you expect a stressful situation to occur or when one has just occurred.

In the last chapter of this book, commit yourself to a separate contract for relaxation or stress protection. Determine what you will do to prevent and treat stress in your life. Write it on the form in Table 7.2.

References

Cousins, Norman. *Anatomy of an Illness*. New York: Norton, 1981.
Edwards, Betty. *Drawing on the Artist Within*. New York: Simon and Schuster, 1986.
Girdano, Daniel, and Dorothy Dusek. *Changing Health Behavior*. Scottsdale, AZ: Gorsuch and Scarisbrick, 1988.
Girdano, Daniel, and G. Everly, Jr. *Controlling Stress and Tension: A Holistic Approach, 2nd edition*. Englewood Cliffs, NJ: Prentice-Hall, 1986.
Houston, Jean. *The Possible Human*. Los Angeles: Tarcher, 1982.
Jacobson, Edmond. *You Must Relax*. New York: McGraw-Hill, 1976.
Ornstein, Robert E. *The Psychology of Consciousness*. New York: Harcourt Brace Jovanovich, 1977.
Rowland, N., and S. Antelman. "Stress-Induced Hyperphagia and Obesity in Rats: A Possible Model for Understanding Human Obesity." *Science* 23 (1976): 310–311.
Selye, Hans. *The Stress of Life*. New York: McGraw-Hill, 1956.
Suzuki, D. T. *An Introduction to Zen Buddhism*. New York: Grove Press, 1964.

Suggested Readings

Benson, Herbert. *The Mind-Body Effect*. New York: Simon and Schuster, 1980.
Benson, Herbert. *Beyond the Relaxation Response*. New York: Berkeley Books, 1984.
Breznitz, S. (ed.). *The Denial of Stress*. New York: International Universities Press, 1984.
Eliot, R., and D. Breo. *Is It Worth Dying For?* New York: Bantam, 1984.
Gillespie, P., and L. Bechtel. *Less Stress in 30 Days*. New York: Plume, 1986.
Hanson, P. *The Joy of Stress*. New York: Andrews, McMeel and Parker, 1985.
King, Serge. *Imagineering for Health*. Wheaton, IL: Theosophical Publishing Co., 1982.
Kriegel, R., and M. Kriegel. *The C Zone*. New York: Fawcett, 1983.

TABLE 7.2 Your Stress Protection Program

	Evening	*Afternoon*	*Morning*
Sunday			
Monday			
Tuesday			
Wednesday			
Thursday			
Friday			
Saturday			

Kushner, Harold. *When Bad Things Happen to Good People*. New York: Schocken, 1983.

Lerner, H. *Stress Breakers*. Minneapolis: CompCare, 1985.

Mathews-Simonton, Stephanie, et al. *Getting Well Again*. New York: Bantam Books, 1980.

Meichenbaum, D. *Stress Inoculation Training*. New York: Pergamon, 1986.

Ogilvie, L. *Making Stress Work for You*. Waco, TX: Word Books, 1985.

Shaffer, M. *Life After Stress*. Chicago, Contemporary Books, 1986.

8 NUTRITION RECALL: A DIET DIARY

ALTHOUGH any of the following maladies could reflect some very serious disease, they could also be early symptoms of vitamin or mineral deficiency. Do you:

Bruise easily?
Have recurrent canker sores?
Have cracks at the corner(s) of your mouth?
Feel irritable much of the time?
Feel depressed often?
Have swollen and sore joints?
Heal slowly after a cut or an infection?
Catch colds easily?
Have recurrent cold sores?
Feel tired and run down much of the time?
Fail to find humor in life?
Have recurrent diarrhea?
Feel nauseous often?
Get nosebleeds easily?
Have bleeding gums?
Have poor digestion?
Have trouble falling asleep?
Have bad breath?
Have tender gums?
Have scaly, itchy, flaking skin?
Have skin rashes?
Have uncommon hair loss?
Suffer from constipation?
Get dizzy often?
Have labored breathing?
Experience emotional instability?

Before reading about how nutrition is related to these maladies, you'll want to know what your eating habits are really like. Check yourself on the following items to get some idea of what you know and what your eating style is. For each "yes" answer, give yourself one point, except with questions 8, 9, 10, and 19 (marked with an asterisk) give yourself one point for a "no" answer. Total your points at the end.

YES/NO

1. I always avoid eating refined sugars. ______
2. I eat raw fruit or vegetables at least twice a day. ______
3. I know how much protein I should have daily and eat that amount. ______
4. I know how much fat should be in my diet and don't go over that limit. ______
5. I eat breakfast, lunch, and dinner and very rarely skip meals. ______
6. I have small snacks between my meals. ______
7. I avoid becoming really starved. ______
8. I sometimes crave certain foods so much that once I get them, I can't control the amount I eat. ______*
9. I eat cookies/candy/other favorite food by myself in a place or at a time when others won't see me eating. ______*
10. Sometimes I start eating and just cannot stop myself. ______*
11. I eat high roughage (fiber) foods daily (fresh fruits, bran, raw vegetables, whole grain products). ______
12. I avoid eating refined flour products (cakes, pasta, cookies, and so on). ______
13. I eat breakfast every day. ______
14. I make it a point to eat whole wheat bread rather than white bread. ______
15. I know that I get my supply of daily vitamins and minerals. ______
16. I drink herbal tea rather than regular tea. ______
17. I avoid drinking a lot of coffee (more than two cups per day). ______
18. I substitute some vegetable protein for meat in my meals. ______
19. Sometimes at night I "binge" eat. ______*

20. My skin is smooth and healthy looking. ______
21. I don't have more than one cold per year. ______

TOTAL ______

The higher your score here (15 to 21), the more likely that you are already interested in your nutritional health but are having trouble getting some of the other aspects of weight control together. If your score is less than 5, you probably have many food and eating habits that you need to change. If you scored between 5 and 10, your eating habits and food preferences won't earn you a nutrition medal. But a score between 10 and 15 shows that you and good nutrition are not strangers.

Let's take a look now at what you do eat.

Food Intake Recording

The only way to find out if you are getting the vitamins, minerals, protein, unsaturated fats, and so on that you should be getting is to examine what you eat each day. I have found that most people have a food pattern that doesn't vary a great deal, so that one day's food intake can be matched fairly closely to that of most of the other days of the week. Of course, special occasions arise to contribute extra food and special kinds of foods, but most individuals' lives are not an endless special occasion. Each day's intake is normal for that day because it is the intake that you have to work with; what you get is what you eat. To outwit that special or not-normal day, you need to record a number of days in a row.

So record what you ate yesterday on the Diet Record given in this chapter (Table 8.1, Form A). Then on a copy of the form, fill in what you have eaten so far *today* and finish filling it in at the end of the day. If you think the average of these days is not typical for you, keep this record for three to seven days, and then average them at the end of the period. I recommend keeping a seven-day record. *I warn you now,* this is a self-examining exercise that may shock you!

Keeping The Record, Straight

Just recording what you eat on the pages of your Diet Record may help you shed a pound or two if you keep it for the recommended

TABLE 8.1 Form A: Daily Diet Record*

Group	*Food*	*Amount*	*Calories*	*Protein*	*Fat*	*Saturated Fat*	*Unsaturated Fat*
Milk and Milk Products							
Eggs, Meat, Fish, Dry beans, Nuts							
Vegetables, Fruits							
Grains							
Fats, Oils							
Sugars							
Misc.							
Totals							

*Use this model form for each day of your diet.

TABLE 8.1 Continued

Choles-terol	*Carbo-hydrates*	*Calcium*	*Phos-phorus*	*Iron*	*Potas-sium*	*Sodium*	*Vitamin A (IU)*	*Thiamine*	*Ribo-flavin*	*Niacin*	*Vitamin C*	*Total Servings per Group*

week. Any time you scrutinize your diet this closely, you are more likely to change your mind and not eat some foods that you feel are bad for you. If you have to write it down in black and white, then you'll be forced to find out *why* it's bad for you.

Step 1. In recording your intake you must obey two rules: *be honest* and *be yourself*. Eat what you feel is the way you always eat and write down *everything*.

Step 2. On a copy of the Diet Record Form, write down everything you ate and drank yesterday. If you can't remember *everything* you consumed yesterday, start with today.

Step 3. If you are not sure of the quantities, go to your kitchen and get out the measuring spoons and a measuring cup, your favorite coffee cup, drinking glass(es), soup bowl, saucer, and plate. Now do some experimenting:

Take a measuring cup of water and pour it into the following: coffee cup, soup bowl, drinking glass, beer glass, cocktail glass, wine glass, any other receptacle from which you drink or eat. Notice how each relates to one cup (eight ounces) or any fraction of a cup.

Take a teaspoon and measure teaspoons of water into a tablespoon. Then measure tablespoons of water into a measuring cup. Remember those relationships, how much of each fits into the other.

Now take a measuring cup full of dry food (navy beans, macaroni—anything in your cupboard that can be easily handled in your "laboratory" and then returned to storage). Pour a cup of your substance onto a saucer, then onto a plate (notice how it looks like a lot more on the saucer!). Do the same with a half cup. Remember what these amounts look like on your plate or saucer.

Measuring meat servings isn't as easy as measuring servings of beans or mashed potatoes, but with the following dimensions, you can draw yourself some pictures that will help:

1. A hamburger patty that is ⅜ inch thick and 2½ inches in diameter is about 3 ounces.
2. Meat loaf ½ inch thick and about 4 inches in diameter is also about 3 ounces.
3. Round steak ½ inch thick and 3 inches by 2 inches in size is about 3 ounces.

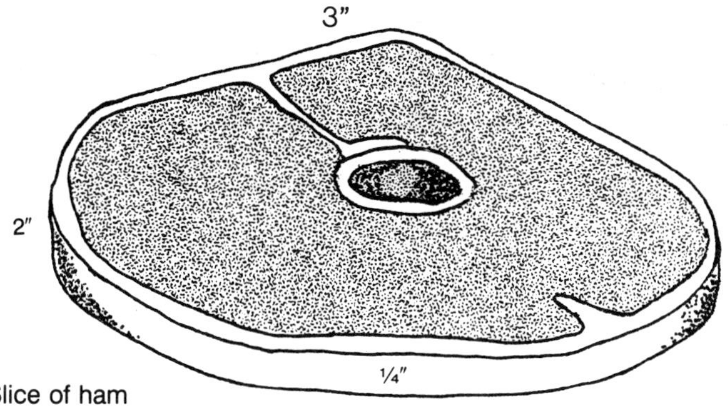

Slice of ham

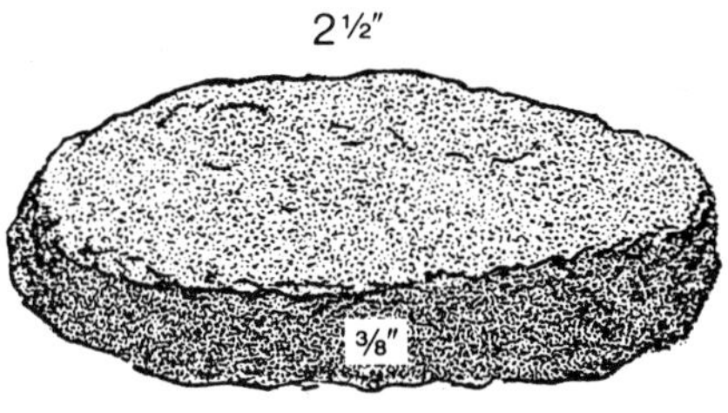

Hamburger patty

4. A veal cutlet 3 inches by 2 inches and ⅜ inches thick is about 3 ounces.
5. Roast beef 2½ inches by 3 inches and ½ inch thick is about 2 ounces.
6. A slice of ham 2 inches by 3 inches and ¼ inch thick weighs about 2 ounces.
7. Roast turkey ½ inch thick and 2 inches by 3½ inches in size is about 3 ounces.
8. A small lean lamp chop ½ inch thick is about 2½ ounces.

You are responsible for measuring the quantity of food that you eat, so if you aren't the shopper/chef at your home, take some kitchen-lab time to acquaint yourself with measurements. If you eat meat, draw the meat pictures and keep the pictures handy until you can tell at a glance how much meat is on your plate.

Step 4. After recording everything you ate and drank for the day in the appropriate places, use Appendix B to record on your Diet Record the nutrients for each amount of food in the columns provided. Using a ruler helps keep you on the correct line. Note the amount before you fill in the figures – the difference between a slice of bread and a loaf of bread is considerable!

Step 5. Add each column and record your totals on Form B, the Daily Diet Record Totals (Table 8.2).

Step 6. Figure your daily average for each nutrient for the days you have recorded. If you record your intake for a week, Form B will be completely filled, your totals will reflect a week's intake of each nutrient, and you will divide each total by 7.

TABLE 8.2 Form B: Daily Diet Record Totals

	Calories	*Protein*	*Fat*	*Saturated Fat*	*Unsaturated Fat*	*Cholesterol*	*Carbohydrates*
Day 1							
Day 2							
Day 3							
Day 4							
Day 5							
Day 6							
Day 7							
Totals							
Daily Averages							
% of Total Calories							
Your RDA							

TABLE 8.2 Continued

Calcium	*Phosphorus*	*Iron*	*Potassium*	*Sodium*	*Vitamin A (IU)*	*Thiamine*	*Riboflavin*	*Niacin*	*Vitamin C*

Step 7. Look for your RDA for each nutrient in Appendix B (Table B.1), and fill it in on Form B. You'll note that there is no RDA for fat or for carbohydrates, so: First, convert your total and each of the subdivisions of fat into calories by multiplying the number of grams of fat by 9:

1 gram of fat = 9 calories

Second, convert your carbohydrates into calories by multiplying total grams by 4:

1 gram of carbohydrate = 4 calories

Third, determine what percentage of your daily calories was contributed by fat and what percentage was contributed by carbohydrates:

fat calories/total calories = daily percentage of fat calories
carbohydrate calories/total calories = daily percentage of carbohydrate calories

For example, if your week's total calories were 14,000, you averaged 2,000 calories per day. If your week's total fat calories were 7,000, you averaged 1,000 calories of fat per day. By dividing daily fat calories by total calories per day, you find that 50 percent of your diet was fat intake:

1,000 fat calories/2,000 total calories = .50 or 50%

After you find what percentage of your diet was carbohydrate and what percentage was fat, determine what percentage of your diet was saturated fat and what percentage was unsaturated fat. We'll discuss the merits of each in Chapter 9.

When you know what percentage of your diet was carbohydrate and fat, the remaining percentage must be protein, because there are only three basic foodstuffs. However, it is a good idea to check protein percentage the same way you did the other two foods:

1 gram of protein = 4 calories

Some calories are usually lost in the mathematics process; so the total percentages of protein plus fat plus carbohydrate does not always equal exactly 100 percent.

Step 8. This is the *final analysis*. What are you getting out of your food? Put a red circle around each average daily intake that shows a deficiency when compared to your RDA. Note that you need 800 *milligrams* of calcium (which is the same as .8 *grams* listed in the RDA chart).

Perhaps you take a vitamin pill every day. Well, that no doubt helps, but just because it brings you up to or over your RDA limit, the pill doesn't increase the value of the foods you are choosing. Add only the nutrients in your food in your total figures.

Of the hundreds of students and private individuals I've helped with their total fitness, I have seen only a handful of them who meet their RDA's in all columns and match the recommended percentages of fat, carbohydrate, and protein daily. Americans are frightfully malnourished—mainly due to their food choices and eating schedules. These generally lead to consumption of "empty calories" and fat storage efficiency.

Now that you have recorded and totaled the various nutrients that you are getting in the foods you eat, go on to Chapter 9, which will help you analyze your diet. Chapter 9 contains the recommendations for daily dietary intake and also shows you how to formulate a diet that is healthy for you in case you have found deficiencies or overabundances in your diet.

9 ANALYZING YOUR DIET AND PLANNING A NEW, HEALTHY MENU

EACH COLUMN on Form A in Chapter 8 (Table 8.1) gave you information regarding your food intake, your eating choices, and your health. For each category given there, compare your results with the knowledge and new insights you gain from the information in this chapter.

Nutrition

This is really a chapter on nutrition, and it's included in this book because nutrition is one of the four main foundations of holistic health. You may not like to think in terms of being what you eat ("you are what you eat"), but what you do eat and at what intervals you eat are basics in getting your body in shape. The better you are at establishing new, lasting nutritional and eating behavior, the more likely you are to be healthy, maintain your ideal weight, and stay healthy for a lifetime.

When you see the word *nutrition* you may feel that something "good" is being discussed, something that someone who has studied biochemistry and/or read about additives and organic gardening and bran and wheat germ does to be super-healthy. Another feeling you may have about nutrition is that it's much too complicated to understand. All those vitamins and minerals and beriberi and scurvy are too boring to study and not applicable to you and most people you know. For example, recently at a housewarming for some of my friends I was talking with the host. He asked me what I'd been writing about lately, so I told him I was writing about nutrition. And this very "with-it" fellow says, "Well, that's something I don't know anything about!" I realize now that I should have said that I was writing about food and eating, and his comment would have probably been. "Well, that's something I know plenty about. Want to interview me?"

Perhaps the most unfortunate thing about nutrition is that people can't eat it! Margaret Mead once told a U.S. Senate Hearing Committee on Nutrition and Human Needs, ". . . people don't eat nutrition. They eat food." And so this chapter is going to be about food and eating if you're a realist, and about nutrition if you deal with the abstract.

RDA

Before you read about foods and their nutritive value, a few words should be said about the Recommended Daily Allowances (RDA). The amounts recommended are established by the National Academy of Sciences-National Research Council's Food and Nutrition Board, and are periodically updated according to current nutritional knowledge.

There are some obvious drawbacks to the RDA; the most obvious is that not all people are alike. I am far more active than many professional women of my age, but theoretically we all have the same RDA. The RDA table (in Appendix B) suggests that we all weigh 128 pounds, which we don't. Bigger (especially more muscular and therefore heavier) people need more nutrients. You can use the RDA table, however, to give you a baseline figure of the nutrients you need (plus a margin of safety).

It would be great to know *exactly* how much of each nutrient each person needs, but the process of measuring vitamin and mineral levels in the body is not yet available in cost and time to most individuals. For instance, there is a lingual ascorbic acid (vitamin C) test made by MineraLab, Inc. (MineraLab, Inc., 1978) and Medical Diagnostic Services (Thie and Perry, 1978) that involves application of an indicator dye on the tongue. If the body reacts within a certain time period (seconds), a satisfactory tissue ascorbic acid level is indicated. A starter kit may cost in the range of $50 and can be used to test hundreds of people, but it isn't something many people would want to buy to check their need for just one vitamin.

Another example of testing nutrient level is hair analysis. Hair, or mineral, analysis is becoming popular in many holistic health care centers, and many articles have been and are being written regarding the merits of hair analysis. Proponents of hair analysis argue that the hair best represents the mineral storage in the body. The blood shows minerals in transport, while urine shows the minerals the body is choosing to eliminate. But neither hair analysis nor blood and urine analysis is inexpensive at this time.

So the RDA table, which gives figures for persons of average height, weight, and "light" activity, is used. Keep Form B (Table 8.2) handy so you can look at each column and compare what you are getting in your diet with what is recommended in the RDA table.

Amount of Food

Just by looking at how much writing you do on each day's food intake record, you may get a general feeling of how closely you meet your nutrient recommendations. If you have only a few items in each category, you may suspect that you are not meeting your vitamin, mineral, and protein requirements through the foods you eat. I have looked at hundreds of such recalls, and it's obvious that those who are reducing food intake are also limiting their chances of meeting their nutritive needs.

Calories

As you know, the calorie is a unit of energy, and ideally, you should eat no more calories than you expend if you want to maintain your weight. To reduce weight, energy output must be greater than the number of calories you take in.

The number of calories recommended in the RDA table is based on the "average" American who engages in "light" activity; that is, each day he or she gets eight hours of rest, eight hours of sitting activity, four hours of standing activity, two hours of walking purposefully, and two hours of energy cost greater than walking. If you are at a maintenance weight and engage in lots of exercise, your necessary caloric intake may be greater than that shown in the RDA table.

The "average" weights for adult men and women stabilize at age 25 in the table because, again theoretically, there should be no weight gain after 25 in a healthy person. For an overly fat person, the calories and nutrients taken in should be those given in the table because those amounts are actually based on lean body mass (muscle) rather than body weight.

The Food and Nutrition Board suggests that the recommended caloric consumption for the 25-year-old be decreased by 5 percent in the decades between 35 and 55 years, by 8 percent for the years between 55 and 75, and by 10 percent for 75 years and older. Your metabolism slows as you grow older.

On your daily intake records review the calorie column and determine what *five* foods you have listed gave you the greatest number of calories. Are they also high in nutrients? If not, you have fallen into the "empty calorie" syndrome.

Although calorie counting of food alone is not a way to reduce your weight and then maintain it, it is an important aspect to be compared with how much and what quality of activity you're engaging in. I used to daydream of starting a camp where children would come to lose weight. They would earn food tokens in relation to their daily activity. For instance, an hour of tennis would earn them a 250-calorie token. Then they would pay for the foods of their choice at the cafeteria with their tokens. With a little guidance, they could learn some good food and exercise choices while they were young.

It would simplify matters if weight reduction involved just calorie counting. But remember, efficiency in taking off pounds or putting them on also includes some other factors:

1. How much food is eaten at *any one time*
2. What *kind* of food is eaten daily and at each meal
3. How *long* is the time between meals
4. How *little* food is eaten (starvation shuts down metabolism)
5. *Energy level* (a continuum from hyperactive to depressed)
6. *When* the overweight condition occurred and how long it has lasted

The full diet recall record suggested in Chapter 8 is a good way to count calories because it lets you know what you get in your food besides calories.

Protein

Look back at your daily Diet Record: Are you getting enough protein daily? There is an obligatory amount of protein that each person should eat each day to keep the body from breaking down structural protein, that is, muscle and other tissue. Extreme cases of emaciation, such as those that occur in prison camps or even anorexia nervosa, are the result of using the only protein the body has in order to stay alive. Day-to-day cellular function depends on enzymes, transport of substances, and other transient uses of protein such as energy which, if not supplied by food, will be supplied by body stores.

STARVATION

During starvation the body first uses up available carbohydrate stores (excess blood glucose and then stored liver and muscle glycogen). This occurs during the first day of starvation, and during that day increasing amounts of protein and fat are metabolized for energy. While protein stores are still ample, the liver changes protein into glucose so the brain will have something to burn for energy. If you have gone on a "starvation diet," you may have experienced headaches in the first day or two. This occurs because the blood glucose level is not as high as it usually is, causing some central nervous system irritability. After protein stores have been partially depleted at the onset of starvation, the body starts the fat-utilization mechanism. Protein is then protected again until the fat stores are almost totally depleted and the only source of energy left in the body is protein. A 154-pound person with 20 percent body fat could live about two months on fat stores.

PROTEIN AND WEIGHT

The properties of protein are such that water adheres to it; so each pound of protein in the body comes complete with about a pound of water. Glycogen is kept in osmotic balance in liver and muscle cells with water, as is glucose in the blood (the greater the number of molecules of glucose or glycogen, the greater the amount of water to balance them osmotically). Perhaps you understand now how a starvation diet causes rapid initial weight loss: When glucose and glycogen stores are used, the water used to balance them is lost. Then when the early depletion of protein occurs, water loss also occurs.

PROTEIN AS FOOD AND ENERGY

The combination of ingested amino acids must be about the same as those used by the body tissues. The most complete forms of protein that you can eat are eggs, meat, and dairy products because each contains all the *essential* amino acids (the amino acids that the body cannot synthesize for itself). The body must have all the essential amino acids for healthy growth and replacement of tissues and enzymes. If the concentration of one essential amino acid is low, other amino acids will become unusable because the cell forms either complete proteins or none at all.

Many vegetables and fruits are incomplete protein foods; they do not contain all the essential amino acids. But with careful consideration of a mixture of fruits, vegetables, and grains, you can get all the essential amino acids necessary for healthy growth and maintenance. Frances Moore Lappe's book, *Diet for a Small Planet* (1982), is a helpful guide for non-meat eaters. You'll want to review your Diet Record to determine whether you are eating complete or incomplete protein foods.

Americans have come to regard protein, especially meat (a juicy T-bone, prime rib, leg of lamb), as a sign of affluence and eat more protein than they need. When more protein is taken into the body than it needs, the body converts it to glucose, glycogen, or fat. It seems paradoxical, after looking at how the body spares protein until the very end in starvation, that after a meal, animal protein is one of the first foodstuffs to enter the bloodstream and be used for energy. Humphrey Sassoon in his article, "Time Factors in Obesity" (1973), showed that the order of appearance of foodstuffs in the bloodstream is:

1. Sugars
2. Animal protein
3. Vegetable protein
4. Carbohydrates (long-chain)
5. Short-chain fatty acids
6. Long-chain fatty acids

Sassoon explained that large amounts of sugar or *easily available amino acids* flood the body with too many calories all at once, and the body is forced to store them. Also, when high levels of protein must be converted into glucogenic (glucose) or lipogenic (fatty) substances in the body, the nitrogen on each amino acid must be processed. For those prone to gout, a high protein diet is not recommended because nitrogen contributes to the uric acid level, and high uric acid levels exacerbate a gouty condition. High protein diets are also inadvisable for anyone with liver or kidney disease. Even for those without such diseases, high protein diets require an increased water intake to keep the kidneys flushed out.

HOW MUCH PROTEIN?

There is a recommended amount of protein intake per day given in the RDA table. A *minimal* level of .4 grams of protein per kilogram body weight should be eaten each day, but .9 grams per kilogram body weight is recommended. Your diet should be about 15 to 20 percent protein.

Fats

If more than 30 percent of your daily calories are contributed by fat, you are eating too much of it. The 30 percent of your diet that is fat intake should be in a ratio of two grams of unsaturated fat for every gram of saturated fat. Look at your totals of fat intake on your Diet Record to see if you are within these recommendations.

If you are not within these guidelines, you probably need to limit your saturated fats. If you are a meat eater, especially of beef and pork, you are probably contributing heavily to your saturated fat calories through these meats. The solution is to eat only lean cuts of meat or switch to chicken or fish as your source of meat protein. These two foods not only have lower fat content, but what fat they do have is more likely to be unsaturated.

Why eat more unsaturated fatty acids than saturated? Saturated fats are harder to break down and move out of the bloodstream than are unsaturated (or polyunsaturated) fatty acids. If you're confused as to which foods have saturated fats and which have unsaturated fats, remember this simple rule: Saturated fats are usually those that are solid at room temperature, such as lard or the fat on a beef steak or roast. Unsaturated fats are in liquid form at room temperature and generally come from vegetable, nut, or seed sources (for example, olive oil, corn oil, peanut oil, sesame oil).

It has become apparent that fish that are rich in certain polyunsaturated fats called Omega-3 fatty acids actually change blood chemistry to lower the likelihood of cardiovascular disease. As few as 2–4 fish meals a week can significantly reduce the risk of heart disease (Glomset, 1985). Not all fish are high in Omega-3 fats, however, so the diet should include those fish that have the higher level of these fats (see Table 9.1).

To identify foods high in each kind of fat, review your Diet Record and note those foods that contribute high levels of each. Remember

TABLE 9.1 Omega-3 Oil Content in 4 oz. of Fish*

Salmon	
Chinook	3.6 grams
Sockeye	2.3
Tuna	
Albacore	2.6
Mackerel	1.8–2.6
Herring	1.2–2.7
Rainbow trout	1.0
Whiting	.9
King Crab	.6
Shrimp	.5
Cod	.3

*Adapted from *Fish Facts*, Salt Lake City: Gastronomy, Inc., 1987.

which ones are desirable and which ones are not so desirable and incorporate that knowledge into your food choices.

FATS AS GOOD GUYS

The two unsaturated fats listed in your Diet Record, oleic and linoleic, are essential fats (you must have them in your diet because the body cannot synthesize them) and are necessary for the constant building of cell structures. They keep the skin smooth and healthy by preventing dryness, and contribute especially to normal growth and maintenance of arteries, nerves, and blood. It is also becoming apparent that unsaturated fatty acids help to maintain a proper cholesterol level.

Oils that are high in linoleic acid are safflower oil (75 percent linoleic acid), sunflower oil (65 percent), corn oil (59 percent), and soybean oil (58 percent). One way to make yourself a healthier bread spread is to mix soft butter half and half with safflower oil.

Fats are necessary in the body as carriers of the fat soluble vitamins (A, D, E, and K), and they aid the absorption of vitamin D, which makes calcium available to bones, teeth, and other tissues that must have calcium. Fats are also necessary to change the vegetable precursor of vitamin A (carotene) into vitamin A.

In the fight against fat, dieters tend to forget that fat stores can and do protect and hold in place the internal organs such as the liver, heart, and kidneys; and subcutaneous fat acts as an insulator against cold temperatures.

There has been much controversy surrounding fat in the diet, and some have reacted by eliminating almost all of this highly caloric food from their diet. However, the satiety value of fat is quite high because fat slows the emptying of the stomach. So a limited amount of the right kind of fat has its place in every diet.

FATS AS BAD GUYS

There is merit to eating some fat, but cautionary measures should be taken to ensure the proper ratio of unsaturated to saturated fatty acids, and to ensure that the menu is not overloaded with fat. Diets higher in fat may be acceptable for highly active individuals, but the commercial high fat fad diets have been attacked by many health experts because of a number of possible health dangers (Wycoff, 1986).

First, a diet rich in only one of three foodstuffs is contrary to nature. If the human body was not meant to ingest carbohydrates and protein, it would not have the elaborate systems for breaking them down into energy. You need a widely varied diet to get the vitamins, minerals, fiber, and so on that a healthy body requires.

A second argument against a high fat diet is that fat and cholesterol intake have been related to atherosclerosis (plaquing of the arteries) by leading scientific research for many years. It is also noted in obesity research that very overweight persons (and those who have had a recent heart attack) have a slow clearance rate of fats from the bloodstream. That is, after a fatty meal, healthy, active individuals clear fats out of the blood much faster than sedentary, or fat, or coronary-prone individuals. If, indeed, this has an implication for plaquing of artery walls, which leads to heart disease, you would be wise to maintain a moderate intake of fats and especially to stay away from high fat fad diets.

Third, the medical world has also noted that when a person is on a diet of fats, the fatty acid and ketone (breakdown product of fatty acids) levels increase, causing an acidic condition in the body. In persons with cardiovascular disorders such as coronary artery disease or cerebrovascular disease, this acidity may in turn cause irregular heartbeat with eventual fatal consequence.

Fourth, diets heavy in fat can also cause diarrhea. When this occurs, the body loses water, vitamins, minerals, and other elements necessary for good health. A marathoner friend of mine, upon learning that fats provide good energy for the "long haul," ate a whole stick of butter the night before a marathon. Fortunately he was a medical doctor, because he had to prescribe himself something to counteract his subsequent case of diarrhea!

A high fat diet, then, in defying nature's law of moderation, can be dangerous to the very susceptible, and bring about a measure of unhealthiness in anyone who continues the diet for more than a day or so.

Cholesterol

One of the popular ways of assessing risk of heart attack is to measure the cholesterol level in the blood. The measurement is given in milligrams of cholesterol per deciliter of blood serum. It is recommended that you maintain a cholesterol level below 200 mg percent. A level of 150 or less is ideal (Farquhar, 1987).

Triglyceride (saturated fat) serum level is also an indication of cardiovascular health. A high level of saturated fat contributes to high levels of cholesterol in the blood. A diet high in saturated fats and cholesterol is commonly linked to both heart disease and cancer.

Two other blood components that are becoming household words related to cardiovascular health are LDLs (low density lipoproteins) and HDLs (high density lipoproteins). These lipoproteins carry fats from one place to another in the bloodstream. LDLs and VLDLs (very low density lipoproteins) carry fats from the liver to the cells. When there is a high level of LDLs in the blood, there is greater risk of heart disease. On the other hand, when the HDL level is high in comparison with the level of LDLs, fats are being carried to the liver to be stored, and heart disease risk is lowered. An excellent way to increase the HDL level in the blood is to partake in regular vigorous exercise (Haskel, 1984). The average level of HDLs for females is 55 mgs and the average level for males is 45 mgs.

There are three main steps to lowering or maintaining a healthy cholesterol level: (1) Eat cholesterol-lowering fibrous foods such as oat bran; (2) Avoid high cholesterol foods such as dairy products, red meat, and high fat bakery items. The American Heart Association recommends that cholesterol intake be kept below 300 mg. daily. The information that you put in your Diet Diary will give you a good indication of the amount of cholesterol in your diet. (3) Switch from high cholesterol foods to lower cholesterol foods such as low fat dairy products and fish rather than meat.

In order to find out what your cholesterol, triglyceride, and lipoprotein levels are, you must have a blood lab draw and analyze a sample of your blood. Tests done in fitness laboratories, wellness centers, and health fairs may provide you with blood chemistry items such as these.

Carbohydrates

What's left to eat? There are only three foodstuffs that will supply your energy needs: proteins, fats, and carbohydrates. If you eat an excess of one, the other two will not contribute as much energy. If you eat too little of one, the others will automatically have to make a greater contribution to your diet. Many students who have eliminated carbohydrates from their diets are dismayed to learn about some of the health dangers of eating too much protein and the drawbacks of eating too much fat. "What else is left to eat?" they ask.

They soon realize that a good "diet" balances the three foodstuffs by providing at least obligatory protein intake (or about 15 percent of the diet), no more than 30 percent of the daily calories as fat, and the remainder of the intake as carbohydrates. Of these carbohydrates, at least 80 percent should be complex, or long-chain, carbohydrates and 20 percent or less should be taken in as sugar.

CARBOHYDRATES AND ENERGY

Most books on nutrition will tell you that carbohydrates are instant energy suppliers and that carbohydrates provide most of your energy throughout the day. Both of these statements are partially correct. Since the discussion of each may give you greater insight into food choices and weight loss habits, we'll take a look at both.

Instant Energy. First of all, dietary carbohydrates come in different sizes in a chain formation. Most of the sugar you consume is in the shortest chain (only two molecules), while starches are the longest chains (such as in potatoes or rice). There is also cellulose, which is indigestible for humans, so of course it would be the most resistant to supplying energy in the human body.

An enzyme in saliva begins the digestion of carbohydrates in the mouth. So sugar, only a two-molecule chain, *is* instant energy. In fact, it's so instant, it can be dangerous if a large amount is taken into the system at once or if a person is exceptionally susceptible to sugar intake (such as a person with diabetes or hypog floods the bloodstream and stimulates a strong ir the pancreas. The insulin then floods the blood blood sugar be quickly transported into musc the result of this process is the rebound sugar—the individual who just ate or drar an hour or so. The technical name for ce- mia"—low blood sugar as a reaction d sugar causing a massive insulin response, as depict e 9.1.

So the kinds of carbohydrates that are good to have in the diet are those that occur in a long chain. For instance, it takes an hour to two hours for carbohydrate from pasta to be available for energy. That is not exactly "instant energy." With long-chain carbohydrates the system receives a steady supply of energy as the chain is broken down and there is little instant-high or reactive-low blood glucose level.

Delayed Energy. If your body is running mainly on carbohydrates, then you aren't using fat or protein to any measurable extent. In order to switch your energy source from carbohydrates to fats you need to sustain some kind of physical activity or refrain from eating. The former is encouraged by weight control experts. As you begin to perform physical activity, you use carbohydrates almost entirely for your fuel, but as you sustain your activity (12 to 15 minutes or more), you burn increasing amounts of fat and protein. On a weight reducing regimen, it is highly important to get your body to burn fat, but to do it in a manner that changes the body from an efficient fat storage habit to an efficient fat removal system. To do this (as this book

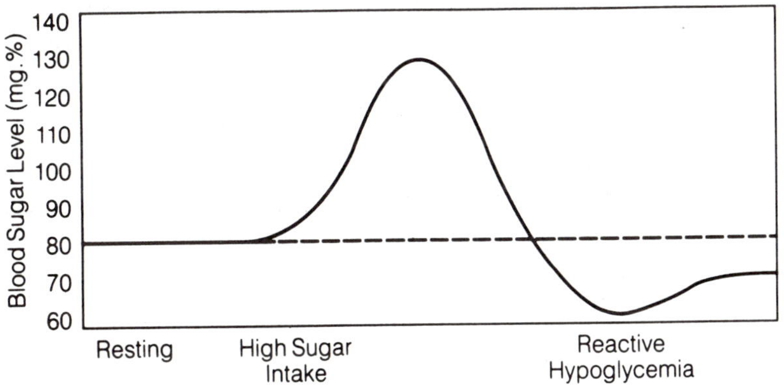

FIGURE 9.1 Reactive Hypoglycemia: The Result of Flooding the System with "Instant Energy"

details), you must feed yourself small meals of the right foods regularly throughout the day. This way the fat stores have to be used a little bit almost constantly. If for some reason you want to maintain a very efficient fat storage system, eat one meal that has a good amount of sugar and alcohol daily. You may coax fat off your system this way if caloric intake is small enough, but when you go off your diet, your weight will rebound because of your storage efficiency.

REFINED SUGAR

If 20 percent of your diet is table sugar (sucrose), you must get 100 percent of your nutrients from 80 percent of your food. Table sugar has no saving grace. It gives you nothing but calories and may lead to eventual trouble with vitamin deficiencies, dental caries, hypoglycemia (which may lead to hyperglycemia, or diabetes), obesity, and a host of maladies related to the problems mentioned here. Pick up any current nutrition book and you will read about the dangers of sugar consumption.

Fruit sugar (or fructose) is a somewhat different story in that when taken in its natural form it doesn't flood the system and cause the same kind of reaction that sucrose does. Figure 9.2 shows the blood sugar reaction to the ingestion of an apple (in red, ripe, natural form), apple juice, and apple cider. Notice that the apple in its natural state does not cause as much of a rise in blood sugar level as the two processed products. The apple also does not cause the rebounding hypoglycemia that the others produce.

It is not surprising then that nature did not plan sucrose to be part of the human diet. Instead, the natural sugars or starches are contained in cellulose or in long-chain carbohydrates that do not contribute to glucose intolerance as refined sugar does.

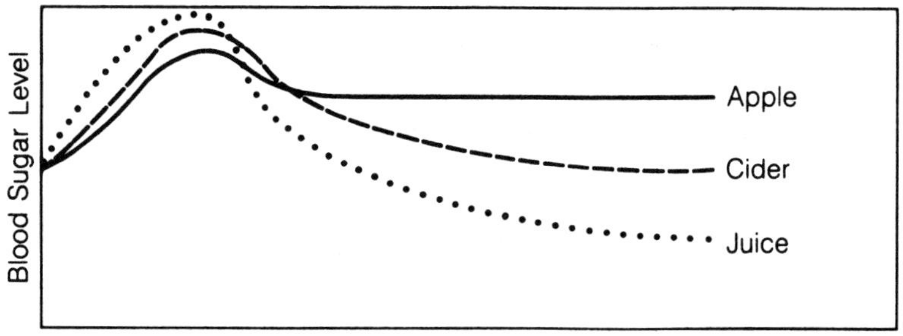

FIGURE 9.2 Blood Sugar Response to an Apple, Apple Cider, and Apple Juice

Hidden Sugars. It is a fact that the incidence of diabetes and hypoglycemia in this country has increased phenomenally in the last few decades, and sugar is highly implicated. Americans have increased their per capita intake of sugar from about 30 pounds per year to more than 100 pounds per year in the last 80 years. You may say, "But I don't use that much sugar—someone else is eating mine." You may be quite conscientious about not putting sugar in your coffee or tea, but if it's instant coffee, there may already be sugar or some other sweetener in it, and many nondairy creamers are presweetened, too. So many of the sugars you eat are hidden in processed foods.

Look at the products in your cupboard in a treasure hunt for sugar—chances are, you'll find it (or a just-as-harmful cousin) listed as an ingredient on more products than you would expect. Look at the following ingredients and try to guess what each product is. (The sugar item in each product is listed in italic.)

INGREDIENTS LISTED ON PACKAGE, IN ORDER OF CONCENTRATION	*PRODUCT*
1. Salt, sodium silicoaluminate, *dextrose*, potassium iodide	________
2. Iodized salt, spices, MSG, garlic, dried onion, *sugar*, artificial color, propylene glycol	________
3. Peanuts, *sugar*, hardened vegetable oil, salt, molasses, mono- and diglycerides	________
4. *Corn syrup solids*, vegetable oil, sodium caseinate, mono- and diglycerides, dipotassium phosophate, artificial flavor, artificial color	________
5. Tomatoes, vinegar, *corn sweetener*, salt, onion powder, spice	________
6. Tomatoes, *sugar*, food starch, wheat flour, salt, *dextrose*, onion powder	________
7. Tomatoes, onion, vinegar, *sugar*, bell pepper, salt and spices	________

8. Soybean oil, vinegar, *sugar*, food starch, egg yolk, *corn syrup*, salt, paprika ____________
9. Flour, vegetable shortening, *corn syrup*, solar salt, butter, soda ____________

Answers: 1. Table salt; 2. Seasoned salt; 3. Peanut butter; 4. Coffee creamer (nondairy); 5. Catsup; 6. Tomato soup; 7. Meat relish; 8. Salad dressing; 9. Pretzel Nubs.

These, of course, are only some of the products you might not expect to contribute to your sugar intake. After you recover from this project, look for some products you know contain sugar. Such packaged foods as sugar-coated breakfast foods may show the *first* ingredient to be sugar! This means that there is a greater concentration of sugar than any other ingredient in that product. Table 9.2 identifies some products that you know have sugar in them. But did you know how much sugar they contain?

A good habit to develop is to read all ingredient labels: if sugar is within the first four ingredients, don't eat the product. Good places to find foods without added sugar content are in the produce, dairy, fresh meat, and seafood sections of your grocery store. Natural grains, nuts, and seeds are also not tainted with sugar. Then if you want to add sweetness when you prepare these foods, use a natural sweetener such as fruit juice concentrate.

TABLE 9.2 Sugar Content of Various Products

Food	*Sugar Content (teaspoons)*
1 average chocolate bar	7
1 marshmallow (60 to 1 lb.)	1½
1½-inch square chocolate fudge	4
1/12 chocolate cake (2-layer with icing)	15
1/12 angel food cake	6
plain doughnut, 3-inch diameter	4
½ cup sherbet	6–8
½ cup ice cream	5–6
1/6 pumpkin pie	10
1/6 cherry pie	14
1/6 apple pie	12
6 oz. cola	4–5
6 oz. ginger ale	3–4

(100 grams = 20 teaspoons = ½ cup = 3½ oz. = 400 calories; or 1 teaspoon = 20 calories)

Nutrient Robber. Besides the fact that sucrose plays havoc with blood sugar, it also robs the body of nutrients needed to break the sugar down for energy. Most natural foods provide vitamins and minerals that help metabolize each food, but not sugar. Since sugar has no nutrients, the body must donate vitamins (especially thiamine and other B vitamins) to break down the sugar so it will do the one thing it can do—provide energy. If the body is already short of nutrients due to an inadequate diet, the sugar robbing the body of the B vitamins may result in such symptoms as indigestion, heartburn, and/or nausea when carbohydrates cannot be properly metabolized.

Advertised Sugar. When you see or hear an advertisement for a candy bar or other high-sugar content food product, be aware that the advertisement is there merely to sell the product. It is not concerned with your good health any more than a cigarette advertisement is. Advertisers of sugar products usually resort to the word *energy* to hook you. And it's true, sugar will provide you with energy. But the ad will not tell you the possible hazards of sugar, nor will it suggest foods that may be more nutritious snacks with an equal amount of energy. Think about what the *real* message is when you see the next candy commercial, and determine what the *implied* message is. Defend yourself from Madison Avenue.

ARTIFICIAL SWEETENERS

"If I can't eat sugar, how can I satisfy my cravings for sweetness?" This is a question I hear from nearly every student. The dangers of cyclamates have been advertised. Brown sugar is as bad as white—both have all impurities and all nutrients removed. Honey and molasses, although having some vitamin, mineral, and protein content, also have sucrose content and may not be advisable sweeteners for those who are hypoglycemic and others with glucose intolerance.

The artificial sweeteners when compared with table sugar would probably be less dangerous. But it is much healthier to be less addicted to the artificial sweetness of sugar or cyclamates and to depend on natural fruit sugars to satisfy a taste for sweetness.

PROCESSED FLOUR

Another caution you may want to take in choosing carbohydrates is to look for and avoid processed flour. Processed flour, just as refined sugar, is not the natural way to get carbohydrates. When flour is processed, virtually all the vitamins and minerals are removed so that what are left are calories. Nearly all flour processors or subsequent flour-product processors try to correct what has been undone by fortifying their products; they put in thiamine, riboflavin, and niacin—and perhaps iron. But there is no way they can synthetically restore the nutrient content of the original grain. Processing takes out *at least* 22 elements and puts back parts of four elements!

Instead of stone grinding grains (which was done for centuries), people now rely on a process that generates heat, which in turn destroys protein, wheat germ, and its oil. This process of milling also removes the outer coating of the grain, and thus most of the remaining nutrients are lost as well as the fiber that they would naturally give. Then the flour is bleached, aged, and preservatives are added. The product that remains is pure starch.

Ninety percent of the vitamin A, 77 percent of vitamin B_1, 80 percent of B_2, 81 percent of vitamin B_3, 72 percent of B_6, 77 percent of B_{12}, 90 percent of vitamin D, 86 percent of vitamin E, 76 percent of iron, 77 percent of potassium, and from 30 to 90 percent of other vitamins and minerals that the body needs (and that the flour needs in order to be metabolized)—all are stripped from natural wheat grain in processing. White flour is an unhealthy choice.

Fight White. One product you probably choose in your daily diet is bread or other bread products such as rolls, muffins, and biscuits. If you choose to eat bread products, eat products made of whole wheat or rye or other whole grains such as corn, rice, or oats. When you eat breakfast in a restaurant, order whole wheat toast—almost every restaurant has it, but they would usually rather give you white bread. There is now a whole array of English muffins that are much more interesting and nutritious than the plain old white ones. And if you haven't tried whole wheat or bran biscuits, it's probably the only reason you're not hooked on them. If you like to bake, try some whole grain recipes. Your enjoyment of baked goods will be greatly enhanced, and you will be doing your entire family a favor.

White rice, just like white flour, has been stripped of its nutritive value but "enriched" by the processors. To get food value from rice, switch to brown or wild rice. Wild rice has twice the amount of protein, four times as much phosphorus, eight times the thiamine, and twenty times as much riboflavin as white rice.

Alternative Choices. If you avoid refined sugar and processed flour, you will need to replace these items in your diet. In almost all instances you can substitute whole grain flour for "enriched" white flour. You can buy whole grain spaghetti and macaroni made from spinach or whole wheat. You can add wheat germ, bran, corn meal, sesame seeds, powdered milk, or other nutritive ingredients to recipes that you feel must have white flour. One standard way of adding nutrients to your white flour products is to add a tablespoon of soy flour, a tablespoon of powdered skim milk, and a teaspoon of wheat germ per cup of flour. Or add a tablespoon of sesame seeds, a tablespoon of cornmeal, a tablespoon of powdered milk, and a tablespoon of bran to each cup of flour. Both of these combinations replace some of the nutrients processing has removed, and they also help provide bulk.

If you want cookies in your diet, make the ones with oatmeal, granola, or some other health-producing ingredient rather than white flour. Substitute natural sweeteners for sugar, and try carob instead of chocolate.

FIBER

It is suspected that the increased incidence of cancer of the bowel, colitis, gastroenteritis, impacted colon, and other disorders of the large and small intestines is related to the decreased amount of fiber in the daily American diet. Meat, cheese, processed flour, refined sugar, overcooked fruits and vegetables—none provides the body with necessary fiber. Fiber not only aids digestion and elimination, it also provides satiety value—a great asset for those who are watching their weight but always seem to be hungry.

Fiber can easily be gained by adding whole grains (in the form of pasta, breads, or other baked goods, breakfast cereals such as granola or others that contain bran), raw fruits, and raw vegetables. Every meal should (and can easily) provide fiber for your diet. For example (fiber items are italicized):

Breakfast	*Fresh orange* Egg *Whole wheat toast* or *bran cereal* with milk Tea or coffee
Snack	*Sesame wafers* with peanut butter Milk

Lunch	*Fresh green salad* with shrimp *Rye crackers* Cheese Ice tea
Snack	Milk and *granola cookie*
Dinner	*Stir fried vegetables* on *brown rice* *Tomato* on bed of *lettuce* *Fresh fruit* and cheese Tea or coffee
Snack	*Popcorn* with herbs Tomato juice

A diet that contains at least 25 grams per day of fiber can prevent or treat conditions that may be brought on by eating too many refined foods (Girdano, et al., 1985). Table 9.3 contains a list of foods that provide 2 grams of fiber per serving.

TABLE 9.3 Selected Foods that Provide 2 Grams of Fiber per Serving

Fruits	
apple (1 medium)	banana (1 medium)
cherries (10 large)	strawberries (½ cup)
orange (1 medium)	peach (1 medium)
pear (½ small)	plums (2 small)
Breads/cereals	
whole wheat, rye (1 slice)	grapenuts (3 tablespoons)
shredded wheat (½ biscuit)	wheat bran (1 teaspoon)
corn flakes (⅔ cup)	
Vegetables	
broccoli (½ stalk)	carrots (⅓ cup)
celery (1 cup)	green beans (½ cup)
lettuce (2 cups shredded)	potatoes (1 medium)
tomato (1 raw)	
Miscellaneous	
peanuts (10)	pickle (1 large)
peanut butter (2½ teaspoons)	
Meat, Eggs: virtually no fiber content	

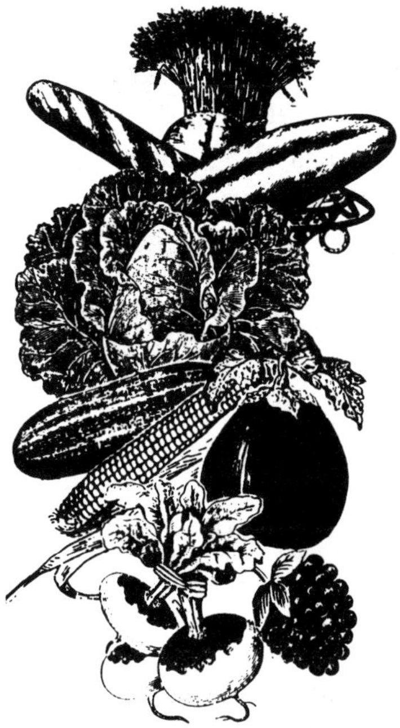

LOW CARBOHYDRATE DIETS

A number of popular diets seek to reduce carbohydrates to a bare minimum or omit them completely from the diet. Unless you are medically assured that you should eliminate carbohydrates of all kinds (not just sugar and processed flour), you should keep some in your daily menu. When carbohydrates are abruptly cut from the diet (for example, going from 100 to 200 grams or more per day to virtually none), it is a shock to your normal blood sugar level. You may experience dizziness (especially when you stand up suddenly), headaches, and irritability. This is due to the central nervous system's response to a lowered blood sugar level. The blood concentration of glucose molecules also helps determine how much fluid is in the bloodstream; so if glucose concentration is down, so is blood volume. This precipitates dizziness due to diminished blood supply to the brain.

Healthy individuals who wish not only to shed weight but also to develop healthy food choice habits that will last a lifetime will continue to use natural grains, fresh fruits and vegetables, seeds, and nuts to add interest, flavor, and nutrients to their diets.

PROCESSED FOODS

Nearly all of the boxed, processed foods you buy at the grocery store now contain one to four basic ingredients: wheat flour, corn, soybean, and/or sugar cane—all of which have been first refined then put through chemical treatment. Next, artificial ingredients are added, and the final product might turn out to be a frozen pizza! The crust, of course, is basically white flour, the tomatoes may be artificial (coal tar dyes, artificial flavoring, and sugar added for taste), the cheese may be artificial, and the meat may be artificially made from soybeans. If this pizza is made from processed foods, it lacks some essential amino acids and major minerals that were lost in processing. The nutritional content of this pizza might appear to be high (as is a pizza made with whole wheat flour, real tomatoes, vegetable oil, real cheese, and real meat), but most of the time the average consumer assumes the packaged food is real food. Next time, look at the ingredient label before you buy.

A person reduced to a diet of processed foods that contain basically only four ingredients is defying nature and a healthy, natural past. The diet should include a wide variety of natural grains, fruits, vegetables, milk products, and meats.

Bernard Jensen, nutritionist, in his address to the World Symposium on Humanity in April of 1979 suggested that everyone eat five different kinds of grains and reduce wheat intake because it is becoming apparent that some people do not process the gluten in wheat easily. According to Dr. Jensen this may be a reason for carbohydrate intolerance in some individuals. The grains he suggested that should be added to everyone's diet are rice (brown), rye, oats, soy, and corn (Jensen, 1979).

CARBOHYDRATES SUMMARY

The carbohydrates you choose to eat should provide bulk, variety, nutrients, and be easy on the blood sugar level. Therefore, follow these guidelines:

1. Eliminate refined sugar from your diet.
2. Also eliminate processed flour in favor of whole grain cereals.
3. Eat most of your fruits and vegetables raw or quick-cooked.
4. Choose a wide variety of natural grains, fruits, vegetables, nuts, and seeds to fulfill your carbohydrate needs.
5. Never eliminate carbohydrates completely from your diet unless so prescribed by a knowledgeable physician or nutrition expert.

Vitamins and Minerals

CALCIUM

If you do not drink milk or use other milk products, your Diet Record probably showed that you fell short of your RDA for calcium. You should be getting 800 milligrams of calcium *per day* to supply your continuing need for healthy maintenance of bones, teeth, blood, and nerve conduction. If you are pregnant, the necessity for calcium intake is even greater (1,200 milligrams) because a pregnant mother must supply calcium for the growing fetus and for herself. If that calcium is not supplied by the diet, it is taken from the body's (mother's) calcium stores (bones, teeth), leaving the body unhealthily depleted of calcium.

Because of the prevalence of osteoporosis (a condition where the bones become porous and empty-looking, making them susceptible to injury), many nutrition specialists are recommending 1,000 to 1,200 mg per day, and 1,500 mg per day for postmenopausal women.

There is a common misconception that once you reach adulthood you don't need calcium any more because your teeth and bones are formed. Much to the contrary, though, with age the requirement for calcium may actually increase because the rate of absorption diminishes. Normally, only about 20 to 30 percent of ingested calcium is absorbed—the rest is eliminated from the body. In order to be absorbed and utilized by the body, calcium: (1) must be in water soluble form, (2) needs acid in some form in the body, (3) depends on the presence of vitamins A, C, and D, (4) must be matched at least one for one with phosphorus, and (5) must be accompanied by magnesium. Calcium is poorly absorbed if these conditions are not met. Also if calcium foods are ingested at the same time as (or in) foods that contain oxalic acid (such as spinach, rhubarb, and chocolate) or phytic acid (cereals and grains), the calcium is bound by the acid and passed out of the body. Calcium can also combine with excessive amounts of fat and thereby become nonabsorbable and lost from the body, too. It makes you wonder how Popeye got his super energy from a can of spinach!

You wouldn't suspect that bones are constantly in flux, but the bone structure you have today is not the same you had yesterday nor what you will have tomorrow. Calcium and phosphorus are continually being broken down and eaten away, and more calcium and phosphorus (in the presence of vitamin D) are made into bone. It's like having a constant, fresh supply of bone. Tooth enamel has a longer turnover time because it is more dense than bone, but calcium there is also constantly being spent and replaced. In some disease states where calcium is not in sufficient supply, the breakdown of bone is greater than its deposition and the bones become porous and fragile. Osteoporosis is an example of this. Rickets is also an example of inadequate calcium supply or inadequate utilization of calcium due to vitamin D deficiency.

Since calcium is necessary for nerve conduction and muscle contraction, two of the earliest signs of calcium deficiency are muscle cramps and numbness of the extremities. Moderate calcium deficiency may also be indicated by symptoms such as joint pains, tooth decay, excessive nervous irritability, or impaired growth. If calcium deficiency becomes extreme, it may result in retarded blood clotting time (or even hemorrhage) and brittle bones.

Calcium Food Choices. Milk and milk products rank at the top of the list of high-calcium content foods. In fact, one pint of milk supplies three-quarters of the adult RDA, while two servings of meat, four servings of fruit and vegetables, and four servings of bread together supply only about one-quarter the adult RDA of calcium!

As you probably noticed in recording your food intake, one cup of whole milk (3.5 percent fat content) contains 233 milligrams of calcium. So, three eight-ounce glasses of milk per day will easily meet the RDA. You might have also noticed that skim milk (0 percent fat content) has a higher calcium content than whole milk (296 milligrams), and one cup of partly skimmed milk (2 percent fat content) with nonfat milk solids added provides 352 milligrams of calcium. The latter kind of milk is your best bet for calcium and caloric intake.

The calcium equivalent of a cup of milk can be one and one-half ounces of cheese, one and one-half cups of cottage cheese, or one cup of yogurt. But if you don't eat dairy products, some nondairy foods high in calcium are:

3 oz. sardines with bones	372 mg.
1 cup cooked broccoli	354 mg.
¼ cup whole sesame seeds	348 mg.
½ cup red salmon with bones	259 mg.
½ cup cooked mustard, turnip greens, collards, or kale	140 mg.
1 artichoke	102 mg.

The last resort for those who for some reason cannot get their calcium RDA through their food intake would be to use a calcium supplement such as bone meal. For those who can't use bone meal, calcium gluconate or calcium lactate (easily absorbed natural derivatives of calcium) might be taken.

PHOSPHORUS

Next to calcium, phosphorus is the mineral found in greatest abundance in the body. Healthy bones maintain a ratio of 2.5 parts of calcium to one part phosphorus. This mineral is necessary in every cell of the body. It helps the body utilize carbohydrates, fats, and proteins for growth and development. It is necessary for muscle contraction (including the heart muscle). It helps in the digestion of niacin and riboflavin, and is necessary for proper skeletal and tooth growth, kidney function, and nerve impulse transmission.

This mineral is easily absorbed in the presence of vitamin D and calcium. Absorption can be thrown off by large amounts of iron, aluminum, and magnesium in the diet. White sugar disturbs the calcium-phosphorus balance, and a high fat diet also disturbs this balance by increasing the absorption of phosphorus in the intestines while decreasing calcium absorption.

Foods rich in phosphorus include fish, poultry, whole grains, nuts, and seeds. The adult RDA for phosphorus is 800 mg.

IRON

It has been my experience that about 95 percent of my students in weight control do not meet their RDA for iron daily. Women, because of the loss of blood and therefore iron loss during their menstrual period, need more iron than men do. The adult RDA for women is 18 milligrams, while it is only 10 milligrams for men.

Uses of Iron. There are many uses of iron in the body, but its most important use is probably its role as oxygen carrier in the blood. Each hemoglobin molecule in the blood has four atoms of iron in its structure, and oxygen has an affinity for this iron. As the blood circulates the iron releases the oxygen to the tissues of the body. Besides this macroscopic use of iron for respiration, it is also needed at the cellular level for final use of oxygen to produce energy.

Anemia occurs when there is a lack of iron to fulfill the oxygen-carrying need. Symptoms of iron deficiency anemia may include lifelessness (lack of energy), difficulty in breathing, constipation, or brittle nails.

Iron Absorption. Iron, just as calcium, is absorbed in the small intestine, and only a very small percent is actually used (2 to 4 percent). Vitamins C and E aid in the absorption and utilization of iron, and the iron found in animal protein is generally absorbed better than that found in vegetables. Again, as with calcium, oxalic acid and phytic acids should not be ingested at the same time as iron because they deter iron's absorption. Increased motility of the intestines also cuts down on the absorption of iron, just as lack of hydrochloric acid or high intake of cellulose, coffee, or tea will inhibit this process. All of this information should be kept in mind when making food combination choices and/or taking an iron supplement.

Iron in Foods. Again, Popeye has tricked us into thinking his energy came from spinach, one of the foods that contains oxalic acid, which makes absorption of the iron within spinach most difficult.

Probably the one best source of iron is liver (lamb liver has twice the iron content of beef or chicken liver—about 13 milligrams compared to 6 milligrams). Six to ten raw oysters provide about 6 milligrams of iron, and meats such as three slices of rib roast (lean or medium fat) or one pork chop have about 2½ milligrams of iron as does one-half cup of soybeans. Other than these foods, there are few foods that have more than 1 or 2 milligrams of iron per serving, although there is a little iron in many foods from each food group. Milk and unenriched white bread, however, contribute little iron to the diet. The following list includes the iron content of some foods:

2 slices lamb liver	13.4 mg.
2 slices beef liver	6.6 mg.
1 pork chop	2.5 mg.
1 large hamburger	3.0 mg.
3 slices rib roast	2.6 mg.
½ cup baked beans, pork, molasses	3.0 mg.
½ cup soybeans	2.5 mg.
½ cup lima beans	2.0 mg.
½ cup raw oyster meat	6.5 mg.

Also, some packaged breakfast foods are fortified with iron and may contain the RDA.

POTASSIUM AND SODIUM

Potassium and sodium are discussed together here because it is the relationship between these two minerals that occurs in all cells of the body to regulate water balance, nerve conduction, muscle contraction, and the acid-alkaline balance (pH) of the body. A good deal of attention has recently been given to the possible hazards of high salt intake. It appears that in susceptible individuals, water retention due to high salt intake may put a greater load on the cardiovascular system. Potassium-sodium imbalances may also result in irregular heartbeat, nervous disorders, constipation, and muscle damage.

Foods high in potassium include all vegetables, especially green, leafy ones, whole grains, oranges, and bananas. Sodium is found in virtually all foods, especially sea or table salt, but is also more concentrated in seafoods, carrots, poultry, beets, and meat.

There is evidence that sea salt is a better choice than regular table salt because it contains other trace minerals that are necessary in the body (Kushi, 1983).

VITAMIN A

Although the RDA for iron may be somewhat difficult to fulfill, the recommended allowance for vitamin A is quite easy to satisfy. When vitamin A appears in a food, it seems to appear *en masse*. With the RDA set at 5,000 I.U.'s, you can meet your goal daily by including a variety of vegetables and fruits or adding liver to your diet.

Uses of Vitamin A. This vitamin helps form visual purple, a substance in the eyes that help recover vision at night after light has struck the retina. Vitamin A is also constantly required for growth and repair of all body tissues, especially mucous membranes of the respiratory and digestive systems and those that line the bladder and kidneys. The skin must also have vitamin A to keep it clear, smooth, and disease resistant. The digestion of protein is also aided by vitamin A.

Vitamin A deficiency, then, is indicated by symptoms such as night blindness, rough and dry skin, fatigue, eye problems such as sties or the more serious conditions of xerosis or corneal ulcers, softening of bones and teeth, or loss of appetite.

Vitamin A versus Carotene. When you see the units of vitamin A listed for a carrot, what is really meant is the *vitamin A activity*. Carrots and other vegetables do not form vitamin A themselves, but rather contain the precursor of vitamin A, *carotene* (also called provitamin A). Carotene is changed into vitamin A in the body; so we do get preformed vitamin A from animal products such as liver, fish liver oils, cream, and butter. Not all carotene is changed into vitamin A in the body, however. About one-quarter of the carotene in root vegetables such as carrots becomes vitamin A, while up to one-half the carotene in leafy vegetables undergoes conversion. One reason for this is that the "packaging" of the carotene differs from vegetable to vegetable. It may also depend partly on how the vegetable is prepared or eaten (for example, cooked or raw). Some carotene is also stored as such in the fat tissues of the body, but unabsorbed carotene is eliminated from the body.

Vitamin A Toxicity. Too much preformed vitamin A can be toxic to the system, but the body won't overdose on *carotene* to the point of toxicity. Very high carotene intake, however, may result in *carotenemia*, where the skin and the whites of the eyes take on a yellowish tinge.

Vitamin A toxicity is indicated by hair loss; dry, itchy, flaky skin; nausea; vomiting; loss of appetite; headache; or other such symptoms. Prolonged, excessive intake could cause skeletal difficulties such as fragile bones and deep bone pain, skin rashes, and abnormalities of the mucous membranes in general. Toxicity can occur by taking 100,000 I.U.'s of preformed vitamin A daily for many consecutive months.

Food Choices for Vitamin A. The food with the highest concentration of vitamin A is liver. If you're not a liver eater, however, there are many fruits and vegetables that will easily supply daily requirements of vitamin A activity.

Carrots, especially mature ones that have been cooked (rather than young raw ones), have high vitamin A activity—about 10,000 I.U.'s per two-thirds cup of cooked, diced carrots. One medium baked sweet potato is worth about 9,000 I.U.'s of vitamin A activity. One-half cup of cooked green leafy vegetables supplies about 8,000 I.U.'s. One-half of a canteloupe supplies about 7,000 I.U.'s. From these examples it should be apparent that yellow, orange (and red) vegetables and fruits are good suppliers of vitamin A, but green vegetables are good sources, too. You might suspect any food of deep orange color will provide vitamin A activity: egg yolk, butter, cheese, apricots, and so on.

Low Calorie Foods and Vitamin A. An attractive aspect of vitamin A foods is that most of these fruits and vegetables are *very* low in calories. One cup of tomato juice, for instance, is only 46 calories, has about 2,000 I.U.'s of vitamin A activity, and also provides about 40 milligrams of vitamin C—not a bad breakfast or snack suggestion. One cup of cooked leafy green vegetables may be as little as 30 calories, but will provide your RDA of vitamin A and contribute other vitamins and minerals, also. These are not expensive foods, either.

A Suggestion. Look back at your Diet Record and find the foods you like to eat that have high vitamin A content. Then make sure you continue to put them in your diet regularly. Also take some time to look through Appendix B of nutritive values of foods, paying attention to the vitamin A column. Find some new foods to try and check your recipe books to find some appealing ways to fix them.

THE B VITAMINS

Before discussing the three separate B vitamins, we should note that the B complex vitamins (B_1, B_2, B_3, B_6, B_{12}, B_{13}, B_{15}, biotin, choline, folic acid, inositol, and PABA) usually appear in a functional relationship together. All the B vitamins naturally occur in brewer's yeast, whole grain cereals, and liver. Since these vitamins appear as a complex in nature, it is apparent that they should be introduced into the body as a complex rather than as isolated vitamins, unless prescribed otherwise. I have also often found that when someone is deficient in one of the B vitamins (such as thiamine), they are also deficient in the others (riboflavin and niacin). The editor of *Prevention* magazine refuses to allow pharmaceutical houses or other manufacturers of vitamins to advertise single B vitamins in his magazine because he is so dedicated to the idea that the B vitamins should be taken as a complex.

THIAMINE (VITAMIN B_1)

Dr. Cheraskin (Cheraskin and Ringsdorf, 1974) calls thiamine the "laughing vitamin" because when patients appear with a thiamine deficiency they are moping, depressed, serious, and rarely laugh. Thiamine has also been called the "morale" vitamin because of its apparent effect on attitude, perhaps due to its contribution to a healthy central nervous system.

All adults need 1 milligram or more of thiamine every day. This is a water soluble vitamin (as are all the B vitamins and vitamin C), so any thiamine that the body does not need is excreted in the urine. It is not stored in the body like the fat soluble vitamins, so intake must be constant. Thiamine toxicity does not occur, as excess amounts are not kept in the body.

What Does Thiamine Do? One of thiamine's main jobs in the body is to help change pyruvic acid into acetyl coenzyme A. This chemical change is necessary for the final breakdown of carbohydrates. The need for thiamine is related to how much carbohydrates you eat (and also how much alcohol you drink). The National Research Council recommends an intake of .5 milligram of thiamine for every 1,000 calories eaten daily.

Sugar and alcohol are considered "robbers" of thiamine because they must have thiamine for their metabolism, but they contribute nothing to the body except calories. Smoking also depletes the thiamine level in the body.

Thiamine Deficiency. A vitamin B_1 deficiency makes it impossible for the body to break carbohydrates down completely, so the pyruvic acid level rises, and symptoms develop from this acidity: oxygen loss and thus labored breathing, fatigue, mental fuzziness, irritability, and perhaps emotional instability. Besides the central nervous system effects, cardiovascular health is impaired, and gastrointestinal symptoms such as anorexia and indigestion may also occur. The combined syndrome of gastrointestinal, cardiovascular, and central nervous system effects of thiamine deficiency is called "beri-beri."

Thiamine Food Choices. Probably the richest source of thiamine is brewer's yeast (1.6 milligrams in one tablespoon). Another noted source is pork (.63 milligram in three and one-half ounces of pork chop; .75 mg. in three ounces of pork roast). Nuts and whole grains make a good contribution, too.

Again, you should look at the foods you eat to see which ones supply the most thiamine for you and keep them in your regular diet. Also, peruse the thiamine content of all kinds of foods in Appendix B to see which ones you could add to your diet—especially if you show a thiamine deficiency.

RIBOFLAVIN (VITAMIN B_2)

This B vitamin is necessary in the diet every day in the amount of 1.5 to 1.8 milligrams depending upon age and sex. In pregnancy the daily requirement is 1.8 milligrams and if lactating, the requirement is 2 milligrams. If you are not meeting your RDA for riboflavin you will want to do some research into what foods contain this vitamin and then put the appropriate ones in your diet.

How the Body Uses Riboflavin. This water soluble vitamin is a "must" in the body in order to break down the foodstuffs in final energy. It contributes to a hydrogen carrier in the body called flavoadenine dinucleotide (FAD). Without FAD the body could not completely break down fats, carbohydrates, or protein. So when the diet is deficient of riboflavin, all cells suffer from not being able to produce energy and thus cannot maintain their structure and functions. In this way riboflavin is necessary for healthy skin, eyes, nails, and hair.

Riboflavin Deficiency. When there is a vitamin B_2 deficiency, the first symptom to appear is cracking at the corners of the mouth. In my early teaching days I taught junior high school children from low income families, and it was not uncommon to see the symptoms of vitamin deficiency. Cracking at the corners of the mouth was quite obvious and prevalent. It was also not uncommon to see these children walking to school eating a breakfast of cola, candy bar, and/or doughnut!

Some of the other symptoms of riboflavin deficiency are swollen red tongue; burning of the eyes and other eye disorders such as light sensitivity; scaling of the skin around the nose, ears, and mouth; lesions on the lips; lack of energy; vaginal itching; hair loss; and retarded growth. Pellagra is caused by riboflavin deficiency, also.

Riboflavin Toxicity. Because there is no storage of vitamin B_2 in the body, toxicity does not occur. But again it is important to take a B complex vitamin if one particular B vitamin supplement is taken. If, for instance, one takes a riboflavin supplement in large dosage, there may be high urinary loss of all the B vitamins in the body. Therefore, a high supplemental dose of vitamin B_2 could cause a loss of all the other B vitamins.

Riboflavin Food Choices. A caution to remember about riboflavin is that it is highly susceptible to ultraviolet light, so foods containing riboflavin should not be exposed to the sunlight. If you have milk delivered in bottles to your door, make certain that the milk delivery person puts them inside a box or some other container that will keep out sunlight.

Brewer's yeast is probably the best source of riboflavin, but this vitamin is found in many foods. However, vitamin B_2 is totally lacking in sugar and fats (foods that must use this vitamin in their breakdown).

Beef liver is again a winning choice (2.37 milligrams of riboflavin per two ounces of fried liver), and so are milk products (40 to 50 milligrams per cup of milk depending on the kind of milk you drink). Milk supplies about half the riboflavin consumed in the United States. If you aren't a milk drinker, then, you should eat enough liver and other organ meats, leafy vegetables, whole grains, nuts, or dry beans to supply your required riboflavin.

NIACIN (VITAMIN B_3)

Niacin is one of the vitamins that the body can produce itself if the amino acid tryptophan is supplied by the diet. Sixty milligrams of tryptophan yield 1 milligram of niacin. The daily requirement of niacin is between 13 and 18 milligrams depending on age and sex. Pregnant and lactating women need 15 to 20 milligrams respectively. During illness, during growth periods, and after physical exercise, dosage should be increased. This is true of all the vitamins.

Uses of Niacin. The role of niacin is much like that of riboflavin; it contributes to the formation of nicotinamide adenine dinucleotide (NAD), a close relative of FAD made from riboflavin. NAD is also a hydrogen carrier that accepts hydrogen as it is broken off fatty acids, amino acids, or glucose in the metabolism of the three foodstuffs. Without niacin, NAD cannot be made and therefore the cells cannot produce energy to carry out proper functions or maintain and repair structure.

Niacin is a vasodilator and has been used medically for persons with poor circulation. It is also vital for nervous system function, maintenance of skin and digestive system tissues, and sex hormone synthesis.

Niacin Toxicity. As with the other water soluble vitamins there is no toxicity because unused niacin is eliminated from the body. Large doses (for example, 100 milligrams or more) cause flushing, tingling sensations, and perhaps itching due to the vasodilation this vitamin causes.

Niacin Deficiency. There are many symptoms of niacin deficiency, from lack of energy to a full-blown case of pellagra (dermatitis, dementia, and diarrhea). Mild deficiency might be indicated by symptoms such as canker sores, insomnia, nausea, tender gums, depression, or bad breath. Prolonged deficiency may cause pellagra.

Niacin Food Choices. Niacin is not as naturally abundant in many foods as are thiamine and riboflavin. Meats are the best sources of niacin, but seeds and nuts also contribute to niacin intake or manufacturing. Chicken, liver, and fish have high niacin value (three ounces of chicken have 11 milligrams of niacin; two ounces of liver have 9 milligrams of niacin; and three ounces of tuna have 10 milligrams of niacin). Vegetables have very little niacin activity, so vegetarians must look mainly to nuts and seeds for their niacin (one-half cup of peanuts has about 15 milligrams of niacin). Brewer's yeast is again a good contributor: about 4 milligrams of niacin per tablespoon of yeast.

VITAMIN C (ASCORBIC ACID)

Vitamin C has received much publicity since the megadose research of Linus Pauling (1971) and the self-cure of Norman Cousins (1977). Many nutritionists suspect that there is more to vitamin C than is known at this time. The RDA is listed as 60 milligrams for adults, but Pauling has suggested that the optimum daily intake should be much higher than this.

Uses of Vitamin C. Because vitamin C is vital to so many tissues of the body, it does far more than merely prevent scurvy by maintaining healthy collagen tissue. Vitamin C plays a role in healing wounds and fighting infection, aids in the metabolism of some amino acids, and protects many of the other vitamins and tissues in the body because it is an anti-oxidant.

Under stressful conditions, the body uses up vitamin C more quickly, just as it does in illness, when the lungs are polluted with cigarette smoke or other pollution (exhaust fumes, insecticides, gas fumes); in fever, in fatigue, during blood loss, when taking aspirin, barbiturates, antibiotics, or cortisone.

Vitamin C Deficiency. If adequate vitamin C is not taken, symptoms such as nosebleeds, bleeding gums, slow healing of wounds, bruising, poor digestion, lowered resistance, and swollen joints may occur. Serious prolonged vitamin C deficiency results in scurvy.

The half-life of vitamin C is 16 days, so it does take the body some time to become depleted. Depletion is hastened by baking soda, sulfa drugs, smoking nicotine, sweating, and drinking large amounts of water, coffee, or tea.

Vitamin C Food Choices. Most fruits and vegetables contain some vitamin C. The citrus fruits (especially oranges and grapefruits) are popular sources of vitamin C, as are tomatoes, green leafy vegetables, and melons. One glass of orange or grapefruit juice will supply more than the RDA for adults.

OTHER VITAMINS AND MINERALS

There are many vitamins and minerals that are not listed on your Diet Record. Omission of them is certainly not because they aren't important to your health. Part of the rationale for choosing those presented here is that RDA's have been established so you can compare your diet with the National Research Council's standards. If all the vitamins and minerals were on your Diet Record, you would still be recording them even now!

Some vitamins, such as vitamins D and K, are not topics here because they generally are supplied by the diet and/or are synthesized by the body, and so you don't need to concentrate on them. The other B complex vitamins (those not mentioned here) usually accompany thiamine, riboflavin, and/or niacin in your foods.

Therefore your daily Diet Record shows the items that may be most susceptible to deficiency. For a discussion of the other vitamins and minerals, a number of nutrition books are recommended sources in the Suggested Readings section at the end of the chapter.

How Did You Fare?

No matter how you fared on your Diet Record, you should put together some of these good food choices for yourself so that you can eat healthily for the rest of your life.

Nobody else's diet plan can work for you because you *must* eat what you like to prepare and what you can fit into your lifetime menu. Somebody else's "diet" may be interesting and helpful for a while, but you'll always come back to being "you" and making your own food choices and combinations.

If your food choices haven't been very good for you, *now* is the time to start changing them. If you want to eat a high-sugar content diet, at least now you know the consequences. Hopefully, however, you will reduce your sugar intake and your intake of processed flour.

As a summary and for ease in making food choices, here are some main foods in which you'll find the principal vitamins and minerals:

Calcium – milk products
Iron – liver, shellfish, greens
Vitamin A – yellow fruits and vegetables
Vitamin C – fruits and vegetables
Thiamine – pork, nuts, whole grains, dried beans

Riboflavin — milk, whole grains
Niacin — meats

Looking at these, you may notice that in order to get the vitamins and minerals that you need, you must eat what are called the *basic four*: milk products, meat and fish, fruits and vegetables, and whole grain cereals.

Adults should have each day two servings from the milk group; two servings of meat, fish, poultry, dry beans, peas, nuts or seeds; four servings of fruits and vegetables (preferably 60 percent to be eaten raw); and four servings of whole grain cereals.

In the interest of weight control, you'll want to find foods that you enjoy that give you the most food value for the least amount of calories. For instance, fish or chicken will supply niacin as well as (or better than) other meats, and they will give you fewer calories. Two percent milk has more calcium than whole milk and is less caloric. You have the tools to build yourself a good menu, so try it.

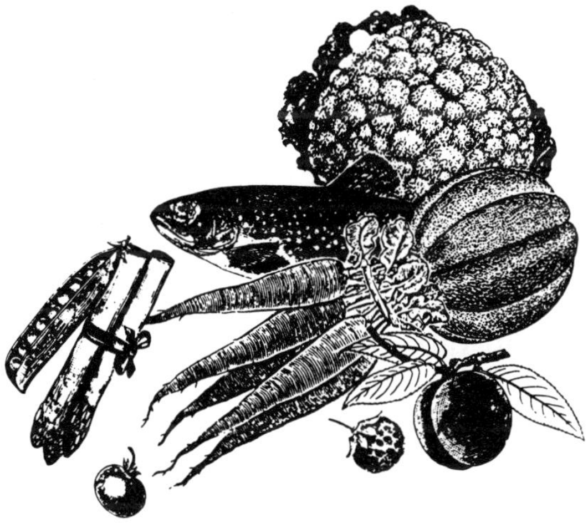

Don't Go On A Diet!

One thing that you should not do to reduce your weight now is put yourself on a "diet." What you need to do is adopt a fitness eating style that you will continue for the rest of your healthy life.

I've mentioned before that you shouldn't starve yourself by eliminating too many calories or by eating most of your calories at any one time and then starving yourself the rest of the day. Your body will react by slowing its metabolism and by becoming more efficient at

TABLE 9.4 Foods You Could Enjoy

Milk and Milk Products	*Meat, Fish, Poultry, etc.*
Fruits and Vegetables	*Whole Grain Products*

storing what you *do* eat. So eat your calories spread through six small meals a day. If you find it impossible to plan for three between-meal snacks a day, you can incorporate your snack foods into the preceding meals.

In Table 9.4, write down the good foods you could enjoy for a lifetime in each of the four food groups. Then set up a week's menu for yourself in Table 9.5, paying special attention to the servings you should have from each group. Then spread your foods throughout your day: breakfast, midmorning snack, lunch, midafternoon snack, dinner, bedtime snack. Compare this menu with the one you made in Chapter 5.

Summary

In my many years of shopping in supermarkets I have become aware that there are two general categories of shoppers: (1) those who load their carts with mainly fruits, vegetables, and whole grain products, and (2) those who have large supplies of cookies, bags of potato chips and dips, cake mixes, and sugar-coated breakfast foods. With great

TABLE 9.5 Your Week's Menu

	Monday	*Tuesday*	*Wednesday*	*Thursday*	*Friday*
Breakfast					
Snack					
Lunch					
Snack					
Dinner					
Snack					

objectivity I can say that I generally find those who are obviously overweight to be the latter kind of shopper. Those who are really serious about healthy lifestyles reflect it in their food choices, and conversely, the shoppers who have obvious weight control problems reflect part of their problem in their shopping cart contents.

Incorporating nutrition into a total healthy lifestyle takes a little knowledge, desire, and discipline. Make your food work for you. You have only one body and the better you feed it, the more you can enjoy its good health. When you start feeding it better, you're going to like yourself better. And the more you like yourself, the less chance anyone has to stop you from being who you want to be.

So if you're not feeding yourself right, get to it. And exercise!

References

Cheraskin, E., and W. M. Ringsdorf, with Arline Brecher. *Psychodietetics*. New York: Bantam Books, 1974.

Cousins, Norman. *Anatomy of an Illness*. New York: Norton, 1981.

Farquhar, J. *The American Way of Life Need Not Be Hazardous to Your Health*. Palo Alto: Stanford Alumni Association, 1987.

Fish Facts. Salt Lake City, Utah: Gastronomy, Inc., 1987.

Girdano, Daniel, George Everly, Jr., and Dorothy Dusek. *Experiencing Health*. Englewood Cliffs, NJ: Prentice-Hall, 1985.

Glomset, J. "Fish, Fatty Acids, and Human Health," *New England Journal of Medicine* 3 (1985): 1253.

Haskel, W. "Exercise-Induced Changes in Plasma Lipids and Lipoproteins," *Preventive Medicine* 13 (1984): 23–36.

Jensen, Bernard. "Health and Nutrition." Speech at World Symposium on Humanity, Pasadena, CA April 7–14, 1979.

Kushi, M. *The Cancer Prevention Diet*. New York: St. Martin's Press, 1983.

Lappe, Frances Moore. *Diet for a Small Planet*. New York, Ballantine, 1982.

MineraLab, Inc. *Hair Analysis Plus Nutritional Evaluation Equals a Formula for Better Health*. MineraLab, Inc., 1978, 409 Massachusetts Avenue, Acton, MA 01720.

Pauling, Linus. *Vitamin C and the Common Cold*. New York: Bantam Books, 1971.

Sassoon, Humphrey. "Time Factors in Obesity." *American Journal of Clinical Nutrition* 26 (1973): 776–783.

Thie, John, and Leroy Perry. "Vitamin C (Ascorbic Acid) Testing Methods," *Digest of Chiropractic Economics* (March–April, 1978).

Wycoff, S. "Diet Fads Waste Money, Not Pounds." *Consumers' Research* 69 (1986): 20–23.

Suggested Readings

Asterita, M. *Physical Exercise, Nutrition and Stress*. New York: Praeger, 1985.

Bland, J. *Nutraerobics*. San Francisco: Harper & Row, 1985.

Becker, G. *Heart Smart*. New York: Simon and Schuster, 1984.

Brody, Jane. *Jane Brody's Nutrition Book*. New York: Bantam Books, 1981.

Cancer Facts and Figures. 1986. New York: American Cancer Society.

Diabetes Facts and Figures. 1986. Alexandria, VA: American Diabetes Association.

Ettinger, V. *Recipes for Better Bones*. New York: Perigee, 1988.

Hatfield, F. *Ultimate Sports Nutrition*. Chicago: Contemporary Books, 1987.

Health and Human Services. *Diet, Nutrition and Cancer Prevention*. NIH publication #85-2711. Washington, D.C. Government Printing Office, 1984.

Heart Facts. 1986. Dallas: American Heart Association.

Kirschmann, J. *Nutrition Almanac, 2nd edition*. New York: McGraw-Hill 1984.

Netzer, C. *The Complete Book of Food Counts*. New York: Dell, 1988.

Osteoarthritis. 1986. Atlanta: Arthritis Foundation.

Phillipson, B., et al. "Reduction of Plasma Lipids, Lipoproteins, and Apoproteins by Dietary Fish Oils," *New England Journal of Medicine* 312 (1985): 1210–1216.

U.S.D.A. *Handbook of the Nutritive Value of Foods*. New York: Dover, 1986.

10 EXERCISE: HOW FIT ARE YOU?

A MEDICINE MAN came through the town and was promoting a product that if taken properly was proven and guaranteed to make you stronger, aid in appetite and digestion, help you sleep better, alleviate the harmful effects of emotional stress, straighten your bones and posture, increase your oxygen intake and use, aid in medical recuperation, help prevent bodily injury, make you appear younger and more lithe, provide a great emotional outlet, and help you slim down your body.

Was this person arrested? What kind of product could be guaranteed to do all that? Well, the medicine man was a fitness expert, and the product was exercise. Yes, *exercise*.

If you don't do *anything else* outlined in this book to help you slim down, please do yourself a favor by reading and following the prescription for exercise given in the next three chapters (Chapters 11 through 13). This one addition or change to your lifestyle will be more beneficial to you than any one of the other areas, partly because it transcends some of the emotional aspects and is a natural way to alleviate emotional stress and tension. It also makes you feel good. You'll want to do other good things for yourself, such as put the right kind of fuel in your body and reduce your smoking. And exercise is an automatic fat remover.

Maybe you already have an exercise plan that you follow. Generally, I find that overweight people do not have a loving relationship with exercise. I've had some interesting postprogram feedback about exercise habits from a large variety of students. One wrote, "I never learned to appreciate my body and how it moves. I never felt like I had control of it before." Another wrote, "I never exercised because I was so big, it was embarrassing to move in front of other people. I felt like a baby elephant jogging down the road — everybody turned and stared." Still others responded: "I just never learned any sports skills—even how to run or throw or catch." "As a little girl I was discouraged from doing any kind of physical activities—only boys or 'tomboys' did stuff like that!" "I never wanted to exercise because I was afraid my arm and leg muscles would bulge and I'd look like the Incredible Hulk." "I always figured that exercise was bad for me because when I did exercise, I'd get sore muscles or I'd read about how someone just died of a heart attack while they were jogging."

You might recognize yourself in some of those statements. If you don't exercise regularly, you have a good reason tucked away somewhere in your mind. Whatever that reason is, it is probably based on beliefs you used to have, misinformation, and reluctance to experience how good you can feel from exercising. You'll probably want to "reason with that reason" in order to let go and allow yourself to enjoy the benefits and pure pleasure of exercising.

The body is meant to move and it responds healthfully to movement. Exercise is an entropic process—a process whereby using the muscles makes them increase their strength. Many centuries ago the body lost its importance when ancient philosophy branched into a dualistic mentality; that is, the thinking, logical mind became the master while the body and the intuitive mind were tagalong, necessary evils. As this civilization emerges back into a holistic health age, the body and intuitive mind once again have become inseparable from the logical mind, and holistic health scientists are requiring physical activity in an integrated lifestyle. So now it has become all right to move; social approval is being given again. And for each person there is some kind of activity that the person can learn to love as well as enjoy its benefits—there's even an activity for you.

Your Exercise Profile

Before looking for the activities best suited to you (in case you haven't found them yet), take a look at your activity level by answering the following questions with "yes" or "no." Give yourself one point for a "yes" answer on the first eight questions and one point for a "no" answer on the last nine questions.

YES/NO

1. I perform regular cardiovascular activity (running, biking, rope skipping, and so forth). ______

2. Regular physical activity is ingrained in my lifestyle. ______
3. I know my resting heart rate. ______
4. I know my blood pressure. ______
5. I get my heart rate above 150 beats per minute for at least 15 minutes a day. ______
6. I am pretty good in at least one physical activity. ______
7. I like my body and do whatever I can to keep it strong. ______
8. I end most days *without* feeling tired or drained of energy. ______
9. I avoid walking as much as possible (by parking close to the place I'm going, by driving rather than walking to a meeting, the store, and so on). ______
10. I take an elevator whenever possible rather than find and use the stairs. ______
11. I would much rather watch an athletic contest than play in one. ______
12. I don't like to get all hot and sweaty with exercise. ______
13. I've never been an athlete and I probably never will be. ______
14. I'd rather spend my summer vacation sunbathing than hiking or doing something else physical. ______
15. I would like to be physically active, but I'm so clumsy, fat, lazy (one or more of these) that I will probably never participate in physical activity. ______
16. People who participate in most kinds of physical activity build up unsightly muscles. ______
17. When I increase my physical activity to lose weight, I just end up eating more and regaining weight. ______

TOTAL ______

If your total is less than 8, you need to know more about physical activity so you can learn to use and enjoy it. If your total is more than 15, you must be in fairly good shape and are already enjoying being active. Examine your answers to determine if you are merely lacking in knowledge about your body and the benefits of exercise, or if you have some emotional ties to a sedentary life.

Assess Your Fitness Level

There are a few quick tests that you can perform that will give you a rough idea of what kind of physical shape you're in. These exercises test your arm and shoulder muscle strength, your abdominal strength, your hamstring (the muscles at the back of your thigh) flexibility, and your cardiovascular endurance. Can you pass these tests?

1. Women: Can you do 10 sit-ups in one minute? (From a bent-knee position, hands behind your head, touch your nose to your knees as you sit up. It's okay to have someone hold your feet down.)

   Men: Can you do 15 sit-ups in one minute (same exercise as women)?
2. Women: Can you do 10 push-ups (straight body) from your knees without stopping?

   Men: Can you do 10 push-ups (straight body) from your toes without stopping?
3. Men and women: Can you touch your toes and hold that position for three seconds without bending your knees?
4. Women and men: Can you run/walk one mile in 12 minutes or less?

If you can't answer "yes" to each of these questions, you need a fitness program to get yourself into shape.

What Do Muscle Strength and Endurance, Flexibility, and Running Have To Do with Weight Control?

Running or other aerobic exercises discussed in Chapter 13 are what might be called "fat loss" exercises when they are done properly. They burn off many calories, so they are a "must" in a weight control program. To have a completely holistic approach to fitness, you need to move your total body for a long enough period of time. Running is just one example of that kind of movement. Chapter 13 gives you more choices, such as biking and cross-country skiing.

Muscle strength and endurance exercises and stretching activities won't burn as many calories as aerobic exercises will. But in gaining strength in your muscles, you gain control over your body and its movement. The stomach muscles and arm and shoulder muscles are two excellent examples of "feel good" muscles when they are strong. It feels good to be able to tighten your stomach muscles to hold in your tummy and keep your posture in alignment. Being overweight nearly always means a protruding belly that is pulling you off balance and may be causing you low back pain. Shortened hamstrings may be contributing to low back pain, too. To avoid pain and to stay in balance, stretch all muscles that you strengthen through use. You use your hamstrings every time you take a step!

When you feel in control of yourself physically, it helps you know that you can control other aspects of your life as well. Thaddeus Kostrabalas, a well-known San Diego psychiatrist/marathoner, uses physical activity as a successful form of psychotherapy.

How Much, How Soon?

Each of the following three chapters on exercise discusses the amount and intensity of exercise that any exerciser may perform. But generally you will want to run your program at least *three times a week* for *at least one half hour per day.* A good program would include at least three days of aerobic exercises and three days of strength and stretching exercises. These days might be staggered so that on Monday, Wednesday, and Friday you bike or run or do some other aerobic activity, and then on Tuesday, Thursday, and Saturday you stretch and build up your strength. On Sunday you give yourself a day off just to relax or play. Hopefully, you will consider all of your physical activity as play.

Start your program *slowly*. This is one of the most important things to remember. *Never exercise faster than you can talk!* It's a simple way to pace yourself.

Most people adhere to a program more faithfully if they set up an exercise plan and post it in their bedroom or on the refrigerator or in some other obvious spot. It helps to do exercises to music and to vary the kind of exercises you do so you really stay interested in them. Exercising with someone else may also keep up your interest.

Before You Start

As you are getting yourself ready for a good exercise program, check the list of things you should do before you start:

1. Take a pinch of fat on the back of your upper arm. Tighten up the muscle and pinch the fat behind it. How thick is it? Give it a number – ½ inch, 1 inch, and so on.

2. Measure the circumference of your waist, hips, chest, upper arm, thigh, and any other body part you're concerned about. Write it down. A chart for that purpose is given in Chapter 11 (Table 11.3).
3. Take your resting heart rate on several consecutive mornings, before you get out of bed. Average the rates and write the average down. A chart for that purpose is given in Chapter 13 (Table 13.1).
4. Ask your physician if there is any reason why you should not start an exercise program.
5. Read Chapters 11, 12, and 13 in this book.

Exercise Precautions for the Elderly and/or Out-of-Shape

Although it is difficult to draw a line between "young" and "old," it is important to note that the aging process reduces muscular strength, flexibility, and cardiovascular endurance. For those who stay in good physical shape through exercise, the precautions here may not apply until later in life. However, many who are overweight and out of shape should heed these precautions, even if they don't consider themselves "elderly."

1. Always spend a short time (5 to 10 minutes) warming up your muscles before engaging in strength or cardiovascular exercise.
2. Always spend a short time (5 to 10 minutes) cooling down after a workout.
3. In weight lifting use light weights with slow motions.

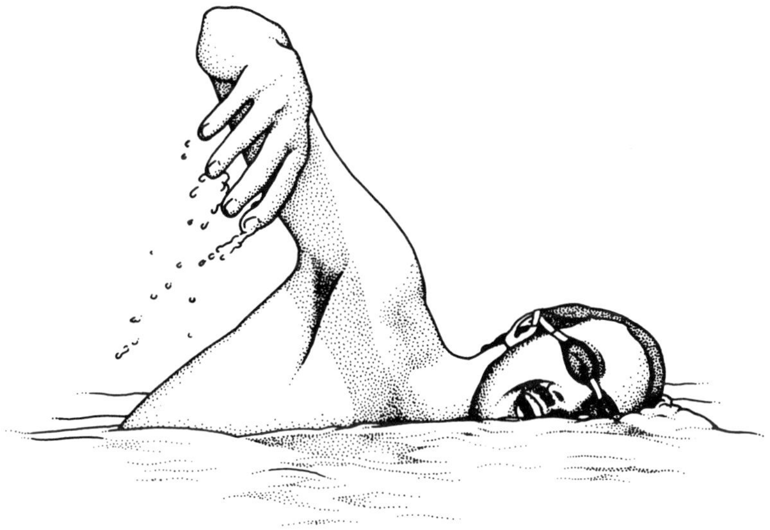

4. Breathe throughout the exercise. Do not hold your breath.
5. If you have arthritis, swim or bicycle rather than jog or run.
6. Do body twisting exercises slowly and in a seated position.
7. Use slow, smooth movements of the head up and down and to the right and left rather than doing head or neck rolls with 360° rotation.
8. Always do slow, steady stretching. Do not bounce or jerk.
9. Do not put your body weight against stiff or locked joints.
10. Avoid straight-leg sit-ups or leg lifts.
11. Perform knee bends with no more than half a contraction.
12. Take a warm shower after a workout.
13. Training heart rate may be as low as 110 to 120 beats per minute.
14. If in doubt about certain exercises or activities, ask a trained health professional.
15. Get a physical checkup and a medical approval to start a physical activity program.

11 MUSCULAR STRENGTH AND ENDURANCE PROGRAM

HAVING *muscular strength* means that you can overcome a resistance with your muscles, and *muscular endurance* means that you can exert that resistance over a period of time. Resistance may come in the form of carrying a bag of groceries, a bale of hay, or a piece of furniture; hitting a ball with a racket; or driving your car off the road safely when you have a flat tire or a blowout. The greater your strength and endurance, the easier you can handle emergencies, the less effort you will have to expend at work or play, and the more energy you will have at the end of the day.

Generally, people who keep their muscles toned and ready to go feel better about themselves. You notice their liveliness and self-assuredness. Doing exercises that increase the strength and endurance of muscles also helps to contour the muscles into graceful curves that most people find becoming on themselves and others.

Women have recently discovered that increasing muscular strength does not mean building "Popeye" muscles. So an ever-increasing number of women are working with weights, weight machines, and weight systems.

The exercises given in this chapter burn up available carbohydrates (blood sugar) in the body, but do not usually cause much fat loss because they don't evoke a high enough heart rate for a long enough period of time. However, these exercises are extremely important in your weight control program because: (1) They can result in loss of inches because toning the muscle takes out the "sag"; (2) they help improve your overall body contour; and (3) they help you feel more aware of your body and in better control of it. All these effects can be important in building self-assuredness.

This chapter presents strength and endurance exercises in two sections. One section will give exercises that can be done with no equipment, and the other section will present exercises that can be done with weights. The exercises done without weights use the resistance of the body to develop strength, whereas with weight training, the resistance is the iron of the weights.

Most of the exercises here are *isotonic*, that is, the exercise takes the body part through a range of motion. In some instances, the exercise will be an *isometric* or static exercise where you do not go through a range of motion, but rather hold a muscle at full contraction against an immovable resistance or against itself.

Developing a Program

If you need to develop a muscular strength and endurance program, sit down and schedule it at least three days per week. Write it down and then stick to your schedule. Fifteen to thirty minutes will be sufficient time for each session.

You don't need any fancy clothes for this exercise program; just wear something that is comfortable and allows free movement of your body and limbs. If you don't know what would be best suited to you, try different clothing and you will soon find the outfit that best suits your workout. If you have an opportunity to try a program with weights, make sure that you have nonskid shoes if you are working with free weights (those that are not attached to a wall or a machine).

As you read the exercise possibilities for each area of the body, choose one or two from each group for your program and place it on the chart in Table 11.1 (for exercises without equipment) or Table 11.2 (for exercises with weights). As you gain strength and endurance, increase the number of repetitions or increase the amount of resistance you work against.

Muscular Strength and Endurance Exercises Without Equipment

The exercises without equipment in this chapter are given in groups for different parts of the body: neck, arms, arms and shoulders, stomach, back, buttocks, thighs, and legs. The exercises given for each body part generally follow a progression of easiest to hardest, but in some instances all of the exercises in the group are about the same difficulty.

TABLE 11.1 Your Muscular Strength and Endurance Program Without Equipment

Body Area	*Exercise*	*Repetitions*					
		Wk. 1	*Wk. 2*	*Wk. 3*	*Wk. 4*	*Wk. 5*	*Wk. 6*
Neck							
Arms							
Arms/ shoulders							
Stomach							
Back							
Buttocks							
Thighs							
Legs							

Start with 10 repetitions of each exercise that you choose (one exercise for each body area). When 10 repetitions are not enough for you to feel that you are benefiting from the exercise, move on to a harder exercise or increase your repetitions (but don't do more than 15 repetitions).

TABLE 11.2 Your Weight Training Program

Exercise	*Part of Body*	*RM*	*Dates*									*Load (_____RM)*
Example:												Set 1
												Set 2
												Set 3
												1
												2
												3
												1
												2
												3
												1
												2
												3
												1
												2
												3
												1
												2
												3
												1
												2
												3
												1
												2
												3

NECK

HEAD LIFT
Starting position: Lie flat on your back, arms to the side.
Action: Lift your head off the floor, pressing your chin to your chest. Hold for six seconds and then return to starting position.

HEAD PRESS
Starting position: Sit comfortably on a chair or on the floor, arms comfortably at your sides.
Action: Let your head fall to the left side as far as possible (ear to shoulder). Place your left hand against your head above the left ear and push your head and hand together for six seconds. Do the same to the right side. Do the same to the back using both hands to resist against. Do the same to the front using both hands.

ARMS

ARM CIRCLES
Starting position: Stand with your feet together, arms straight out at the sides.
Action: Circle both arms in a slow backward circle on the count of four. Then circle both arms forward in the same manner.

ARM RAISE
Starting position: Stand with feet together, arms at sides.
Action: Extend your arms out and up to a 135° angle leading with the backs of your hands. Hold for six seconds. Variation: Repeat this action, but lead with your palms.

TENNIS BALL SQUEEZE
Starting position: Hold a tennis ball lightly in your hand.
Action: Squeeze the ball 10 times; hold the tenth time for six seconds. Alternate hands.

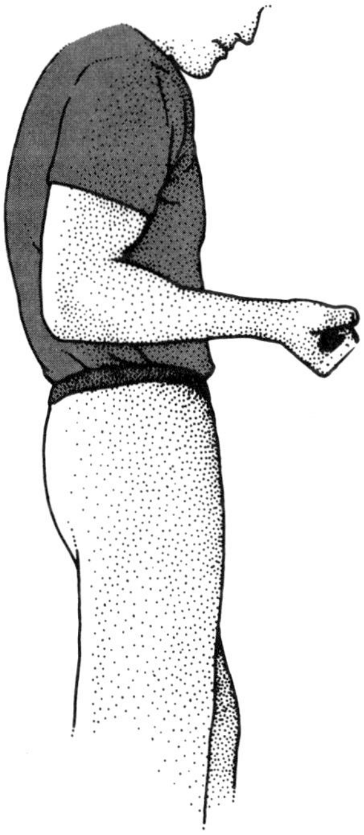
Tennis Ball Squeeze

ARMS AND SHOULDERS

WALL PUSH-AWAY
Starting position: Stand at arm's length from a wall that will support your weight. Place your hands at shoulder height on the wall.
Action: Bend your elbows, allowing the upper body to approach the wall. Push yourself back to the starting posture. Keep your body held straight; don't sag in the rear. Note: This push-away is the least intensive of all the push-ups that follow. If you have some arm strength

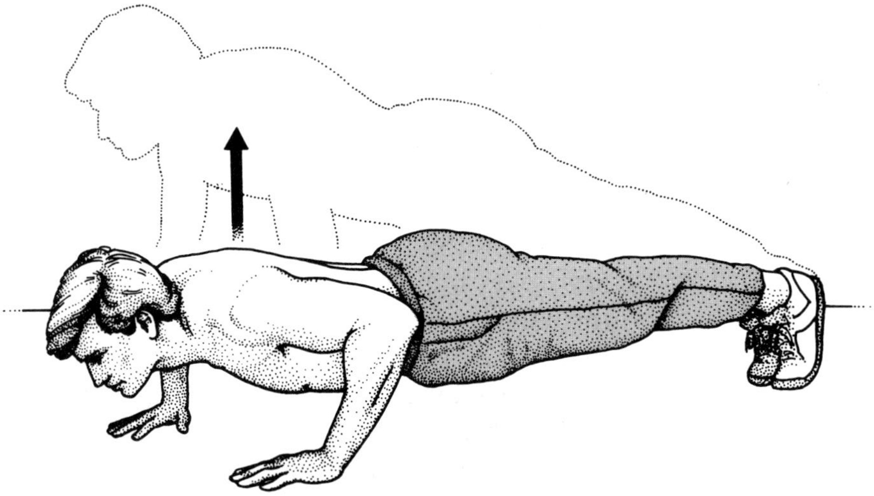

Straight-Body Toe Push-Up

already developed, find a push-up with more resistance in the following pages and add it to your program.

Push-Up Continuum (Easiest to Most Difficult)

SQUARE-BACK PUSH-UP
Starting position: On your hands and knees, knees under hips, hands under shoulders.
Action: Bend the arms slowly, lowering your body to the floor or mat. Straighten your arms as you push back up into the starting position.

STRAIGHT-BODY KNEE PUSH-UP
Starting position: On your hands and knees with the body in a straight line from knees to shoulders, feet up.
Action: Keeping the body straight, lower your chest to the floor or mat and push yourself back up into the starting position.

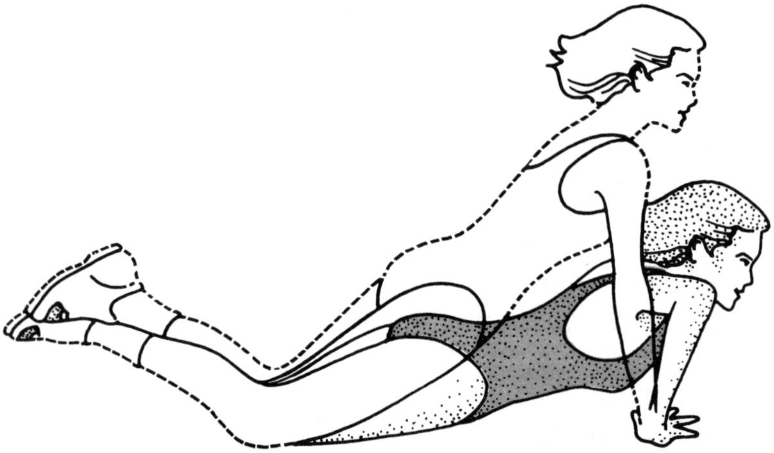

Straight-Body Knee Push-Up

STRAIGHT-BODY TOE PUSH-UP
Starting position: On your hands and toes with your body held straight.
Action: Keeping the body straight, lower the body to the floor or mat until your chest touches. Straighten your arms to return to the starting position.

PUSH-UP FROM ELEVATED SURFACE
Starting position: On your hands and toes with your body held straight, but place your toes on an elevated surface such as a step, a box, or a chair. The more elevated the surface, the more resistance you will feel in your arms and shoulders as you push up.
Action: Keeping the body straight, lower the body to the floor or mat until your chest touches. Straighten your arms to return to the starting position. With your toes on higher surfaces, you may find difficulty in touching your chest to the floor. So just make sure you completely flex your arms (a complete bend at the elbow).

STOMACH

Sit-Up Continuum (Easiest to Most Difficult)

In all sit-ups, especially if you are out of shape, bend your knees, placing your feet flat on the floor or mat in order to isolate the muscles you wish to tone – the abdominal muscles. Have someone hold your feet until you can do the action alone.

CURLS, OR "CRUNCHES"
Starting position: Lie on your back, bend your knees, and place your feet on the floor about the width of the hips apart. Cross your arms on your chest.
Action: Curl your head, neck, and shoulders up until your shoulder blades are lifted. Curl back down to the starting position.

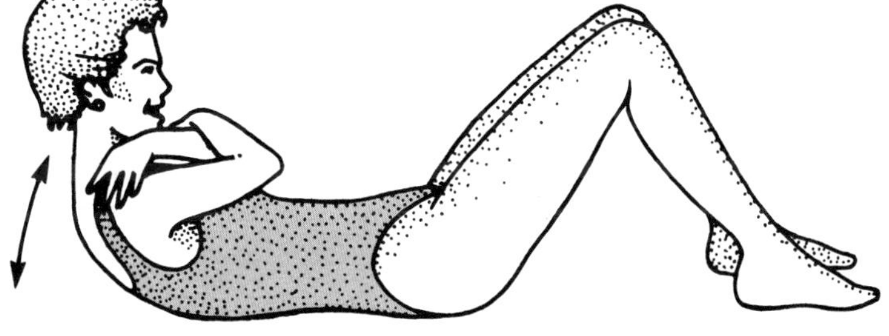

Curls

Crossed-Arm Bent-Knee Sit-Up

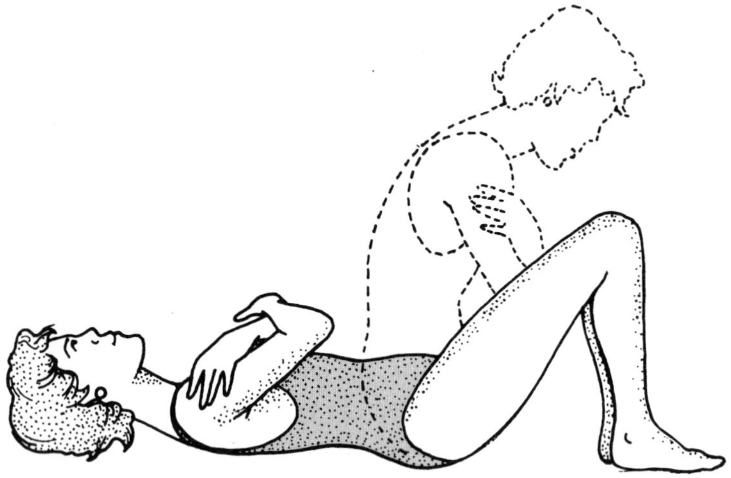

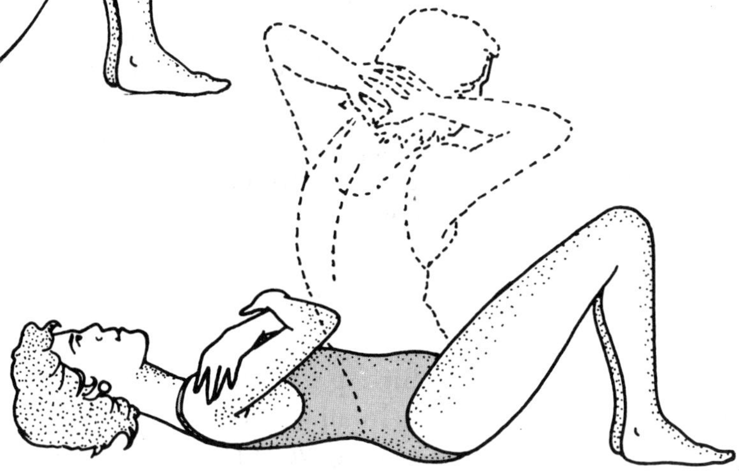

Bent-Knee Sit-Up with Twist

STRAIGHT-ARM CRUNCHES

Starting position: Lie on your back, knees bent. With your hands grasping the sides of your thighs, pull yourself up just until the shoulder blades are off the floor. Then stretch your arms out so that they are parallel with your thighs.

Action: Move your arms and shoulders just ½ to 1 inch forward and back. Do 20–50 of these short movements before returning to the starting position.

CROSSED-ARM BENT-KNEE SIT-UP

Starting position: Same as the curls with arms folded across the chest. This adds more resistance for your abdominal muscles to overcome.

Action: Curl yourself up into a sitting position. Let your arms touch your knees. Curl back down again. You may need someone or something to hold your feet on the floor until your strength develops. Stay with this exercise until you can perform it without help.

BENT-KNEE SIT-UP WITH TWIST

Starting position: The arms are crossed on the chest, knees bent, feet flat on the floor. At first you may need help to hold your feet down.

Action: Curl yourself into a sitting position. Twist body to the left. Curl yourself back down to the starting position. Repeat twisting to the right.

BICYCLING/ROWING

Starting position: Sit with your weight supported by your hands and buttocks (lean back a little on your hands).

Action: Raise your legs in front of you and first bend your knees and bring them to your chest, then extend your legs one at a time in front of you as though riding a bicycle. You may also alternately bend and extend both legs up and out in front of you in a rowing action. Note: As you progress with your abdominal strength, put less weight on your hands, balancing on your seat.

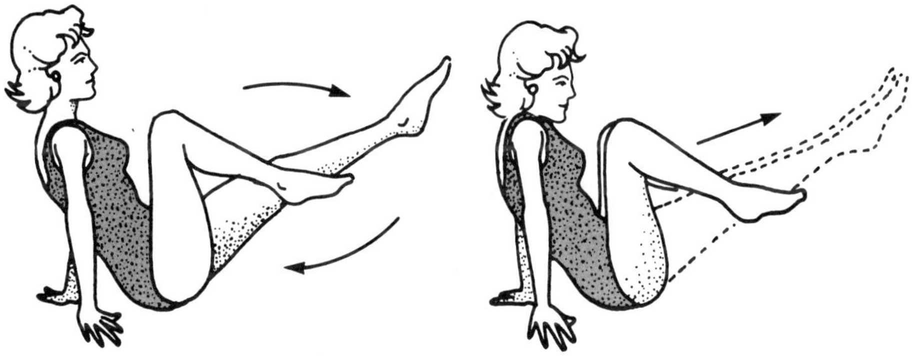

Bicycling/Rowing

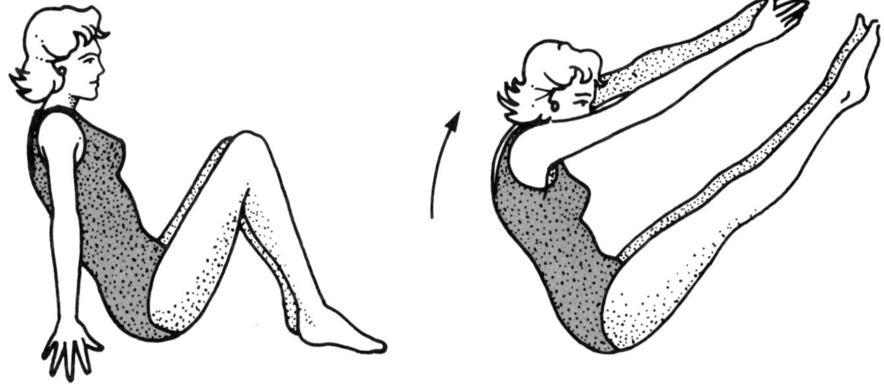

V-Sit

V-SIT

Starting position: Sit on the floor or mat with your knees bent, feet on the floor, hands on the floor behind your buttocks.

Action: Raise your hands up and outward; straighten your legs and your back upward into a V position.

POP-UP
Starting position: Lie flat on your back, arms straight overhead on the floor.
Action: Pop up into a V position; touch your toes with your fingers

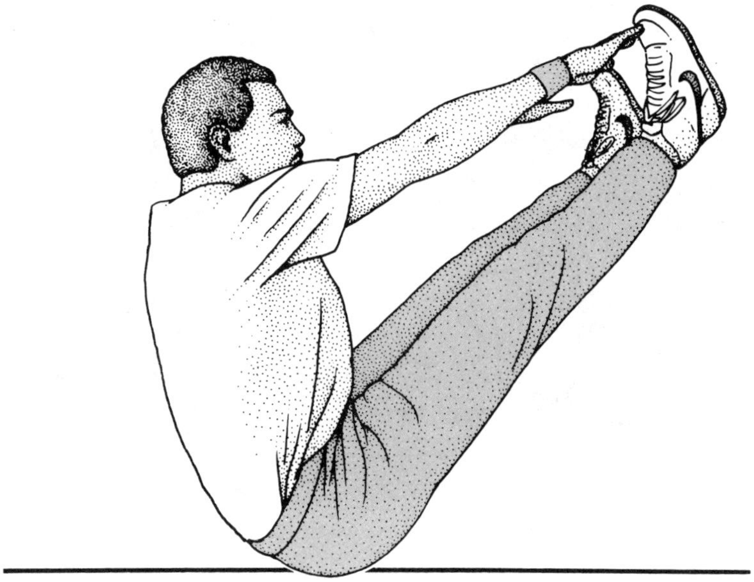

Pop-Up

BACK

WAIST PUSH-UP
Starting position: Lie on your stomach, arms bent with hands under your shoulders.
Action: Push up slowly from the waist, hold your upper body for six seconds, and return to the starting position. Progressively use more back muscle and less arm power to rise and hold the position.

UPPER BODY LIFT
Starting position: Lie face down; clasp your hands behind your neck. Have someone or something hold down your feet and hips.
Action: Slowly raise your upper body off the floor; hold for six seconds. Do not jerk into this position. Slowly lower yourself back to the starting position.

SINGLE LEG LIFT
Starting position: Lie face down, chin resting on your hands.
Action: Slowly raise your left leg; hold it up for six seconds; lower it. Slowly raise your right leg; hold it up for six seconds; lower it.

DOUBLE LEG LIFT
Starting position: Lie on your stomach; turn your face to one side; place your hands under your thighs.
Action: Slowly raise both legs together and hold them up for six seconds. Lower them to the starting position.

OPPOSITE ARM AND LEG LIFT
Starting position: Lie face down, arms extended over the head.
Action: Slowly raise one straight arm and the opposite leg. Hold for six seconds and lower. Repeat on the other side.

BUTTOCKS

LEG LIFT
Starting position: On hands and knees.
Action: Lift your leg and hold it straight behind you for six seconds; lower it. Raise your right leg and hold for six seconds. Return to the starting position.

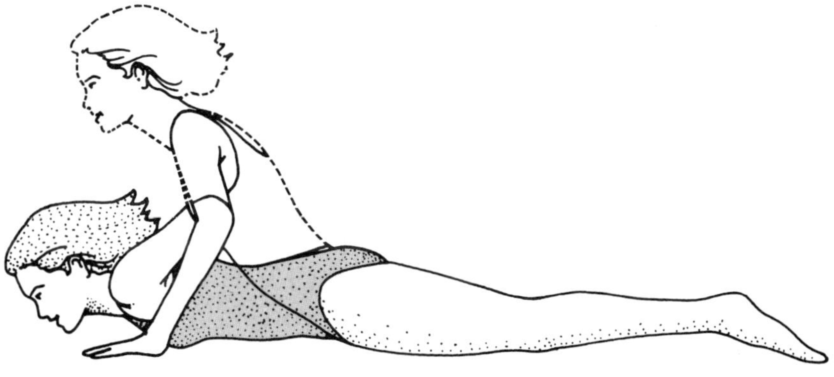

Waist Push-Up

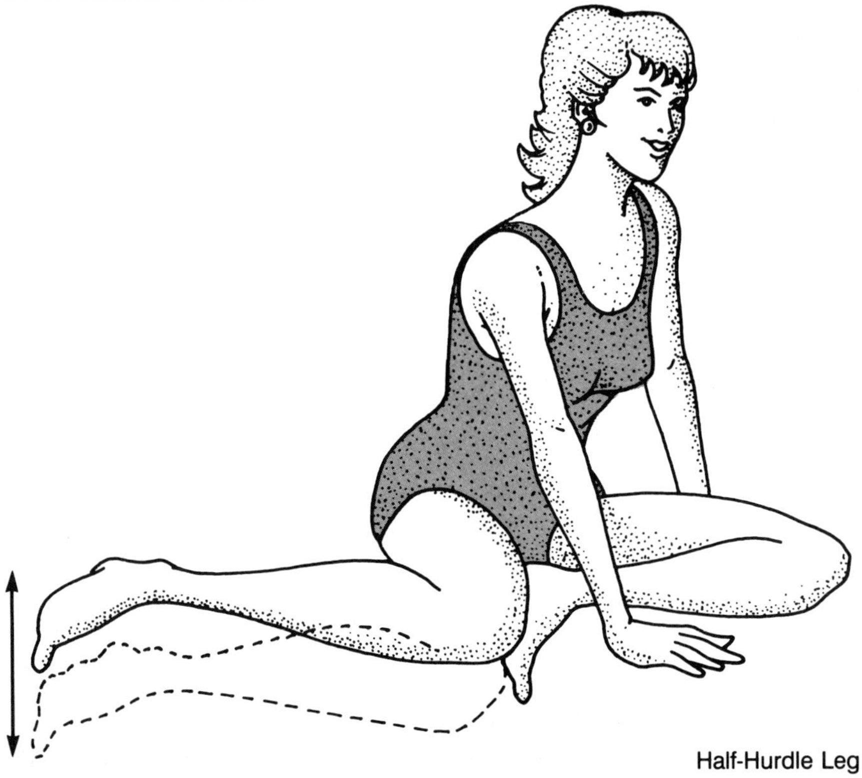

Half-Hurdle Leg Lift

HALF-HURDLE LEG LIFT

Starting position: Sit on the floor in the half-hurdle position: The front leg is bent at the knee with the foot next to the thigh of the rear leg. The rear leg is bent at the knee and ankle into two 90° angles (as the trailing leg over a hurdle would be). Place your hands at the sides on the floor to help support your body.

Action: Raise your rear leg one to two inches off the floor. Hold for six seconds. Do your repetitions on one side, and then change legs and repeat the exercise.

STANDING LEG LIFT

Starting position: Stand, feet together.

Action: Keeping your body erect, arms out at the sides for balance, raise your left leg to the rear and hold it straight out behind you for six seconds. Repeat with the other leg, returning to the starting position between repetitions.

RUNNING, BENCH STEPPING, RUNNING STAIRS

The first two of these exercises are featured in the aerobic or "fat loss" chapter (Chapter 13). Heed all caution statements, and remember to *watch the steps* if you choose to use step running for excellent development of the gluteal muscles.

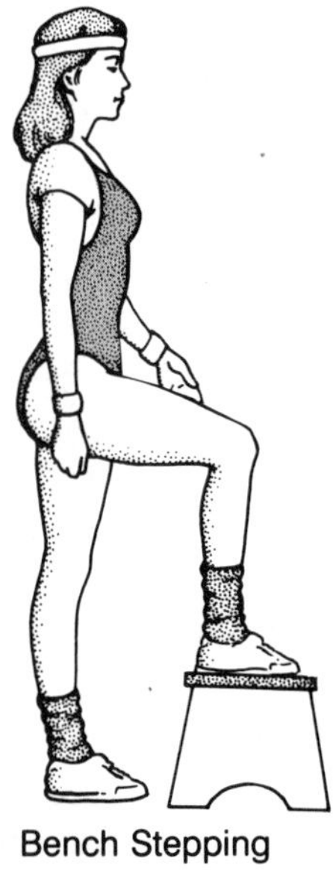

Bench Stepping

THIGHS

SQUAT THRUST

Starting position: Stand, hands at the sides.

Action: Bend legs, place hands on the floor about shoulder-width apart (a squat position). Jump your feet behind you to a full push-up position: You will be supporting your weight on your hands and toes. Jump back into a squat position with your hands still on the floor. Stand erect again.

LINE JUMPING

Starting position: Select a line on the floor or place a tape or flat object on the floor. Stand parallel to the line (not facing it).

Action: Squat slightly and jump sideways over the line, landing in a slight squat (skiing position). Jump from side to side.

BODY RAISE

Starting position: Lie on your back, knees bent, feet on the floor, arms at your sides.

Action: Raise hips until your body is straight from the shoulders to the hips. Hold for six seconds and return to the starting position.

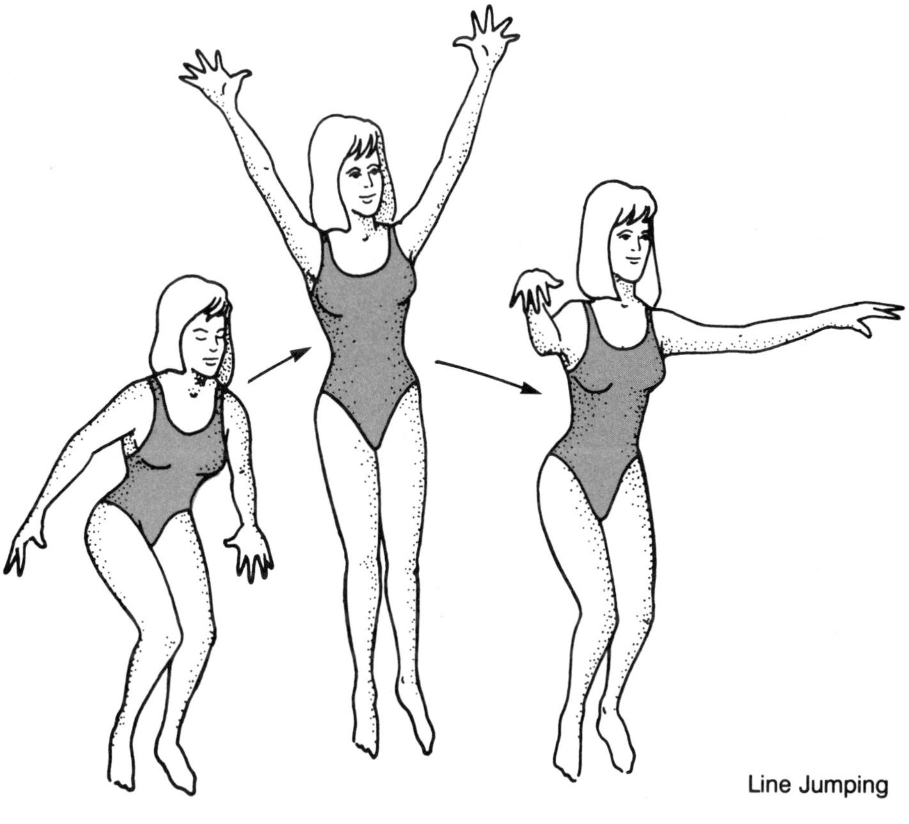

Line Jumping

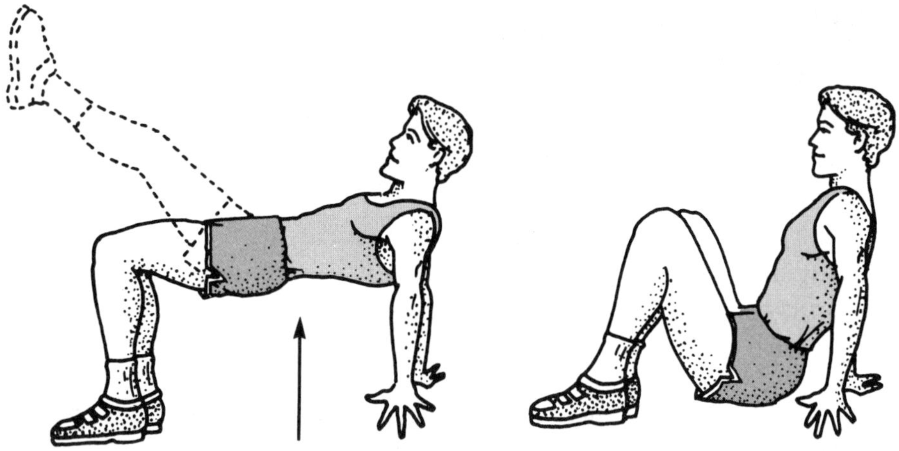

Square-Body Leg Raise

SQUARE-BODY LEG RAISE
Starting position: Sit, knees bent, feet on the floor, hands on the floor to either side of your buttocks, shoulder-width apart.
Action: Raise your trunk to form a "table." Lift your right leg slowly and hold for six seconds. Return it to the floor. Lift your left leg slowly and hold for six seconds. Return it to the floor. Lower yourself into the starting position.

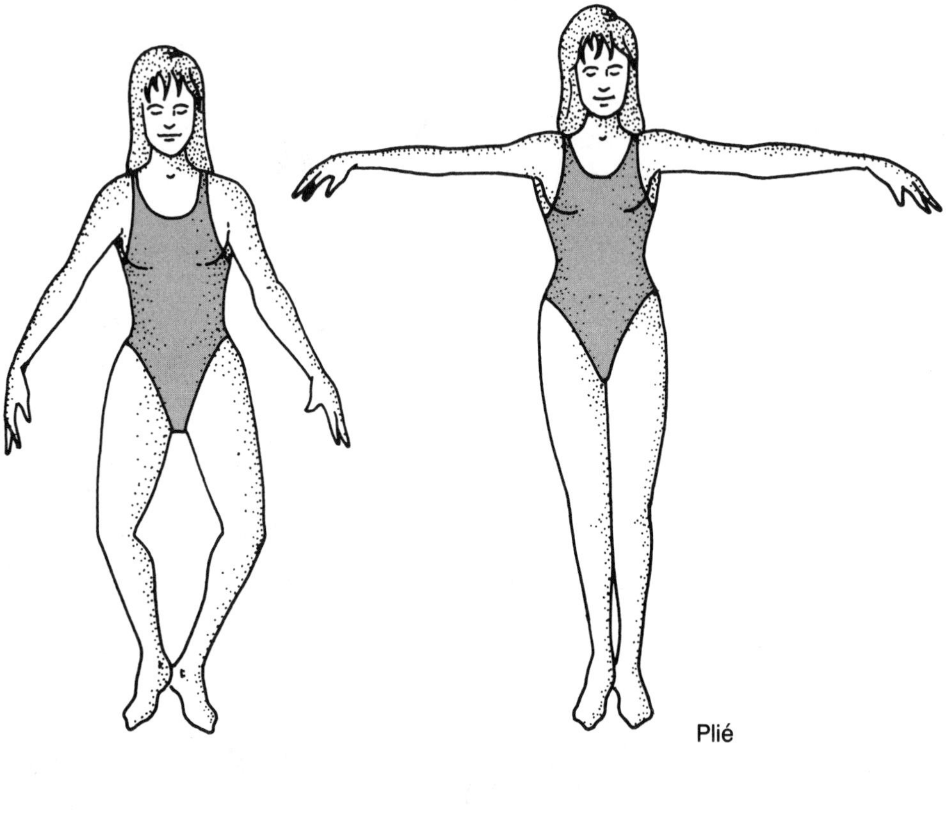

Plié

PLIÉ

Starting position: Stand, feet with toes pointed out at about a 45° angle, heels together, arms extended to the sides.

Action: Keeping your back straight (don't stick out your buttocks), bend your knees to the outside *over your toes*, lowering yourself slowly about one-quarter of the way down. Hold for six seconds. Slowly rise back to starting position.

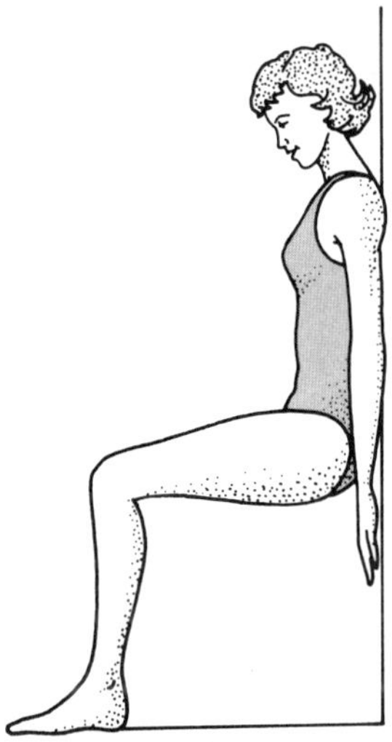

Wall Chair

WALL CHAIR

Starting position: Back up to a wall and stand at thigh's length away from the wall, facing outward.

Action: "Sit down" supporting your back on the wall. Your hips and knees should be at 90° angles. Hold for progressively longer periods. If your shoes do not offer good traction, have someone hold your feet in place. Note: This exercise looks effortless but demands much from the thighs. If you are just beginning to firm up, use some lighter exercises or hold this for only a few seconds.

RUNNING, BENCH STEPPING, RUNNING STAIRS

These are great thigh strengtheners. Again, if you run steps, watch the next one coming up! Chapter 13 provides instruction on running and bench stepping, two aerobic exercises.

LEGS

LEG LIFT

Starting position: Lie on your side, lower arm extended above your head. Hand of upper arm should rest on the floor to help balance you on your side.

Action: Lift your upper leg slowly over a six-second count and lower that leg slowly over a six-second count. Do your repetitions on one side and then repeat on the other side.

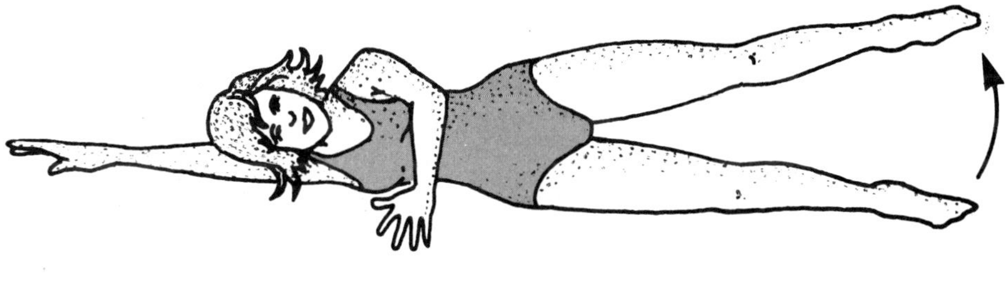

Leg Lift

TIPTOE STAND

Starting position: Stand, feet shoulder-width apart, arms out to the sides for balance.

Action: Rise up slowly onto your toes. Hold for six seconds. Slowly lower to starting position. As you develop strength, stand with your toes on a book and raise your heels from the floor to tiptoe position.

Weight Training

Using a weight as the resistance against which you lift, push, or pull is an effective means of improving your muscular strength and endurance. Weight lifting, however, assumes that you have some kind of weights to lift. Dumbbells and barbells are still common pieces of weight equipment, and a starter set is fairly inexpensive. However, such inventions as the Universal Gym, wall units that are permanently attached to a wall, and the Nautilus system have replaced the free weights in many gyms and clubs. Dumbbells can also be inexpensively made out of plastic jugs and sand, cloth sand bags, or even cans of soup! With sand bags or jugs, you can vary the weight by adding or removing sand. If you do not have access to a gym that has a weight set, you might consider making some of your own or purchasing a small set of weights that can be used on a barbell or as dumbbells.

PRECAUTIONS AND GENERAL RULES IN WEIGHT TRAINING

There are some safety precautions and general rules to follow in a weight training program in order to get the full effect of the program. These are:

1. Begin by using very light weights while you get used to the equipment. Always lift weights off the floor with your legs; squat down beside the bar and with a straight back, lift the weights into position. If you are not working on a machine, get some help on each side of a heavy bar to ensure your safety and that of others around you.
2. Have a friend who knows how to use weights or a qualified instructor help you with your program the first time you use weights.

3. Breathe while you exercise; don't hold your breath. Generally, you will want to exhale during the effort phase, and inhale during the recovery phase.
4. Wear shoes with nonskid soles if you work with free weights or do any inverted leg exercises.
5. For strength, complete one to five repetitions of 60–70% of the maximum weight that you can lift. This is called "repetitions maximum" or RM. Doing six of them at 60% would be 60% RM.
6. For muscular endurance, complete 12–15 at 60–70% RM.
7. Complete three to five sets (that is, go through all of the weight exercises on your program three to five times per session).
8. Work out with weights no less often than three days per week if you wish to see improvement in strength and endurance.
9. Build both muscular strength and endurance by alternating your workouts: two days on strength and one on endurance, then alternate the next week to two days on endurance and one on strength.

YOUR PROGRAM

From the following exercises, choose one exercise for each body area and write that exercise into your Weight Training Program (Table 11.2). Practice three days a week (at least), continuing to increase your weight load as you can.

Muscular Strength and Endurance Exercises with Weights

OVERHEAD PRESS *(arms, especially the triceps; shoulders; upper back)*
Starting position: Stand facing away from the weight machine or hold barbell at the shoulder resting position. Place hands in an overgrip. Make sure that your feet are directly under the hips, shoulders, and the bar.
Action: Extend the arms, pressing the bar above the head until your arms reach full extension. Then bend your arms and lower the weights to your shoulders again.

BENCH PRESS *(arms, especially the triceps; shoulders; chest)*
Starting position: Lie down on the bench with the bar at about shoulder height. Use an overhand grip. The legs can hang over the bench, feet on the floor, or you can bend your legs and place your feet on the bench.

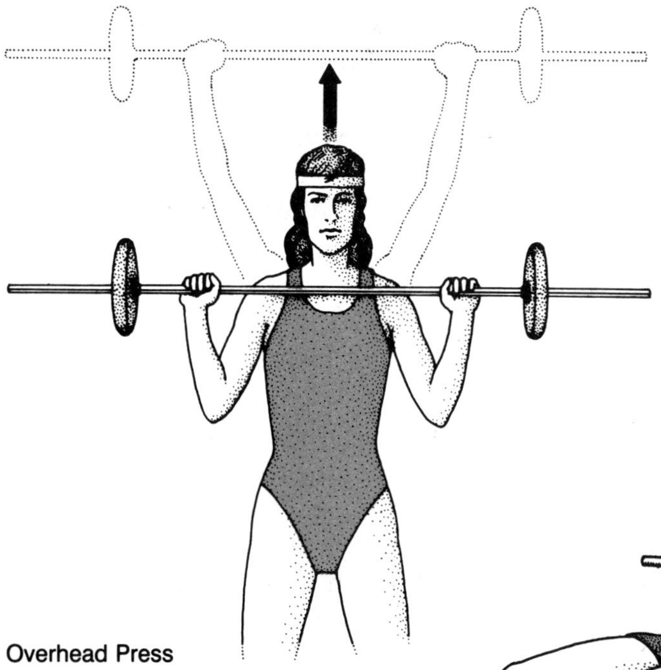

Overhead Press

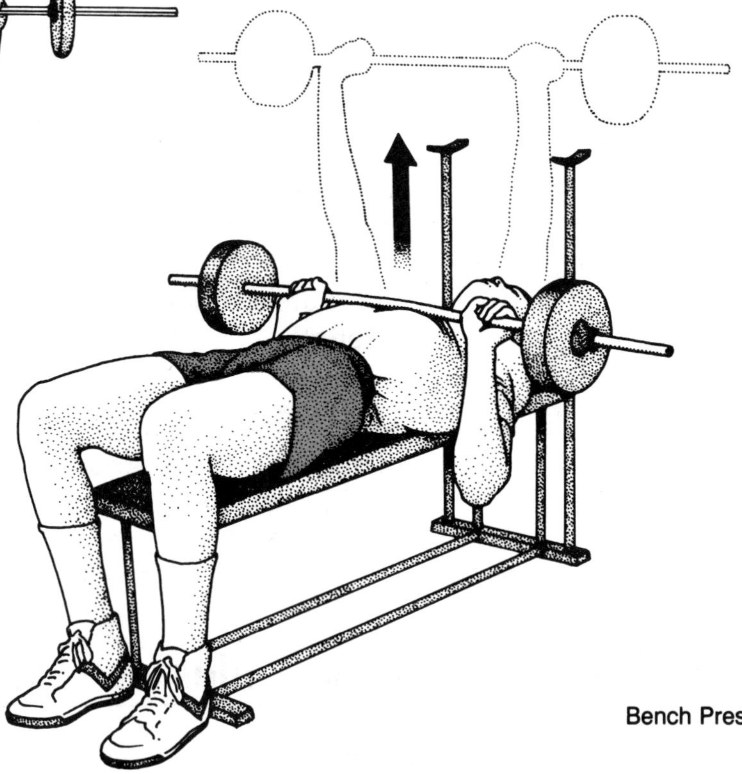

Bench Press

Action: Extend your arms straight up to full extension and then return to the starting position. Keep your back pressed against the bench. Make sure your shoulders are directly under the bar.

BICEP CURL *(bicep muscles of the upper arms)*
Starting position: Stand in front of the machine, or hold dumbbells in one or both hands, or hold barbell in both hands in an underhand grip; backs of the hands with weights in them should rest on the thighs.
Action: Curl the weight up toward the body by flexing the arms at the elbow. Keep the elbows close to the sides. (You can see your biceps at work.) Return to an extended arm position.

HALF SQUAT *(thighs and buttocks muscles)*
Starting position: Stand with the bar resting lightly on your shoulders (behind your neck). Use an overhand grip. Feet are apart, about hip width. Keep your back straight (this is very important to avoid back injury).
Action: Bend the knees to a half squat position (the knee joint is almost at a right angle). Return to the starting position. Take all the weight in the thighs in this exercise.

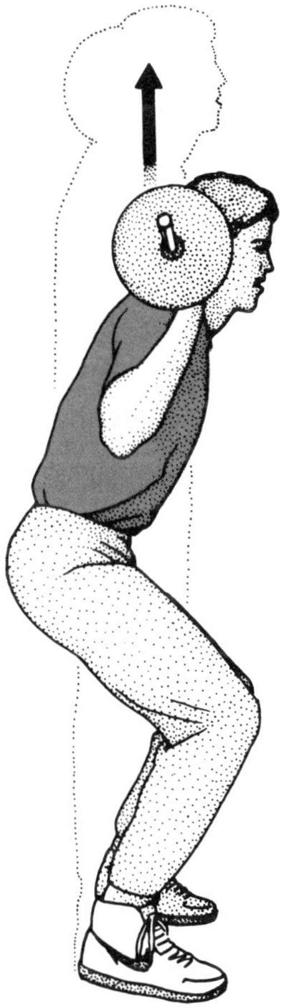

Half Squat

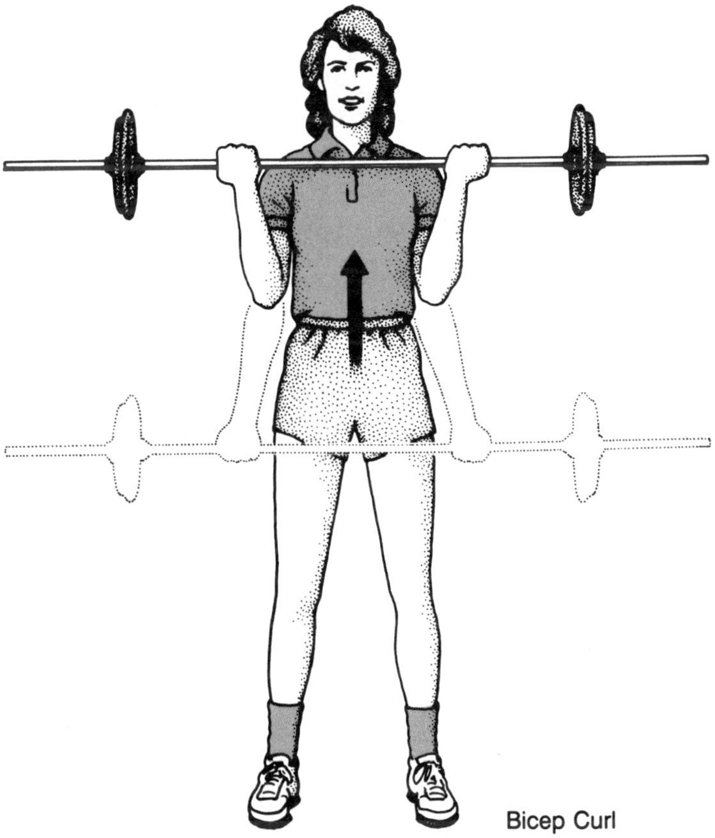

Bicep Curl

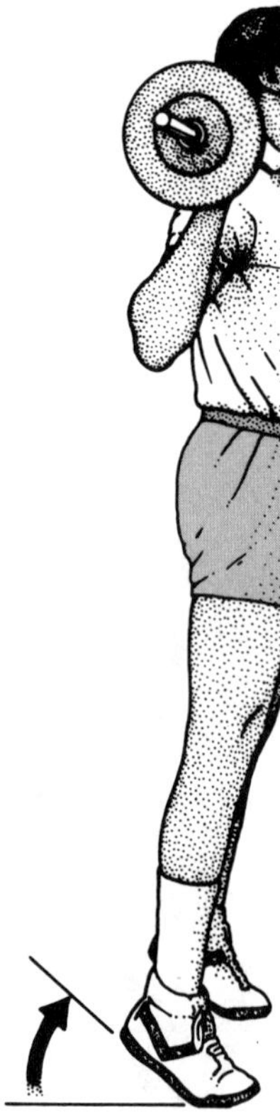

Heel Raise

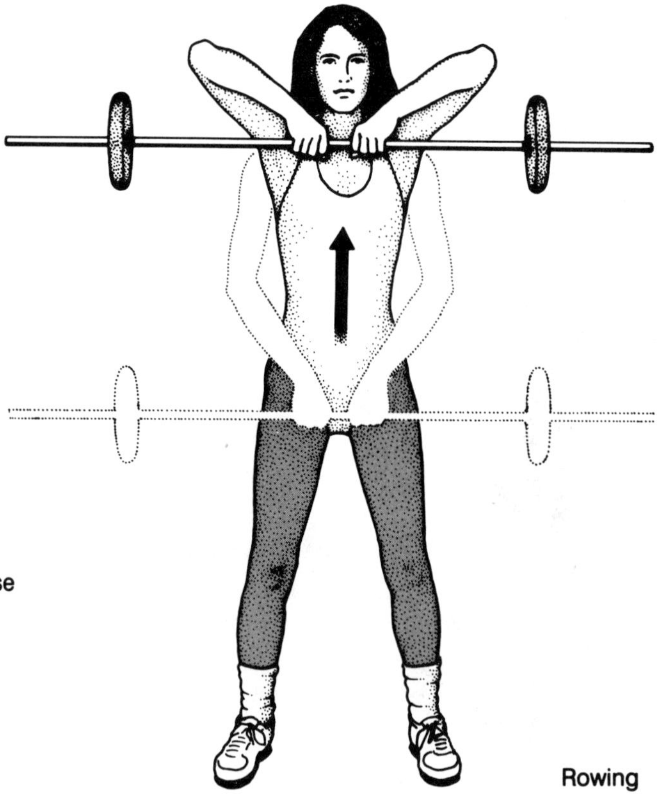

Rowing

HEEL RAISE *(calves, feet)*
Starting position: Same position as the half squat.
Action: Rise on your toes and lower back to the starting position. Again, take all the weight in your legs, not in your back.

ROWING *(upper back, upper arms, and shoulders)*
Starting position: Face the bar; place hands together in an overgrip. Bar is at thigh height.
Action: Lift the bar straight up until it lightly touches the chin. Lower it to starting position.

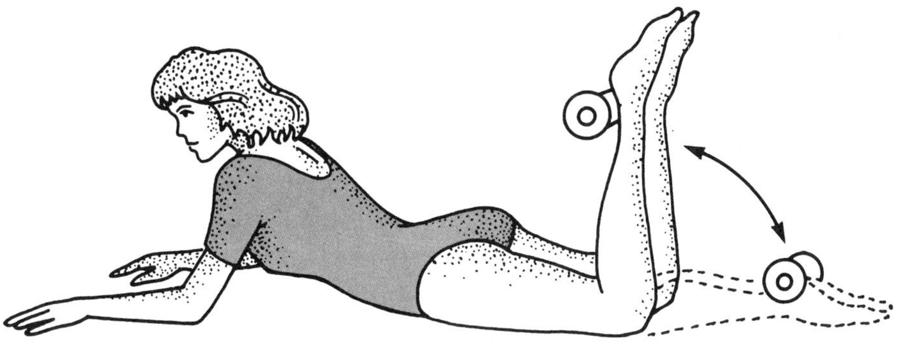

Back Leg Curl

JUMP SQUAT *(thighs and buttocks)*
Starting position: Hold bar on shoulders securely behind the neck. Place hands as far apart as comfortable in an overgrip.
Action: Lower the body to a half squat position and then jump up vigorously into an erect standing position. Note: Begin with light weights as you learn this exercise.

BACK LEG CURL *(hamstrings, buttocks)*
Starting position: Lie on your stomach on the bench with your heels under the pads for back leg curls. Rest on your elbows, grasping the bench with your hands.
Action: Flex the knees to form a right angle. Return to the starting position.

SIT-UP *(stomach)*
Starting position: On a slanted bench, lie on your back with your head downhill, arms folded across your chest, knees bent with feet fastened under the toe strap (or on some benches, with your legs hanging over the end of the bench with your toes tucked under the crossbar).
Action: Curl up just so the shoulder blades (scapulae) come off the bench. Hold for six seconds and return to the starting position. As your abdominal muscles become stronger, add more resistance by holding a weight in your hands across your chest or behind your head. Note: Always keep your back flat on the bench.

Summary

Now that you have reviewed the different types of muscular strength and endurance exercises given here, plan a program that will include the various muscle groups of the body and begin to tone up your body. Keep a chart of your progress (Table 11.3). Even if you perform only one set of exercises on some days, record it. Over a period of weeks you will begin to see how your body is changing. To prove that there is some change, measure now the circumference of your chest, waist, thighs, calves, and upper arms, and record the measurements on the chart in Table 11.3. Take the same measurements once a month and you will find what other exercisers find—you will lose inches as you develop muscular strength and endurance.

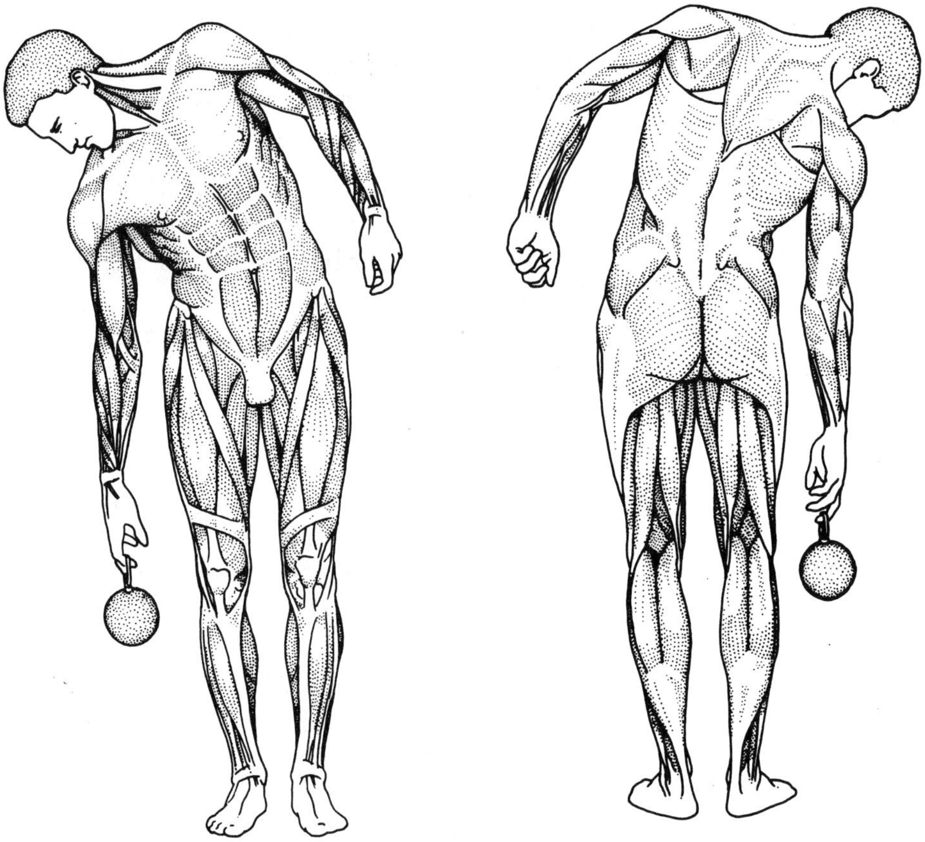

TABLE 11.3 Your Body Measurement Chart

Body Area	*Pre-program Inches*	*Dates*										

12 FLEXIBILITY PROGRAM

EVERY MUSCLE that you strengthen, you must also stretch. This keeps you in good balance and keeps all of your muscles working to their fullest range.

When you stretch a muscle, always apply slow, steady pressure with your other body parts. Do *not* bounce against a muscle and do not have someone else apply the pressure. A sudden jerk on a tight muscle could result in muscle fiber damage. When you stretch, take yourself to a point of mild discomfort, hold your position there, and relax all the muscles surrounding the one you are working on. The discomfort will go away as the muscle and ligamentous tissue elongates. In a short period of time you will see progress.

Try to give your muscles a chance to warm up before you begin stretching. It is easier to touch your toes after a little warm-up activity than it is immediately after you jump out of bed in the morning. You can add your stretching exercises to your muscular strength and endurance workout, but they may be more beneficial in the evening before you go to bed because of their relaxing nature. Several of the stretching exercises that follow are recommended before and after running; these are starred (*) in this section.

Flexibility Exercises

NECK

SIDE TURNS
Starting position: Sit comfortably.
Action: Turn your head slowly to the left and come back slowly to the front. Repeat to right side. Rotate to the point at which you feel a comfortable stretch. Then slowly let your head fall forward to a comfortable stretch and return to starting position. Repeat to the rear.

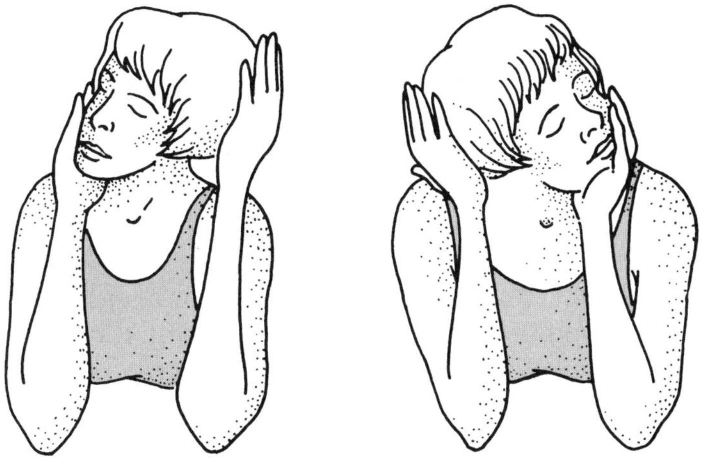

Head Twist

HEAD TWIST
Starting position: Lie on your stomach, support your weight on your elbows. Place your chin in the left palm, place the other hand on your head above the temple.
Action: Slowly twist the head to the left as far as possible by pushing your head with your right hand. Hold for six seconds. Slowly return. Do your given number of repetitions on one side, then change hands and do the same number of repetitions on the other side.

ARMS, SHOULDERS, UPPER BACK, CHEST

ARM FLING
Starting position: Stand, feet together, hands in front of shoulders (elbows bent, out from body).
Action: Throw the arms out gently to the side and return to the starting position.

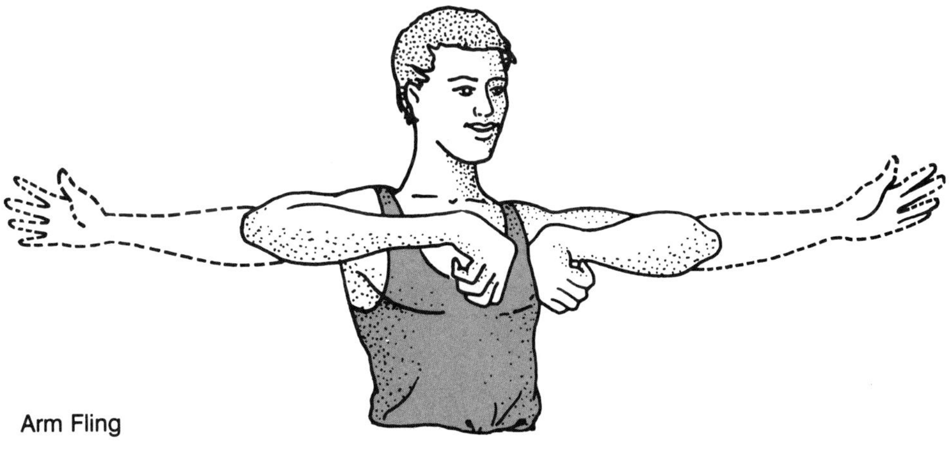

Arm Fling

SHOULDER STRETCH
Starting position: Stand, feet shoulder-width apart.
Action: Reach arms behind you until you can clasp your hands together. Reach up with your arms as far as you can. Hold for six seconds. Then bend forward at the waist, keeping arms behind you. Hold for 10 seconds.

ARM SWING
Starting position: Stand, feet shoulder-width apart, arms at sides.
Action: Swing both arms to the left about shoulder height, then back to the right. Swing back and forth with a nice, easy swing.

ARM CLIMB
Starting position: Stand with feet together, arms straight overhead.
Action: Reach as high as possible with one hand, then the other, as though climbing a ladder. Stretch at the shoulder.

TRUNK

TRIANGLE PROGRESSION
Starting position: Stand with feet shoulder-width apart, arms out to sides.

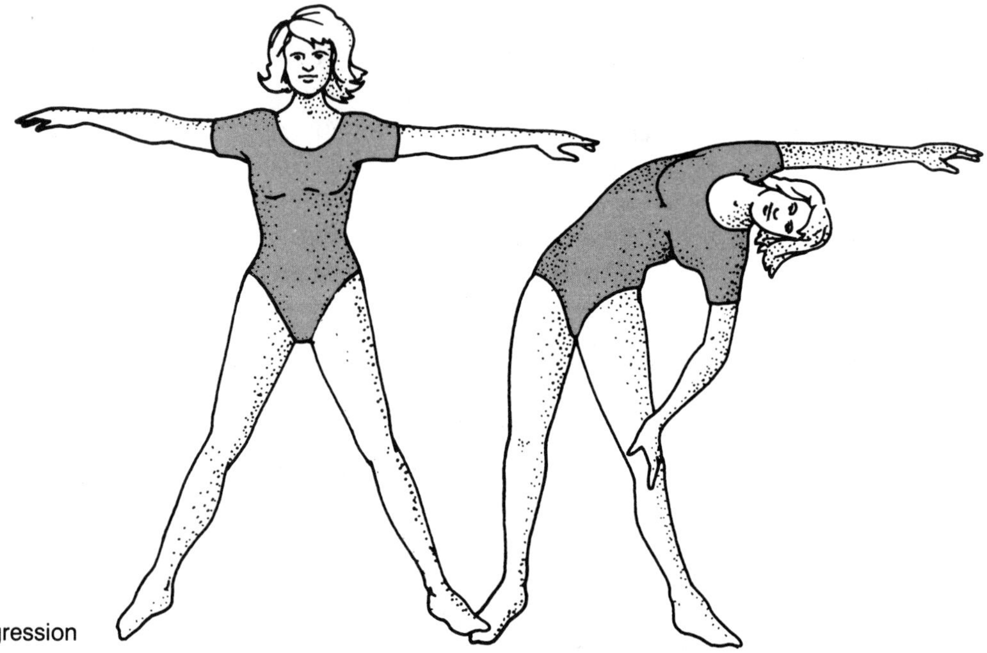

Triangle Progression

Action: Reach down sideways to the knee with one hand and rest your hand there while the other arm comes over the head and reaches out parallel to the floor. Hold for 10 seconds and do the same on the other side.
Progression: As you become more flexible, spread your feet a little farther and support the lower hand on the calf. The last step is to support your hand on your ankle.
Note: On all of the side stretch exercises, keep your body in line, do not twist forward. Feel the stretch all the way down the side.

LEG-OVER
Starting position: Lie on your back, arms straight out from the sides.
Action: Bend the left knee, extend the left foot into the air, twist the trunk as you touch the left foot to the right hand, keeping the shoulders down on the floor. Raise the left leg back up straight, bend the knee, lower the leg to the floor to the starting position. Do the same with the right leg to the left hand.

BODY TWIST
Starting position: Sit cross-legged on the floor.
Action: Slowly twist your trunk to the left and place both hands on the floor to the outside of the left leg. Hold for six seconds. Return to starting position. Do the same to the right side.

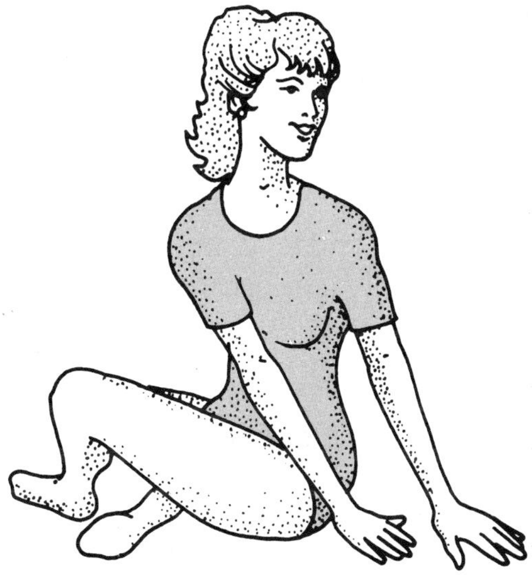
Body Twist

BACK

*ONE-LEG STRETCHER
Starting position: Sit with one leg straight in front, the other bent with foot on the floor, arms crossed behind the back.
Action: Lean body forward over straight leg and hold for ten seconds. Return to starting position. Reverse starting position of the legs and repeat.

SIT-STRETCH
Starting Position: Sit with your legs straight out in front of you, hands at your sides.
Action: Lean forward, hold your knees, and pull yourself forward slowly. Keep your elbows pointed up and out. Find your pain point and hold it 10 seconds.
Progression: Reach for your calves instead of your knees and hold. Reach for your ankles and hold.

SIT-HANG
Starting Position: Sit in a chair that has no arms. Place your feet on the floor.
Action: Lean forward and let your body hang down toward the floor. Let your hands and arms fall forward until your hands dangle on the floor. Hold for 10 seconds and slowly curl back up into a sitting position.

STAND-HANG
Starting Position: Stand with feet shoulder-width apart, arms loose at sides.
Action: Lean forward and let your body hang from the waist. Hold for 10 seconds and slowly curl back up into a standing position.

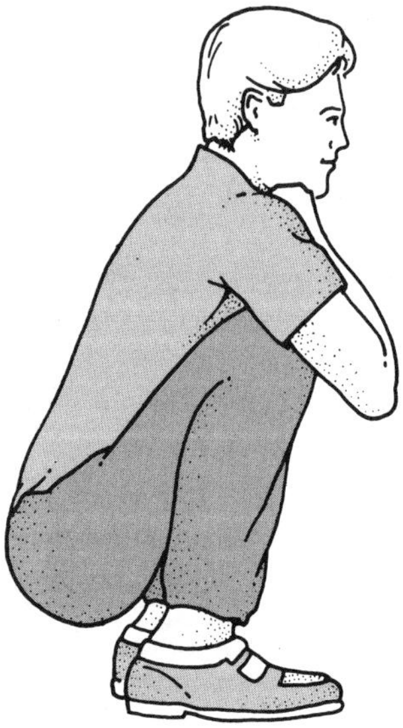
Hunker Squat

*HUNKER SQUAT
Starting position: With feet flat on the floor, squat down with arms resting on the knees.
Action: Hold this position for one or 2 minutes (or longer). If balance is difficult at first, do this exercise with your back toward a wall.

STOMACH

BACK ARCH
Starting position: Stand, feet together, hands at your sides.
Action: Raise your hands and arms forward and up; keep reaching until the back is arched and the arms are slightly behind the ears. Hold for 10 seconds and slowly return to starting position.

BACK LEAN
Starting position: Sit with legs straight out in front of you, arms to sides.
Action: Raise your arms up over your head and extend the body back toward a lying position as far as you can hold it. Hold for six seconds and return to starting position.

HAMSTRINGS

*BENT-LEG HAMSTRING STRETCH
Starting position: Stand facing a surface that is no more than two feet high. Place one foot on the elevated surface. Hands behind the back.
Action: Lean forward, trying to put your head to your knee. Keep your upper knee bent slightly (the other leg can also be bent as it

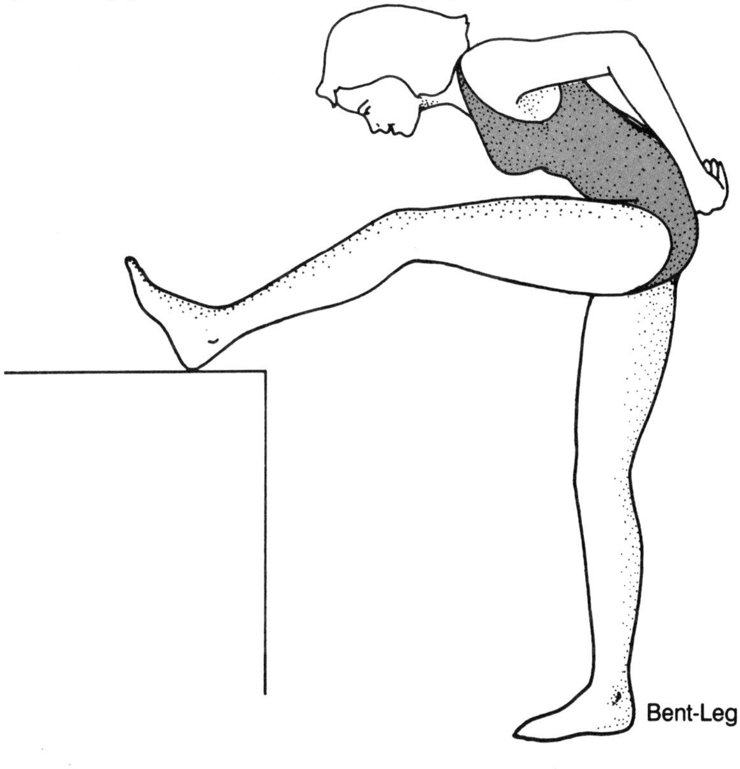

Bent-Leg Hamstring Stretch

supports you). Hold for 10 seconds. Return to the starting position and repeat on the other side. Do this at least six times before and after you run.

SITTING HAMSTRING STRETCH
Starting position: Sit with the left leg straight out in front of you, the right knee bent, with the foot at the crotch.
Action: Lean forward, hold your knee (or calf, or ankle, depending on your flexibility) and slowly lower your body over the front leg. Go down as far as you can and hold for 10 seconds. Return to the starting position and repeat on the other side. This can also be done with a rolled towel, holding one end in each hand with the foot in the middle of the towel.

TOE TOUCH
Starting position: Sit with your legs straight out in front of you.
Action: Reach for the toes (or beyond them) with your hands palm up. At your pain point, hold for 10 seconds. Return to starting position.

LEGS

QUADRICEPS STRETCH
Starting position: Kneel with the tops of the feet flat on the floor, arms down at the sides.
Action: Bring your arms up to reach straight in front of you as you slowly lean back from your knees. Keep the body straight (don't sag in the hips). Hold for six seconds. Return slowly to the starting position.

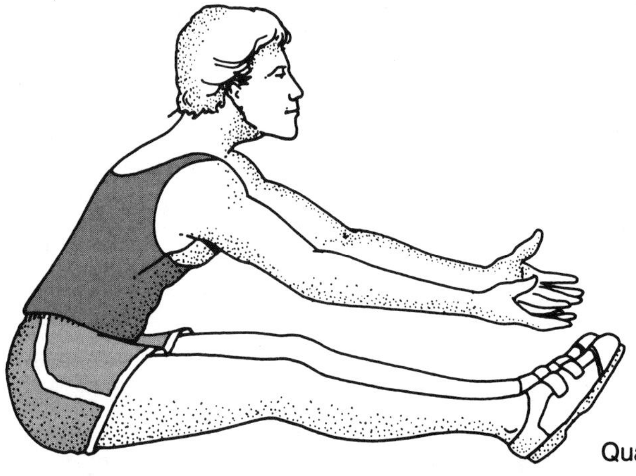
Quadriceps Stretch

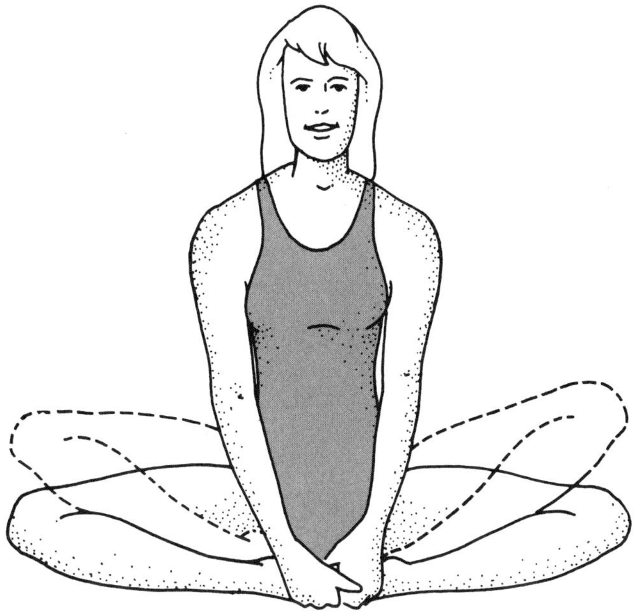

Tailor Stretch

SIDE STRETCH
Starting position: Kneel on the left knee and place the right leg straight out to the side, foot pointed forward.
Action: Place your right hand on your right knee and extend the left arm over the head as you lean your body over the right leg. Feel the stretch on the inside of the right leg. Hold for 10 seconds and return to the starting position. Alternate sides.

TAILOR STRETCH
Starting position: Sit with your soles together, hands holding onto your feet.
Action: Press your knees to the floor and hold for 10 seconds. Return to the starting position.

*CALF STRETCH
Starting position: Stand arm's length away from the wall, facing it.
Action: Place hands or forearms on the wall and lean forward, *keeping your heels flat on the floor*. Feel the stretch in the calves and back of the heel (the Achilles tendon). Hold for 10 seconds and return to the starting position. (Do this at least six times before and after you run.)

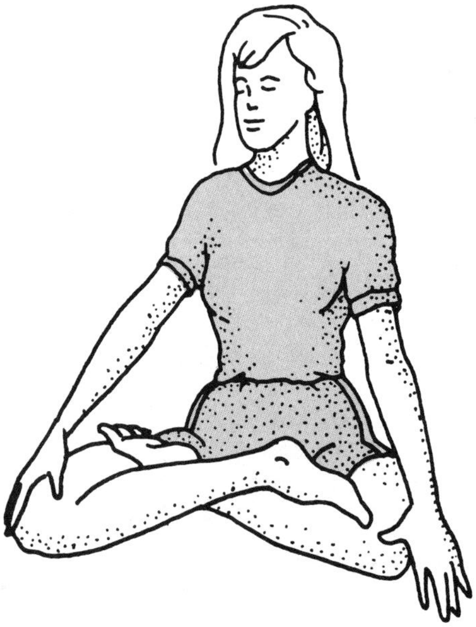

Yoga—Lotus Position

Yoga

If you have an opportunity to take a yoga class or follow a yoga plan such as Hittleman's 28-day plan (1978), you will find that this form of exercise substitutes for a stretching program. The philosophy and relaxation of yoga that go along with the exercises will also blend in very well with the thinness lifestyle suggested in this book.

Summary

Choose at least one stretching exercise from each section given here and do at least three repetitions per session to start out. As you progress, add repetitions until you work up to 10 repetitions. For some exercises you should use the greater stretch position that is given rather than increasing repetitions. In this way time will not become a problem. Write out your flexibility exercise program in Table 12.1.

If you experiment a little with your muscles, you can create other exercises that will give your body a good stretch.

TABLE 12.1 Your Flexibility Exercise Program

Exercise	*Body Part*	*Repetitions/Dates*																

Reference

Hittleman, Richard. *Yoga Twenty-eight Day Exercise Book*. New York: Bantam, 1978.

Suggested Readings

Alter, Judy. *Stretch and Strengthen*. Boston: Houghton Mifflin, 1986.
Lyons, P. and D. Burgard. *Great Shape*. New York: Arbor House/Wm. Morrow, 1988.
Thygerson, A. *Fitness and Health: Life-Style Strategies*. Boston: Jones and Bartlett, 1989.
Tobias, M. and M. Stewart. *Stretch to Relax*. Tucson: The Body Press, 1985.

13 AEROBIC (FAT REDUCTION) EXERCISE PROGRAM

AS A PROSPECTIVE weight reducer you should be able to distinguish which kinds of exercise will use up body fat more efficiently than other kinds. The last two chapters have discussed the kinds of activities that are not very good for fat reduction: muscle strength and endurance exercises and flexibility, or stretching, exercises. Those exercises are generally not strenuous enough over a long enough period of time; thus they burn up available carbohydrates (blood sugar) rather than fats. Even though they provide flexibility and muscle tone that keep the body healthy, safe, and attractive, they burn little fat.

The kinds of activities that will burn stored fat must be of long enough duration that the body goes beyond burning the available carbohydrates and starts pulling fat out of the fat deposits to use for energy production in the muscles. These exercises are commonly called "aerobic" because they make you work hard enough to demand a lot of oxygen. By doing aerobic exercises you increase your ability to take in and deliver more oxygen to all parts of your body, and thus work and play more efficiently. The main benefits are stronger heart, lungs, and vascular system, *and* fat reduction! The side benefits are numerous and were mentioned at the beginning of Chapter 10 as the selling points of the medicine man's product. All these benefits are commonly called the *training effect*.

Generally, aerobic exercises:

1. Must be done for at least 15 minutes per session to get the cardiovascular training effects. Some authorities suggest 12 minutes, but there is a warm-up period in which your heart rate is increasing to the proper intensity; therefore 15 minutes per session is a proper goal.

2. Must be strenuous enough to produce cardiovascular training effects.
3. Must be continuous activity (not stop-and-go, like tennis or bowling).

The principal aerobic exercise forms that will be discussed in this chapter are: dancing, rope skipping, bench stepping, cross-country skiing, bicycling, walking, running, and jogging. Other activities such as handball, racquetball, squash, swimming, and so on are considered by some as aerobic, but it must be remembered that the action should be continuous—not allowing the heart rate to drop below a training rate.

Some Cautions

It is normally advised that if you are not an active person, if you have refrained from regular physical activity for a long period of time, or if you are over 30 years old, you should have a physician's approval to start a cardiovascular fitness program. Another way to ensure a safe program would be to plan it under the supervision of a trained health professional. It is possible for those who have cardiovascular problems or other health problems to engage in some aerobic activity, but it *must be under proper supervision.*

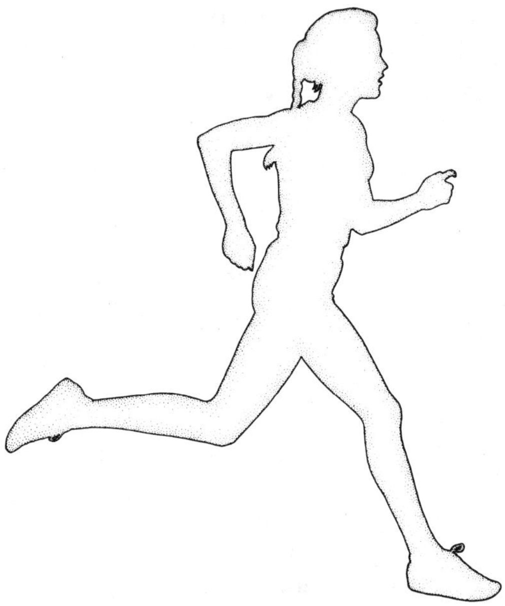

If when you are engaging in an aerobic exercise, you feel faint, become dizzy or disoriented, or feel ill in any way, ease down to a very slow walk, sit down with your head between your legs, or lie down flat on your back. This will help move blood back to your head more easily than if you were just standing.

Plan to do your aerobic exercise in the cool part of the day and when you are slightly hungry, rather than just after you've eaten. If you perspire profusely, consider taking sodium/potassium pills or drinks, and drink plenty of fluids.

Taking Your Heart Rate

This is a skill that should be developed by everyone. Your heart rate is an extremely valuable piece of information for you at all times. So if you do not know how to take your own pulse, you'll want to take some time now to learn. Your heart rate is a key element in cardiovascular fitness.

Every time your heart beats it sends out a "shock wave" that can be felt in most major arteries of the body. The shock wave comes from pushing the blood out of the heart and into the aorta, and it is related to the highest point in your blood pressure reading (your systolic pressure).

There are two major points on the body that are easiest to find your pulse: on your wrist (the radial artery pulse) and on your forehead (the temple pulse).

Put light pressure on the area so you don't shut off the pulse. If you are taking your own pulse you can use your thumb, but in taking another person's pulse use your fingers. Your thumb has a pulse of its own and the fingers do not. So in taking another's pulse, you must use your fingers rather than your thumb so that what you feel will be the other's pulse, not yours. One or both of these two arteries may be buried somewhat, so you may have to probe around a bit to find them.

THE RADIAL PULSE

Using your first two or three fingers on either hand, place the fleshy part of the fingers on the inside of the opposite wrist in the small hollow between the ligament that stands out in the middle of the wrist (running lengthwise) and the outside of your wrist on the thumb side (see Figure 13.1).

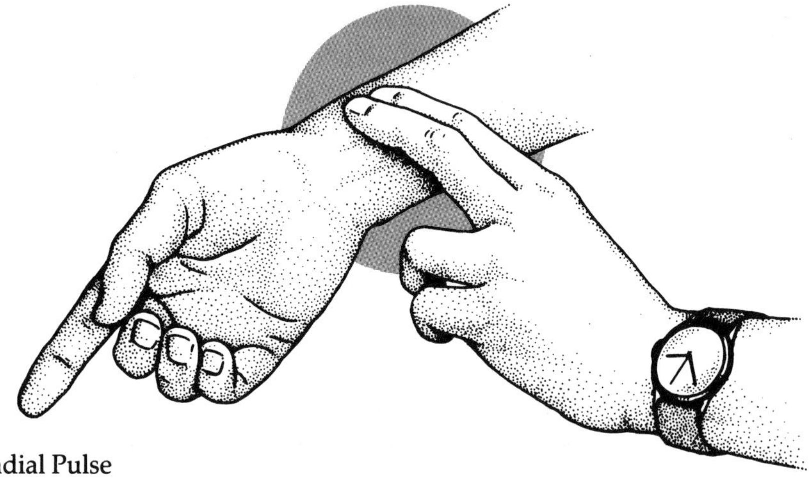

FIGURE 13.1 The Radial Pulse

THE TEMPLE PULSE

One place on the head where an artery is fairly exposed is at the temple. Figure 13.2 shows where to find this pulse. After exercising, place your fingers lightly on your temple and take your pulse while continuing to move slowly. Always start your count with "zero." Although it may be tempting to take your pulse at the carotid artery on the side of the neck, resist the temptation, as pressure at this point causes a reflex slowing of the heart.

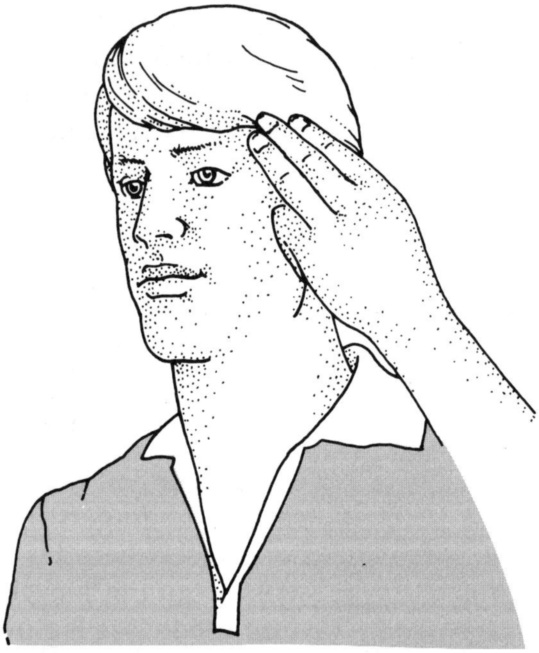

FIGURE 13.2 The Temple Pulse

COUNTING THE PULSE

After you find your pulse in either area, start counting each beat that you feel. Feel the cadence of your pulse while you sit and then stand up, still feeling your pulse. Feel what happens. Run in place for 30 seconds and then feel your pulse.

Now get a watch or clock with a second hand and take your resting, sitting pulse for one minute. Taking the resting pulse for a whole minute is better than taking it for just 10 seconds and multiplying by 6—it gives you a full picture of what is happening for that minute. When you have taken your resting pulse several times while seated, record it on the chart in Table 13.1. Then lie down and take your pulse several times. Record each reading. Do the same after standing still for two minutes, after running in place for one minute, and after a given period of physical activity of your choice, such as 50 minutes of tennis. In the latter case, record what activity you did and how long the exercise period was.

TABLE 13.1 Your Pulse Chart

Activity	*Trials*			*Average*
Sitting resting pulse				
Standing resting pulse				
Lying resting pulse during the day				
Pulse after 1-minute run in place				
Pulse during chosen exercise ___________ exercise _____ min.				
Resting pulse/A.M. in bed				

The last pulse on the chart is to be taken immediately upon awakening in the morning, preferably when you wake up naturally, not to the sound of the alarm or the jar of your child jumping into your bed. This will be your lowest resting heart rate (RHR)—it tells you how often your heart has to pump when there are only basal demands on it. Take it tomorrow morning (if you can), and then record it once or twice a week during your new exercise program. You'll be surprised at what your program can do for your resting heart rate!

The medical physiology textbooks state that the average heart rate for adults is 72 beats per minute. In a highly trained individual the resting heart rate may drop as low as 35 to 40 beats per minute. Imagine the difference between the demand a heart with a resting rate of 60 beats per minute has and the demand handled by a heart with a resting rate of 40 beats per minute has. In one minute, the latter heart would beat 20 times less and rest one-third more of the time. The trained heart is stronger, more efficient, and gets more rest than the untrained heart.

It will be necessary for you to know your resting heart rate in order to calculate your training, or exercise, heart rate.

Intensity and Heart Rate

Virtually all exercisers ask the same question, "How hard should I exercise to get myself into shape?" The answer depends on several factors, such as your fitness level, how fast you wish to progress, and what kind of exercise you can perform. With aerobic exercise the amount of training or improvement you get from your exercise varies with the intensity and duration of your activity. Since intensity of exercise can be determined by your heart rate, it is fairly easy to monitor. A healthy young person (less than 30 years of age) whose heart rate during aerobic exercise increases to only 110 beats per minute would get about the same training effects in three hours that would be obtained in twenty minutes if the heart rate were 140 beats per minute (Cooper, 1982). Younger, healthier, more physically fit people can exercise harder for a shorter period of time, while less fit people should take more time and exercise less strenuously in order to get the benefits of the exercise and see improvement in their fitness.

The American College of Sports Medicine (1986) recommends that adults:

1. Exercise three to five times per week.
2. Exercise to an intensity of 60 to 90 percent of their maximum heart rate reserve.
3. Exercise for periods of 15 to 60 minutes in continuous activity in which the duration is dependent upon the intensity of the activity. The nonathletic adult should engage in lower to moderate intensity for a longer period of time than the athletic adult.
4. Engage in activity that involves large muscle groups and that can be maintained continuously.

To determine the intensity at which you should exercise, you'll want to calculate what is called your "training heart rate." This is the heart rate at which you get all the training effects from your exercises. To calculate this you first determine your *resting heart rate* and your *maximum heart rate*. Earlier in this chapter you assessed your resting heart rate (take it in the morning before you get up and figure the average for several days). Now determine your maximum heart rate.

MAXIMUM HEART RATE

Your maximum heart rate (MHR) is as fast as your heart can beat. For the hummingbird, maximum heart rate is over 500 beats per minute! However, for men and women, it is considerably lower, and it decreases with age. A common method for finding your maximum heart rate is to subtract your age from 226 if you're a female and from 220 if you're a male. The difference in these numbers is based on the difference in maximum heart rate that men and women can achieve. Women's average maximum heart rate is slightly higher than men's. Calculate your maximum heart rate here:

WOMEN	*MEN*
MHR = 226 − age	MHR = 220 − age
Your MHR = ____	Your MHR = ____

TRAINING HEART RATE

Once you know your maximum heart rate and your resting heart rate, you can determine your training heart rate (THR). The following formula will tell you what your heart rate should be to get cardiovascular training effects from your exercise. The .60 in the formula is a suggested 60 percent of maximum heart rate, but the formula is individualized by inserting the resting heart rate (RHR).

$$\text{training heart rate (THR)} = [(\text{MHR} - \text{RHR}) \times .60] + \text{RHR}$$

Let's take an example of a 26-year-old woman who has a resting heart rate of 80. Her MHR is 200 so her training heart rate is:

$$\begin{aligned} \text{THR} &= [(\text{MHR} - \text{RHR}) \times .60] + \text{RHR} \\ &= 200 - 80 \times .60 + 80 \\ &= 120 \times .60 + 80 \\ &= 72 + 80 \\ &= 152 \text{ beats per minute (BPM)} \end{aligned}$$

This means that when she exercises, she should increase her heart rate to 152 and keep it there for 15 minutes to get her training effects.

Training Heart Rate Range. If you are in good cardiovascular shape, your formula for training heart rate can be revised from 60% to 70% or even 80% of maximum heart rate. It is not advisable to go beyond 80% of maximum unless you are a highly conditioned and competitive athlete. One practice that works well for those just starting a cardiovascular program is to find a *range* of training heart rates. Then during exercise, the beginner keeps the heart rate above a minimum and below a maximum. A recommended range for beginners is between 60% and 70% of the maximum heart rate (corrected for resting heart rate) (American College of Sports Medicine, 1986). If you feel that you are really out of shape, you might want to try a range of 50% to 60%. To find the range, use the THR formula with each of the figures you choose. The results will give you the low end and the high end of your range.

To use our same example, the THR at 60% was 152 BPM. Training heart rate for this same woman at a 70% figure would be:

$$\begin{aligned} \text{THR} &= [(\text{MHR} - \text{RHR}) \times .70] + \text{RHR} \\ &= 200 - 80 \times .70 + 80 \\ &= 120 \times .70 + 80 \\ &= 84 + 80 \\ &= 164 \text{ BPM} \end{aligned}$$

As she improves her cardiovascular fitness she will have to work a little harder to get her heart rate to a training level. At this point she may want to upgrade her range from 60–70% to 70–80%. The top of her new range would be:

$$\begin{aligned} \text{THR} &= [(\text{MHR} - \text{RHR}) \times .80] + \text{RHR} \\ &= 200 - 80 \times .80 + 80 \\ &= 120 \times .80 + 80 \\ &= 96 + 80 \\ &= 176 \text{ BPM} \end{aligned}$$

Her new range would be 164 to 176.

If, after weeks of training her RHR went down to 60, she would have to insert that new figure into the formula and her 70–80% range extremes would then be 158 to 172.

Taking Your Training Heart Rate. Finding out what your heart rate is when you do cardiovascular exercise is simple. Once you know how to take your resting heart rate, you have the problem half solved. The other half of the problem is solved by taking a short (6- to 10-second) pulse rate *immediately* after you stop exercising. A caution to heed when finding your postexercise heart rate is to *keep walking slowly* while finding and counting your pulse. You can easily check if you are within your THR range by multiplying your pulse by 10 or 6, depending on how long you wish to take your pulse. When the woman runner of the example started her program, her THR range was 152 to 164. Her 10-second pulse after cardiovascular exercise should be between 25 and 27 BMP (See Figure 13.3). If she took a 6-second pulse count, she would expect the count to be 15 or 16 (152/10 and 164/10) to be within her THR range.

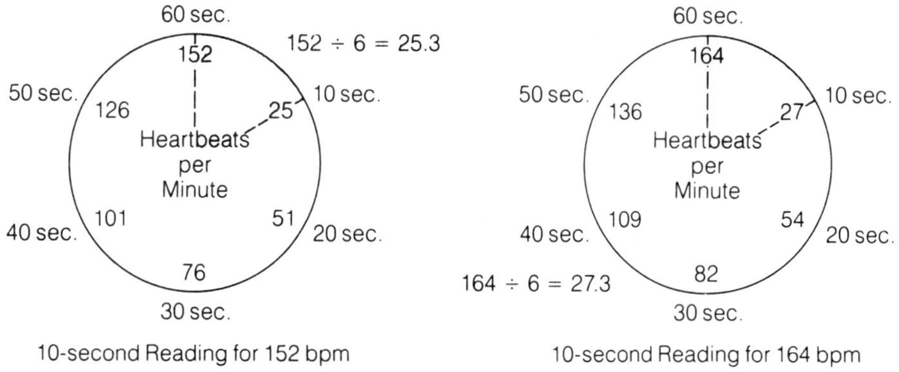

FIGURE 13.3 A Ten-Second Reading for a THR Range of 152 to 164

This is an easy check to see if the heart rate is in the proper range. If it is too low, the exerciser must increase the intensity of the activity. If the heart rate is too high, the intensity should be decreased.

If you are just beginning a cardiovascular program, start out walking briskly for a few minutes and take your postexercise pulse (keep walking slowly as you take it). See what your heart rate is for that exercise. It *may* be high enough for your training rate. If your heart rate didn't go high enough with a brisk walk, alternately jog and walk. If that still does not get you to your THR, jog more than you walk. Always increase the intensity if you are not yet into your range, and decrease the intensity if your heart rate is too high.

One of the most common reasons beginners in cardiovascular programs quit their programs is because they get too tired and say, "It's just not worth it." Usually, these people start their programs with too much intensity and "burn themselves out." You can help make cardiovascular exercise enjoyable for yourself by making it into a heart rate game. Calculate your THR range and monitor it repeatedly at first. Learn what you can do to increase your heart rate and keep it in your range. After a short while you will need to monitor it only periodically to make sure the intensity of your exercise maintains pace with your training effects. You should also take your resting heart rate periodically (at least once a week) and record it. If you are in your THR range and exercise often enough, you will see the difference it is making in your heart rate. A slower heart rate at rest generally means a healthier heart.

If you have initial difficulty in finding or getting to your THR range, be assured that exercise of less intensity will, in fact, help build up your cardiovascular system. Walking is an excellent exercise to start with because it demands less from your body parts, especially your knee and ankle joints. If you feel that you are not ready for a vigorous cardiovascular exercise, just go out and *walk*. A person who is nonathletic can get a significant training effect with a sustained training heart rate as low as 110 to 120 beats per minute (American College of Sports Medicine, 1986).

Aerobic Exercises

Each of the activities that follow can be used effectively for fat reduction if you stay within your THR range for 15 minutes or more. The effectiveness of the exercise is less if you do not reach your training heart rate, but remember that there is some effect, especially if you spend more time doing the activity.

To help you see your progress and meet a cardiovascular fitness goal for yourself, keep a record of your exercises in the chart in Table 13.2. Also, make a reasonable goal for yourself to meet in a specified time; for example, running two miles in 20 minutes, achieving a resting heart rate of 72, and so on.

DANCING

Dancing is a popular activity that is seldom thought of as exercise. But if its intensity and duration are right for you, it becomes a fat-burning exercise. Aerobic dancing is popular in many areas. It consists of doing a pattern of exercises to music, and it is tailored to the fitness of each participant. Any aerobic dancer can tell you it's a great workout. If you cannot join a local aerobic dance class or if you lack creativity in making your own dance, you can buy a book of complete instructions and even video tapes on aerobic dance at many bookstores.

Other kinds of dancing can be fat-burning exercise, too, if you dance nonstop for 15 minutes. Most popular dances are of great enough intensity to qualify as fat burners, and some of the old favorites such as the polka are also good exercises.

If you cannot find uninterrupted music that lasts long enough, tape a 15-minute segment of something you like. You could also make up a "between songs" routine to keep you moving. Compose your own dance routine with hopping, jumping, running, kicks, arm exercises, and so on. Invite a friend to join you—dancing with a partner is more fun.

ROPE SKIPPING

Again, you must skip rope for 15 minutes to get the benefit of burning fat. Make yourself a rope (of nylon, about one-half inch in diameter) with plastic tubing for the handles. Put a knot on each side of the handle so it stays in place. Stand on the rope with it under the balls of both feet. The ends of the rope should come to midchest.

Avoid jumping on both feet together or jumping on a hard surface—it's tough on the feet, shins, and knees. Instead, take a step, then hop on each foot alternately. Or, if you have some space, run as you twirl your rope. Jump on grass, a mat, or something softer than concrete. You can try fancy routines and cross your arms as you

TABLE 13.2 Your Aerobic Exercise Program

Goal	*Date for Goal*			
Date	Activity	Duration (time, miles, etc.)	THR	RHR (A.M.)

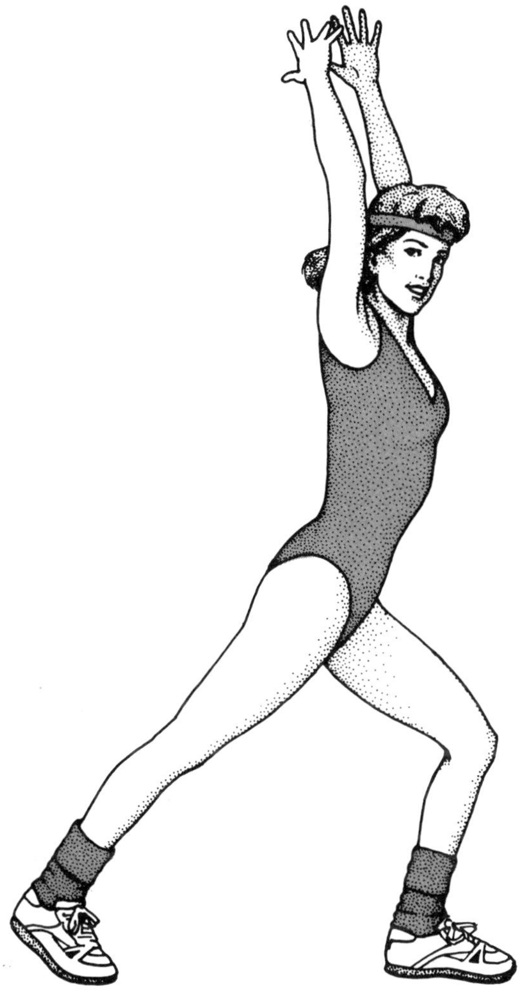

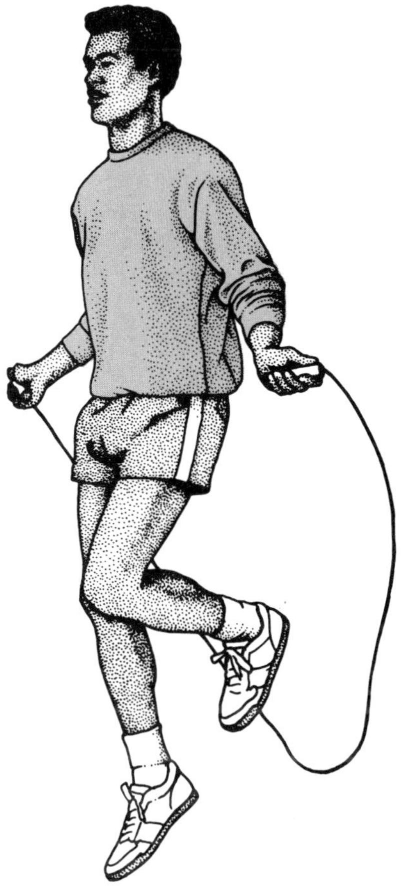

swing the rope. A good way to avoid boredom is to do a number of step-hops, then a few single hops, then a number of crosses—almost like doing your own dance routine. You can do it to music, too, or while you're watching TV.

BENCH STEPPING

The bench step exercise became popular as a form of exercise to test cardiovascular fitness. The Harvard Step Test is familiar to thousands of high school and college students who were asked to step up on a 18-inch or 21-inch bench and back down to the beat of a metronome for three to five minutes. Those who couldn't keep up with the beat

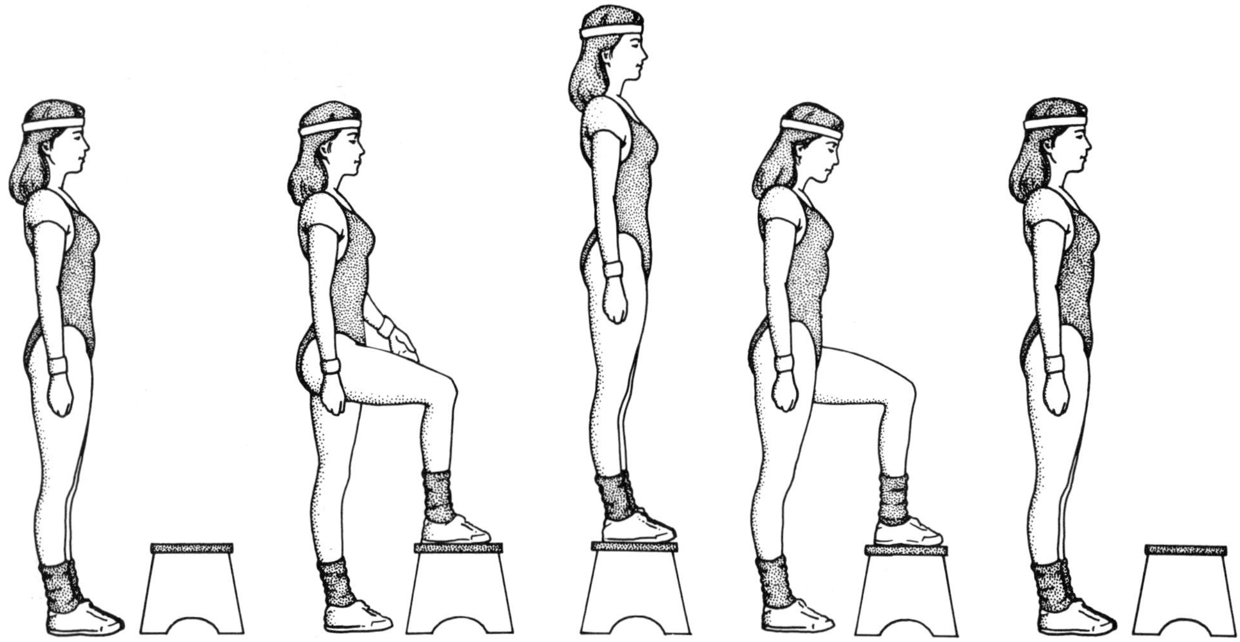

were asked to sit down and their pulse rates were taken at various intervals to see what the heart recovery rate was. The sooner the heart rate decreased to nearly normal, the more fit was the cardiovascular system.

The exercise is simple. Step up on a low bench (that is firm and stable) with your right or your left foot (it doesn't matter which one goes first), then step up with the other foot. Step down with your lead foot, then bring the other foot down, and stand on the floor. If you start with your left foot, the sequence will be "up with your left, up with your right, down with the left, and down with the right." Continue this for 15 minutes at an intensity rate that is right for you.

CROSS-COUNTRY SKIING

This is an exercise that combines skiing, skating and hiking. Although seasonal, it is a great form of exercise. It is easy on the knees and ankles because you glide rather than bring your body weight down on your feet as you do in walking or running. It's easy to cross-country ski for 15 minutes—in fact, it's hard to stop at just 15 minutes. If you live where it snows, you'll probably want to try cross-country skiing.

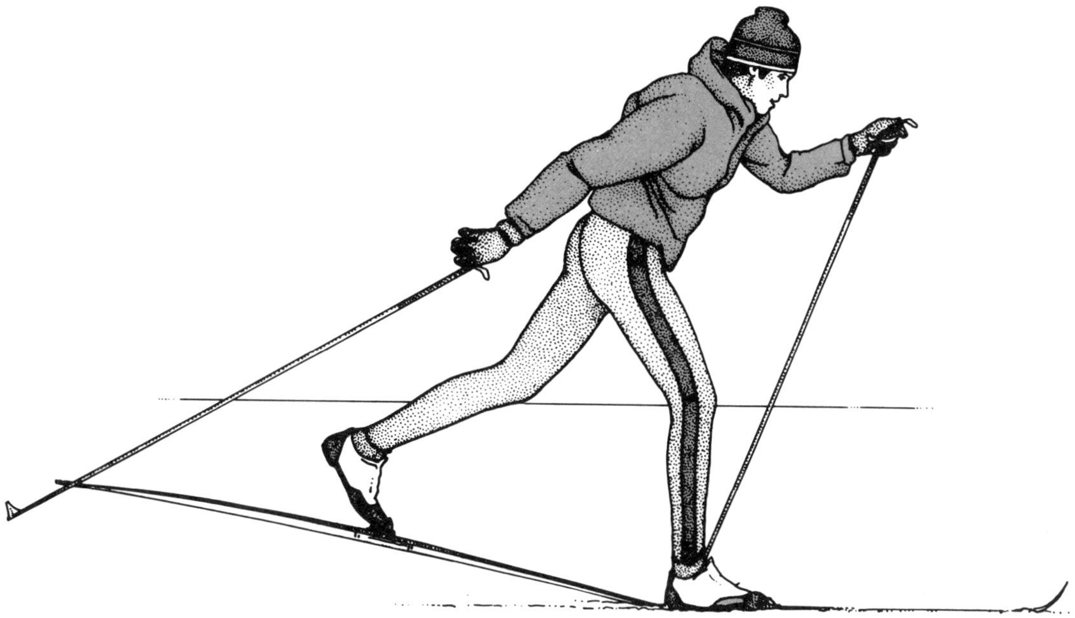

It is relatively easy to master the art of cross-country skiing in a short period of time. The diagonal stride consists of pushing off and gliding on one foot while swinging the opposite arm forward vigorously after having planted that pole in the snow and pushing off on it. Racers also skate on their skis. This activity will cost a certain amount for boots, poles, and skis, but like running, your exercise area can be the wide open spaces. Track fees at commercial cross-country ski areas are usually only a few dollars for all day.

BICYCLING

Whether stationary or moving, a bicycle gives you great fat-burning exercise that is easy on the joints. Of all the exercises presented here, bicycling may be the most expensive in equipment. A good stationary bike will cost at least $100 and you may pay $500 or more for a top-of-the-line model. You need one that is stable, allows you to add resistance to the wheel, and has a speedometer. An odometer also provides great motivation as you can see how many miles you have ridden and you can focus on tenths of a mile as they click by. Also, for a more interesting ride, if your radio, TV, or stereo has earphones or ear plugs, enjoy your favorite show or music without the noise of the bike.

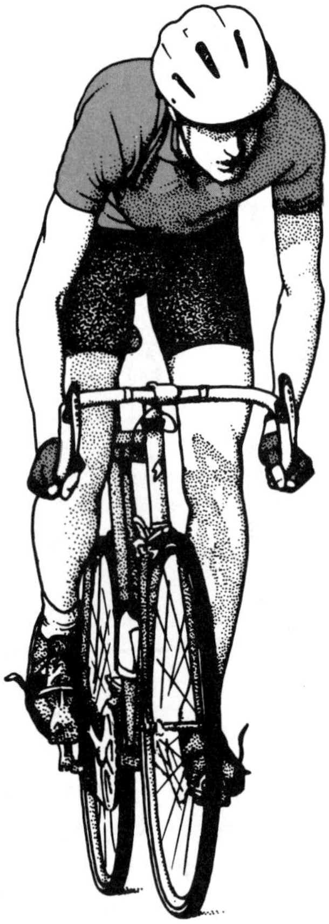

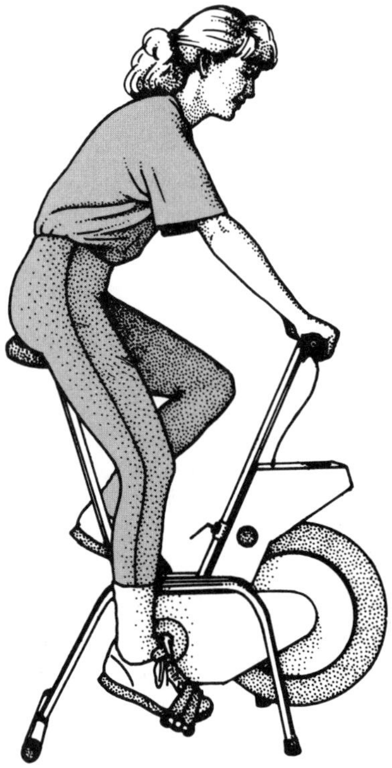

A caution for stationary bike riders is to avoid cranking the resistance up too high too soon, straining the knees and forcing the heart rate too high.

For a regular, ride-around-town bike, you should have at least a five-speed. This allows you to keep the intensity of exercise constant over flat terrain and up hills. Find some interesting bike paths and enjoy being out in the fresh air while you slim down. If you must ride in automobile traffic, invest in a rear view mirror and be sure you know the safety rules and skills involved in biking.

WALKING

This exercise is the easiest and cheapest. A good pair of walking shoes (or running shoes) must be worn, but you don't need the extra shock absorbent quality of a running shoe. However, many walkers become joggers or runners, so putting money into a good pair of shoes at this point would be worthwhile. After you have been in a walking program for a while, you will find your walks must be faster to maintain the intensity of exercise you need. When walking will no longer give you enough intensity, you will have to switch to some other fat-burning exercise.

I had a 52-year-old student in my program a few years ago who chose walking as her exercise and lost more than a pound a week for the 15 weeks of the program. She also grew to love her walking time. She would look forward to investing some time in herself each day, a time when she did not have to worry about taking care of the rest of her family.

If safety is a problem in your neighborhood, walk with a friend and/or in the daylight hours. A friend in Wyoming has started a

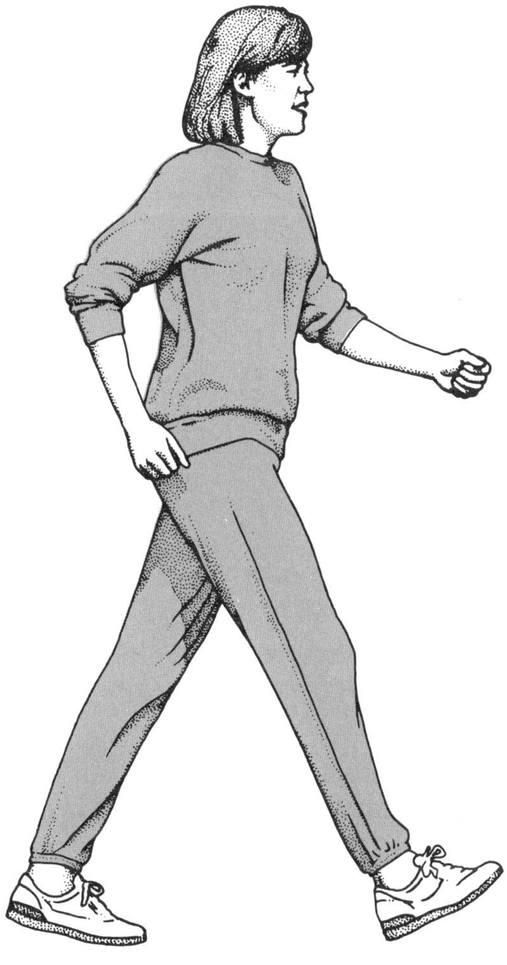

"walking club" with her friends. Nearly everywhere I go, I see former students and their children, spouses, family dogs, and/or others out for their morning or evening jaunt. Surely there is a Zen of walking.

RUNNING AND JOGGING

These activities can be discussed together, for the main differences between them are speed and the mechanics of speed. Good running shoes are a *must* in this activity—they provide support and protection for your feet, and the heel thickness absorbs some of the shock of your weight hitting the ground. Jogging and running may jar the ankle and knee joints in susceptible individuals, but good shoes, proper running form, good warm-up, and preparation for a running program help make running a favorite activity of millions of Americans.

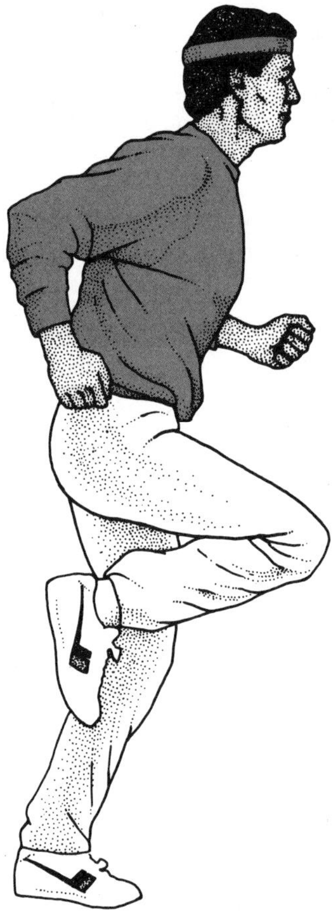

Running at the proper intensity for you will burn off your fat, flatten your stomach, and strengthen your buttocks and leg muscles, not to mention all the other benefits of aerobic exercise. A conditioning program that helps strengthen your posture muscles will help your running, making it easier to hold yourself erect. In holding a relaxed, upright posture, you conserve energy and feel in control of your movement. I watched a runner one day in the suburbs of a small Texas town. He was loping along toward me, easy, upright, relaxed, when suddenly he made a great leap sideways and kept on running. Such agility comes from being in shape and in control! As I approached the spot of his sideways jump, I found what I suspected to be the cause of that agile leap—a dead rattlesnake!

To avoid shin splints, a pulled Achilles tendon, and sore calf muscles, a good combination of stretching exercises should be done before and after running. The exercises I recommend to all beginning runners are the crossed-arm bent-knee sit-up, or crunches, sitting hamstring stretch, calf stretch, hunker squat, and push-ups. All of these exercises are described in Chapters 11 and 12 on muscular strength and endurance and stretching exercises.

A young woman in my program started a running program on her own, but after two days of her new program she hobbled in complaining of sore shins and calf muscles. Joyce, the young woman, explained that she got up at her regular time in the morning, jumped into her new running suit, had a quick cup of coffee, and ran out to do her exercise. On the first day of her program she covered a full mile, running as fast as she could until she was exhausted, then walking, and finally ending with a brisk walk. Her fast run, using the calf muscles to push off on her toes, was too much too soon for her muscles. She did no stretching before she ran, and she ran her mile on city sidewalks. She didn't monitor her heart rate to prevent total exhaustion. No wonder she wasn't having any fun!

I reviewed proper running technique with Joyce: Hit on the heel with the knee directly over the heel, rock to the ball of the foot and push off from the toe for the next step. (This is probably the most natural way to run and proves to be the least tiring. Running on toes is great for sprinting, but sprinting is not considered fat burning because a person can't sprint for that long.) After setting her pace at her proper intensity, adding some stretching and conditioning exercises, correcting her running mechanics, and running on a regular running path, Joyce became a fan of running and began losing weight and collecting the other benefits of running.

Summary

Choose an aerobic exercise that your body most prefers, but beware, you may become addicted to it! Millions of Americans have joined running or jogging clubs, cross-country skiing groups, or bicycling groups and have found such enjoyment in the life it has brought them that they feel restless and unhappy when they don't get their exercise.

Again, as with the strength and stretching exercises, keep a chart of your progress (Table 13.2). The change in your resting heart rate will tell you quite a story as your endurance improves. But also keep track of body measurements, a mental image (or actual pictures) of how you physically look now, and how the scores change on your Readiness Profile (Chapter 1), your Nutrition Profile (Chapter 8), your Exercise Profile (Chapter 10), and your Stress Profile (Chapter 7) that you have taken in this book.

References

American College of Sports Medicine. *Guidelines for Exercise Testing and Prescription*, 3rd edition. Philadelphia: Lea & Febiger, 1986.

Cooper, Kenneth. *The Aerobics Program for Total Well-Being*. New York: Bantam Books, 1982.

Suggested Readings

Baitch, S. "Aerobics Dance Injuries," *JOPERD*, (May–June, 1987): 57–58.

Cantu, R. *Exercise Injuries: Prevention and Treatment*. New York: Stone Wall Press, 1983.

Cooper, Kenneth. *The Aerobics Program for Total Well-Being*. New York: M. Evans, 1982.

deVries, H. *Physiology of Exercise*, 4th edition. Dubuque, IA: W.C. Brown, 1986.

Fonda, Jane. *Jane Fonda's New Workout and Weight Loss Program*. New York: Simon and Schuster, 1986.

Kashiwa, A., and J. Rippe. *Fitness Walking for Women*. New York: Perigee, 1987.

Katz, Jane. *Fitness Works!* Champaign, IL: Leisure Press, 1988.

Lawrence, R., and S. Rosenweig. *Going the Distance*. Los Angeles: Tarcher, 1987.

Matarazzu, et al. (eds.). *Behavioral Health: A Handbook of Health Enhancement and Disease Prevention*. New York: Wiley, 1984.

Prudden, Bonnie. *Bonnie Prudden's After Fifty Fitness Guide*. New York: Ballantine, 1986.

Schwartz, L. *Heavyhands Walking*. Emmaus, PA: Rodale Press, 1987.

Sutton, R. *Body Worry*. New York: Penguin, 1988.

Zugibe, F. *14 Days to a Healthy Heart*. New York: Avon, 1986.

14 PUTTING IT ALL TOGETHER

WHAT DOES IT TAKE to learn a total fitness lifestyle? You must *adopt* it as your own.

Adapt the self-responsibility lessons to your background and experience so you can grow more independent, spontaneous, assertive, and self-assured.
Take what you can from the knowledge and lessons about eating and apply this to your life.
Begin physical exercise as a regular and integral part of your lifestyle.
Protect yourself against stress so that your life runs more smoothly.

Do you notice something missing from this list? Perhaps you are thinking of starving yourself, following a silly fad diet for a short while, or focusing on how much you weigh? These things are not necessary to get fit. Total fitness is a result of carefully putting self-responsibility, good food and eating habits, regular exercise, and stress protection techniques into your life. Your weight will take care of itself!

This book has presented some choices and suggestions for how to do each of these lifestyle activities. However, you have one thing left to do—*commit yourself*. To help you do this, the following pages contain four contracts you will want to make with yourself. Each contains the main components necessary for effective learning of the fitness lifestyle proposed in this book (Crockford and Marks, 1980; Ostrander and Shroeder, 1978).

The first of these learning components is *intention*. Acting in a certain way is a quality of intention. Once you intend to do anything, it is the main factor in being able to do it. Merely picking up this book and reading it is an act of intention. The only thing that can stop you now is a little thought in the back of your mind that says, "I can't." *You can* effectively change your lifestyle to one of total fitness. Chapter 1 pointed that out repeatedly.

A second important component is the attitude that *"I am already doing it"* (where "it" is some kind of exercise program, some good eating habits, behaving in a self-responsible way, and performing some relaxation techniques). Each time you miss your exercises it proves that you are *already* doing something (that there *is* something to miss). The statement, "I have a fitness program," is a prerequisite to being physically fit—not a result of a successful fitness program. Affirm that you have it, and you have it!

The third component that is necessary in learning sometimes hurts the ego. The component is *being willing to accept whatever happens in your program,* no matter how much social or physical discomfort (which translates into psychological discomfort) there is in it. Accept your experiences as they happen. They may be embarrassing and you may make mistakes, feel stupid or clumsy, feel like you are wasting time, and so on. But none of these feelings have anything to do with your ability at any one point—they are part of the process, part of the experience you are having while you learn the fitness lifestyle. How can you learn if you don't make mistakes? Suppose you didn't exercise at all today and you ate two pieces of chocolate cake. Now you know how that feels. Mistakes are okay. Your feelings of being unsuccessful come from your past experience—not from what is happening *right now.*

The fourth component is *commitment.* You'll want to put a commitment *in writing* so that not only can you see your success in learning about the fitness lifestyle, but you can also see when you are actually putting it into practice. When you look back at your weekly history, you can be proud that you're a *doer.* The more specific the commitment, the more effective it will be.

To aid you in your commitment, charts have been provided throughout this book so that you may commit yourself in writing to an exercise program, to greater readiness and self-responsibility in those areas of your life that you wish to change, to successful eating practices and menus, and to a relaxation training program.

So now it's time to *do it.* You have all the equipment you need. Read and sign the contracts in this chapter (have a witness if you wish this to be a public commitment), and commit yourself via the charts and schedules given throughout this book. Doing this, you will already be living a lifestyle of fitness. Good luck!

Self-Contract 1: Readiness and Self-Responsibility

I AGREE TO APPROACH MY READINESS TO TAKE ON GREATER SELF-RESPONSIBILITY FROM THE FOLLOWING POINT OF VIEW:

1. The *intention* to be ready to take on greater self-responsibility is the main factor in being able to do it. The only thing that can stop me from doing it is the thought that "I can't." I am willing to assume that if I have the intention of being self-responsible, then I will be able to do so.

2. The attitude "I am self-responsible" is a *prerequisite* to successfully learning how, not the result of such success. I know that if I hold this attitude, mistakes and difficulties become evidence of my *current* skill level rather than being indications of whether or not I *can* become self-responsible.

3. I agree to *accept* whatever happens in the program and *stay with it*, even if it means some discomfort. Discomfort can be in the form of embarrassment, confusion, looking or feeling stupid, making mistakes, feeling awkward, and so on. I am willing to accept that discomfort is a normal and natural part of my learning process and is *not* an indication of whether or not I *can* become self-responsible.

4. Being responsible for myself really means making a *commitment* to use specific techniques to become more self-responsible. The more specific the commitment, the better the result. To make this program truly worthwhile, I will begin—right now—using my Readiness Profile and Readiness History of Change Schedule to help myself become more self-responsible. Specifically, I will set definite times and places to work on all the readiness/self-responsibility skills that I need to work on.

______________________________ __________________

Name | Date

____

Witness (optional)

Self-Contract 2: Eating and Nutrition

I AGREE TO APPROACH EATING AND NUTRITION FROM THE FOLLOWING POINT OF VIEW:

1. The *intention* to eat nutritiously and wisely is the main factor in being able to do it. The only thing that can stop me from doing it is the thought that "I can't." I am willing to assume that if I have the intention of eating nutritiously and wisely, then I will be able to do so.

2. The attitude "I am eating wisely and nutritiously" is a *prerequisite* to successfully learning how—not the result of such success. I know that if I hold this attitude, mistakes and difficulties become evidence of my *current* skill level rather than being indications of whether or not I *can* eat wisely and nutritiously.

3. I agree to *accept* whatever happens in the program and *stay with it*, even if it means some discomfort. Discomfort can be in the form of embarrassment, having to plan ahead, confusion, looking or feeling stupid, making mistakes, feeling awkward, special preparation, and so on. I am willing to accept that discomfort is a normal and natural part of my learning process and is *not* an indication of whether or not I *can* eat wisely and nutritiously.

4. Eating wisely and nutritiously really means making a *commitment* to use the eating patterns and menus I make for myself at home, in restaurants, or while traveling. The more specific the commitment, the better the result. To make this program truly worthwhile, I will begin—right now—using the menu techniques and knowledge in Chapters 5 and 9 to help myself eat wisely and nutritiously. Specifically, I will plan definite menus a week ahead of time and conscientiously shop for, order, and prepare the foods I have chosen.

______________________________ ________________

Name Date

____

Witness (optional)

Self-Contract 3: Stress Protection

I AGREE TO APPROACH RELAXATION TRAINING FROM THE FOLLOWING POINT OF VIEW:

1. The *intention* to learn how to relax is the main factor in being able to do so. The only thing that can stop me from performing relaxation techniques is the thought that "I can't." I am willing to assume that if I have the intention of learning how to relax, I will be able to do so.

2. The attitude "I am relaxed" is a *prerequisite* to successfully learning how to relax, not the result of such success. I know that if I hold this attitude, mistakes and difficulties become evidence of my *current* skill level rather than being indications of whether or not I *can* become relaxed.

3. I agree to *accept* whatever happens in the program and *stay with it*, even if it means some discomfort. Discomfort can be in the form of embarrassment, confusion, looking or feeling stupid, making mistakes, feeling awkward, not seeing immediate progress, and so on. I am willing to accept that discomfort is a normal and natural part of my learning process and is *not* an indication of whether or not I *can* relax.

4. Being relaxed really means making a *commitment* to use the techniques in Chapter 7. The more specific the commitment, the better the results. To make this program truly worthwhile, I will begin—right now—using the Stress Protection Program given in Chapter 7 to help myself to learn to be more relaxed and less emotionally reactive. Specifically, I will set definite times and places where I will use the relaxation techniques given here and others that I have learned.

______________________________ ________________
Name Date

____
Witness (optional)

Self-Contract 4: Exercise

I AGREE TO APPROACH EXERCISE FROM THE FOLLOWING POINT OF VIEW:

1. The *intention* to exercise regularly is the main factor in being *able* to do it. The only thing that can stop me from exercising regularly is the thought that "I can't." I am willing to assume that if I have the intention of exercising regularly, then I will be able to do so.

2. The attitude "I am physically active in an exercise program" is a *prerequisite* to successfully learning how to implement a program, not the result of such success. In the same way, "I am an exerciser" is a prerequisite to, not a result of, learning to exercise. I know that if I hold this attitude, mistakes and difficulties become evidence of my *current* skill level rather than being indications of whether or not I *can* exercise regularly and proficiently.

3. I agree to *accept* whatever happens in the program and *stay with it*, even if it means some discomfort. Discomfort can be in the form of embarrassment, confusion, looking or feeling stupid, making mistakes, feeling awkward, feeling time-pressured, physical discomfort, and so on. I am willing to accept that discomfort is a normal and natural part of my learning process and is *not* an indication of whether or not I *can* exercise regularly and proficiently.

4. Exercising regularly really means making a *commitment* to use the techniques given in Chapters 10 through 13 at home, at school, or wherever I spend time. The more specific the commitment, the better the results. To make this program truly worthwhile, I will begin—right now—using the exercise program charts in this book to help myself become a regular exerciser. Specifically, I will set definite times and places to exercise.

______________________________ ________________

Name Date

____

Witness (optional)

References

Crockford, Phillip, Mary Marks, and Working Miracles. "Teaching Aid." *In Touch for Health*. November 1980, p. 11. (Adapted from Dr. Georgi Lozanov's work in accelerated or "superlearning" techniques.)

Ostrander, Sheila, and Lynn Schroeder, with Nancy Ostrander. *Superlearning*. New York: Delta, 1978.

APPENDIX

A FORMULAS AND NOMOGRAMS TO DETERMINE PERCENTAGE OF BODY FAT

I. Skinfold measurements and formulas for young women (Sloan, Burt, and Blyth, 1962):

A = Skinfold thickness over the iliac crest in midaxillary line (Figure A.1)
B = Back of tricep in midline halfway between acromion and olecranon processes (Figure A.2)

Skinfold thickness measured in millimeters.
Formula for body density:

$$\text{density} = 1.0764 - [(0.00081 \times A) - (0.00088 \times B)]$$

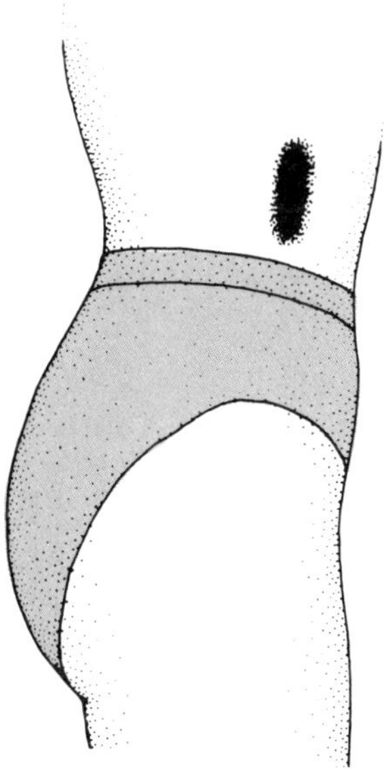

FIGURE A.1 Suprailiac Skinfold

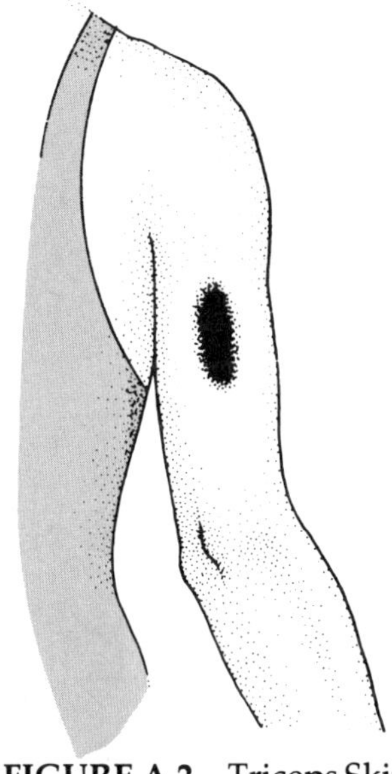

FIGURE A.2 Triceps Skinfold

Formula for percentage of body fat:

$$\text{percentage of body fat} = [(4.95/\text{density}) - 4.5)] \times 100$$

For percentage of body fat in women, see Table A.1.

II. Skinfold measurements and formulas for young men (Sloan, 1967):

C = Subscapular skinfold taken at the bottom point of the shoulder blade (Figure A.3)
D = Thigh skinfold taken in front, midway between the hip and the knee (Figure A.4)

Formula for body density:

$$\text{density} = 1.1043 - [(0.00131 \times C) - (0.001327 \times D)]$$

Formula for percentage of body fat:

$$\text{percentage of body fat} = [(4.570/\text{density}) - 4.142] \times 100$$

Figure A.5 shows a nomogram for determining men's body fat percentage.

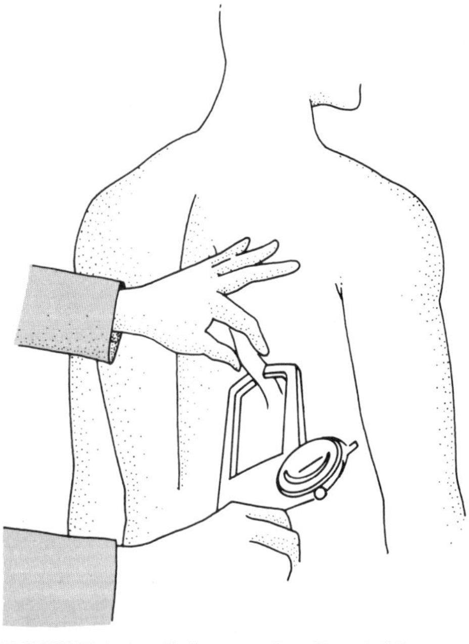

FIGURE A.3 Subscapular Skinfold

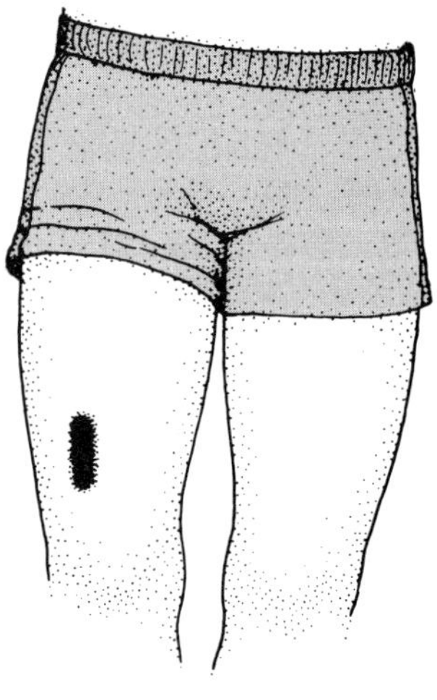

FIGURE A.4 Thigh Skinfold

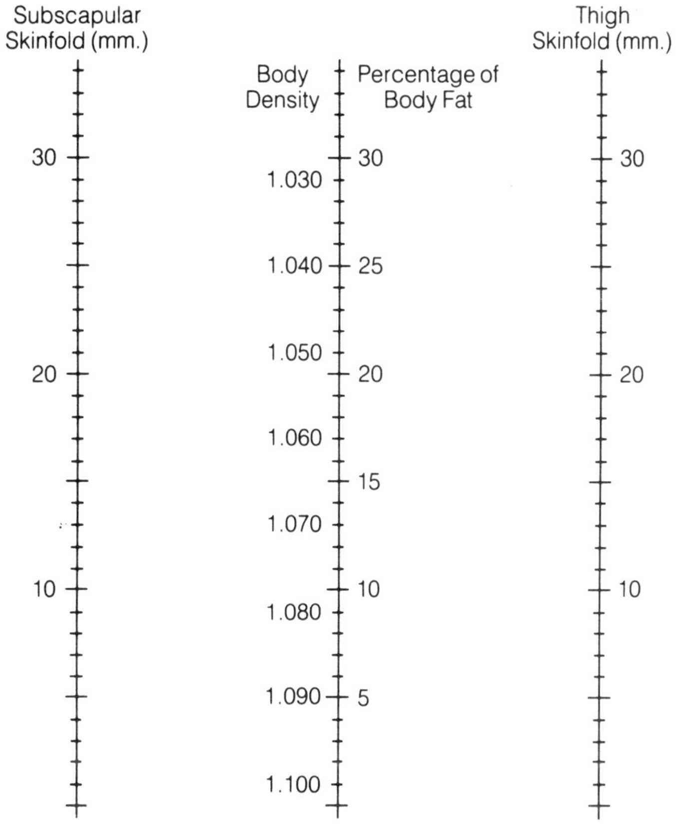

FIGURE A.5 Nomogram for Determining Percentage of Body Fat in Men (using Sloan formula)

Adapted from A. W. Sloan and J. B. Weir, "Nomograms for Predictions of Body Density and Total Body Fat from Skinfold Measurements." *Journal of Applied Physiology* 28 (1970) 221–222. Reprinted by permission.

Directions for Figure A.5: Place a ruler or straight edge of paper across the nomogram so that one point is at your subscapular skinfold measurement and the other point is at your thigh skinfold measurement. Your percentage of body fat is where the line crosses the middle scale.

References

Dusek, Dorothy E. "Percent Body Fat (Women), Iliac Measures 1–50 mm., Arm Measures 1–35 mm." unpublished article, University of Toledo, 1969. Reprinted with permission.

Sloan, A. W. "Estimation of Body Fat in Young Men." *Journal of Applied Physiology* 23 (1967): 311–315.

Sloan, A. W., J. J. Burt, and C. S. Blyth. "Estimation of Body Fat in Young Women." *Journal of Applied Physiology* 17 (1962): 967–970.

TABLE A.1 Percentage of Body Fat in Women (using Sloan, Burt, and Blyth formula)

Suprailiac Skinfold (mm)	*Triceps Skinfold (mm)*																	
	1	*2*	*3*	*4*	*5*	*6*	*7*	*8*	*9*	*10*	*11*	*12*	*13*	*14*	*15*	*16*	*17*	*18*
1	10.7	11.1	11.5	11.8	12.2	12.6	13.0	13.4	13.8	14.1	14.5	14.9	15.3	15.7	16.1	16.4	16.8	17.2
2	11.1	11.4	11.8	12.2	12.6	13.0	13.3	13.7	14.1	14.5	14.9	15.3	15.6	16.0	16.4	16.8	17.2	17.6
3	11.4	11.8	12.2	12.5	12.9	13.3	13.7	14.1	14.5	14.8	15.2	15.6	16.0	16.4	16.8	17.2	17.5	17.9
4	11.8	12.1	12.5	12.9	13.3	13.7	14.0	14.4	14.8	15.2	15.6	16.0	16.4	16.7	17.1	17.5	17.9	18.3
5	12.1	12.5	12.9	13.2	13.6	14.0	14.4	14.8	15.2	15.5	15.9	16.3	16.7	17.1	17.5	17.9	18.3	18.7
6	12.5	12.8	13.2	13.6	14.0	14.4	14.7	15.1	15.5	15.9	16.3	16.7	17.1	17.5	17.8	18.2	18.6	19.0
7	12.8	13.2	13.6	14.0	14.3	14.7	15.1	15.5	15.9	16.3	16.6	17.0	17.4	17.8	18.2	18.6	19.0	19.4
8	13.2	13.5	13.9	14.3	14.7	15.1	15.5	15.8	16.2	16.6	17.0	17.4	17.8	18.2	18.6	18.9	19.3	19.7
9	13.5	13.9	14.3	14.7	15.0	15.4	15.8	16.2	16.6	17.0	17.4	17.7	18.1	18.5	18.9	19.3	19.7	20.1
10	13.9	14.2	14.6	15.0	15.4	15.8	16.2	16.6	16.9	17.3	17.7	18.1	18.5	18.9	19.3	19.7	20.1	20.5
11	14.2	14.6	15.0	15.4	15.7	16.1	16.5	16.9	17.3	17.7	18.1	18.5	18.9	19.2	19.6	20.0	20.4	20.8
12	14.6	14.9	15.3	15.7	16.1	16.5	16.9	17.3	17.7	18.0	18.4	18.8	19.2	19.6	20.0	20.4	20.8	21.2
13	14.9	15.3	15.7	16.1	16.5	16.8	17.2	17.6	18.0	18.4	18.8	19.2	19.6	20.0	20.4	20.8	21.1	21.5
14	15.3	15.7	16.0	16.4	16.8	17.2	17.6	18.0	18.4	18.8	19.2	19.5	19.9	20.3	20.7	21.1	21.5	21.9
15	15.6	16.0	16.4	16.8	17.2	17.6	18.0	18.3	18.7	19.1	19.5	19.9	20.3	20.7	21.1	21.5	21.9	22.3
16	16.0	16.4	16.8	17.1	17.5	17.9	18.3	18.7	19.1	19.5	19.9	20.3	20.7	21.1	21.5	21.8	22.2	22.6
17	16.3	16.7	17.1	17.5	17.9	18.3	18.7	19.1	19.5	19.8	20.2	20.6	21.0	21.4	21.8	22.2	22.6	23.0
18	16.7	17.1	17.5	17.9	18.2	18.6	19.9	19.4	19.8	20.2	20.6	21.0	21.4	21.8	22.2	22.6	23.0	23.4
19	17.1	17.4	17.8	18.2	18.6	19.0	19.4	19.8	20.2	20.6	21.0	21.4	21.8	22.1	22.5	22.9	23.3	23.7
20	17.4	17.8	18.2	18.6	19.0	19.4	19.7	20.1	20.5	20.9	21.3	21.7	22.1	22.5	22.9	23.3	23.7	24.1
21	17.8	18.2	18.5	18.9	19.3	19.7	20.1	20.5	20.9	21.3	21.7	22.1	22.5	22.9	23.3	23.7	24.1	24.5
22	18.1	18.5	18.9	19.3	19.7	20.1	20.5	20.9	21.3	21.7	22.1	22.4	22.8	23.2	23.6	24.0	24.4	24.8
23	18.5	18.9	19.3	19.7	20.0	20.4	20.8	21.2	21.6	22.0	22.4	22.8	23.2	23.6	24.0	24.4	24.8	25.2
24	18.8	19.2	19.6	20.0	20.4	20.8	21.2	21.6	22.0	22.4	22.8	23.2	23.6	24.0	24.4	24.8	25.2	25.6
25	19.2	19.6	20.0	20.4	20.8	21.2	21.6	22.0	22.4	22.8	23.1	23.5	23.9	24.3	24.7	25.1	25.6	26.0
26	19.6	20.0	20.3	20.7	21.1	21.5	21.9	22.3	22.7	23.1	23.5	23.9	24.3	24.7	25.1	25.5	25.9	26.3
27	19.9	20.3	20.7	21.1	21.5	21.9	22.3	22.7	23.1	23.5	23.9	24.3	24.7	25.1	25.5	25.9	26.3	26.7
28	20.3	20.7	21.1	21.5	21.9	22.3	22.7	23.1	23.5	23.9	24.3	24.7	25.1	25.5	25.9	26.3	26.7	27.1
29	20.6	21.0	21.4	21.8	22.2	22.6	23.0	23.4	23.8	24.2	24.6	25.0	25.4	25.8	26.2	26.6	27.0	27.4
30	21.0	21.4	21.8	22.2	22.6	23.0	23.4	23.8	24.2	24.6	25.0	25.4	25.8	26.2	26.6	27.0	27.4	27.8
31	21.4	21.8	22.2	22.6	23.0	23.4	23.8	24.2	24.6	25.0	25.4	25.8	26.2	26.6	27.0	27.4	27.8	28.2
32	21.7	22.1	22.5	22.9	23.3	23.7	24.1	24.5	24.9	25.3	25.7	26.1	26.5	26.9	27.3	27.7	28.2	28.6
33	22.1	22.5	22.9	23.3	23.7	24.1	24.5	24.9	25.3	25.7	26.1	26.5	26.9	27.3	27.7	28.1	28.5	28.9
34	22.5	22.9	23.3	23.7	24.1	24.5	24.9	25.3	25.7	26.1	26.5	26.9	27.3	27.7	28.1	28.5	28.9	29.3
35	22.8	23.2	23.6	24.0	24.4	24.8	25.2	25.6	26.0	26.4	26.8	27.2	27.7	28.1	28.5	28.9	29.3	29.7
36	23.2	23.6	24.0	24.4	24.8	25.2	25.6	26.0	26.4	26.8	27.2	27.6	28.0	28.4	28.8	29.2	29.7	30.1
37	23.6	24.0	24.4	24.8	25.2	25.6	26.0	26.4	26.8	27.2	27.6	28.0	28.4	28.8	29.2	29.6	30.0	30.4
38	23.9	24.3	24.7	25.1	25.5	25.9	26.3	26.7	27.2	27.6	28.0	28.4	28.8	29.2	29.6	30.0	30.4	30.8
39	24.3	24.7	25.1	25.5	25.9	26.3	26.7	27.1	27.5	27.9	28.3	28.7	29.2	29.6	30.0	30.4	30.8	31.2
40	24.7	25.1	25.5	25.9	26.3	26.7	27.1	27.5	27.9	28.3	28.7	29.1	29.5	29.9	30.3	30.8	31.2	31.6
41	25.0	25.4	25.8	26.2	26.6	27.1	27.5	27.9	28.3	28.7	29.1	29.5	29.9	30.3	30.7	31.1	31.5	32.0
42	25.4	25.8	26.2	26.6	27.0	27.4	27.8	28.2	28.6	29.1	29.5	29.9	30.3	30.7	31.1	31.5	31.9	32.3
43	25.8	26.2	26.6	27.0	27.4	27.8	28.2	28.6	29.0	29.4	29.8	30.2	30.7	31.1	31.5	31.9	32.3	32.7
44	26.1	26.6	27.0	27.4	27.8	28.2	28.6	29.0	29.4	29.8	30.2	30.6	31.0	31.4	31.9	32.3	32.7	33.1
45	26.5	26.9	27.3	27.7	28.1	28.5	29.0	29.4	29.8	30.2	30.6	31.0	31.4	31.8	32.2	32.7	33.1	33.5
46	26.9	27.3	27.7	28.1	28.5	28.9	29.3	29.7	30.2	30.6	31.0	31.4	31.8	32.2	32.6	33.0	33.5	33.9
47	27.3	27.7	28.1	28.5	28.9	29.3	29.7	30.1	30.5	30.9	31.4	31.8	32.2	32.6	33.0	33.4	33.8	34.3
48	27.6	28.0	28.5	28.9	29.3	29.7	30.1	30.5	30.9	31.3	31.7	32.1	32.6	33.0	33.4	33.8	34.2	34.6
49	28.0	28.4	28.8	29.2	29.6	30.1	30.5	30.9	31.3	31.7	32.1	32.5	32.9	33.4	33.8	34.2	34.6	35.0
50	28.4	28.8	29.2	29.6	30.0	30.4	30.8	31.3	31.7	32.1	32.5	32.9	33.3	33.7	34.2	34.6	35.0	35.4

Reprinted by permission of the authors.

TABLE A.1 Continued

Suprailiac Skinfold (mm)	*Triceps Skinfold (mm)*																
	19	*20*	*21*	*22*	*23*	*24*	*25*	*26*	*27*	*28*	*29*	*30*	*31*	*32*	*33*	*34*	*35*
1	17.6	18.0	18.4	18.8	19.2	19.6	20.0	20.3	20.7	21.1	21.5	21.9	22.3	22.7	23.1	23.5	23.9
2	18.0	18.4	18.7	19.1	19.5	19.9	20.3	20.7	21.1	21.5	21.9	22.3	22.7	23.1	23.5	23.9	24.3
3	18.3	18.7	19.1	19.5	19.9	20.3	20.7	21.1	21.5	21.9	22.3	22.7	23.1	23.4	23.8	24.2	24.6
4	18.7	19.1	19.5	19.9	20.2	20.6	21.0	21.4	21.8	22.2	22.6	23.0	23.4	23.8	24.2	24.6	25.0
5	19.0	19.4	19.8	20.2	20.6	21.0	21.4	21.8	22.2	22.6	23.0	23.4	23.8	24.2	24.6	25.0	25.4
6	19.4	19.8	20.2	20.6	21.0	21.4	21.8	22.2	22.6	23.0	23.4	23.8	24.2	24.6	25.0	25.4	25.8
7	19.8	20.2	20.5	20.9	21.3	21.7	22.1	22.5	22.9	23.3	23.7	24.1	24.5	24.9	25.3	25.7	26.1
8	20.1	20.5	20.9	21.3	21.7	22.1	22.5	22.9	23.3	23.7	24.1	24.5	24.9	25.3	25.7	26.1	26.5
9	20.5	20.9	21.3	21.7	22.1	22.5	22.9	23.3	23.7	24.1	24.5	24.9	25.3	25.7	26.1	26.5	26.9
10	20.8	21.2	21.6	22.0	22.4	22.8	23.2	23.6	24.0	24.4	24.8	25.2	25.6	26.0	26.4	26.8	27.2
11	21.2	21.6	22.0	22.4	22.8	23.2	23.6	24.0	24.4	24.8	25.2	25.6	26.0	26.4	26.8	27.2	27.6
12	21.6	22.0	22.4	22.8	23.2	23.6	24.0	24.4	24.8	25.2	25.6	26.0	26.4	26.8	27.2	27.6	28.0
13	21.9	22.3	22.7	23.1	23.5	23.9	24.3	24.7	25.1	25.5	25.9	26.3	26.7	27.1	27.6	28.0	28.4
14	22.3	22.7	23.1	23.5	23.9	24.3	24.7	25.1	25.5	25.9	26.3	26.7	27.1	27.5	27.9	28.3	28.7
15	22.7	23.1	23.5	23.9	24.3	24.7	25.1	25.5	25.9	26.3	26.7	27.1	27.5	27.9	28.3	28.7	29.1
16	23.0	23.4	23.8	24.2	24.6	25.0	25.4	25.8	26.2	26.6	27.0	27.5	27.9	28.3	28.7	29.1	29.5
17	23.4	23.8	24.2	24.6	25.0	25.4	25.8	26.2	26.6	27.0	27.4	27.8	28.2	28.6	29.0	29.5	29.9
18	23.8	24.2	24.6	25.0	25.4	25.8	26.2	26.6	27.0	27.4	27.8	28.2	28.6	29.0	29.4	29.8	30.2
19	24.1	24.5	24.9	25.3	25.7	26.1	26.5	27.0	27.4	27.8	28.2	28.6	29.0	29.4	29.8	30.2	30.6
20	24.5	24.9	25.3	25.7	26.1	26.5	26.9	27.3	27.7	28.1	28.5	29.0	29.4	29.8	30.2	30.6	31.0
21	24.9	25.3	25.7	26.1	26.5	26.9	27.3	27.7	28.1	28.5	28.9	29.3	29.7	30.1	30.6	31.0	31.4
22	25.2	25.6	26.0	26.5	26.9	27.3	27.7	28.1	28.5	28.9	29.3	29.7	30.1	30.5	30.9	31.3	31.8
23	25.6	26.0	26.4	26.8	27.2	27.6	28.0	28.4	28.9	29.3	29.7	30.1	30.5	30.9	31.3	31.7	32.1
24	26.0	26.4	26.8	27.2	27.6	28.0	28.4	28.8	29.2	29.6	30.0	30.5	30.9	31.3	31.7	32.1	32.5
25	26.4	26.8	27.2	27.6	28.0	28.4	28.8	29.2	29.6	30.0	30.4	30.8	31.2	31.7	32.1	32.5	32.9
26	26.7	27.1	27.5	27.9	28.3	28.8	29.2	29.6	30.0	30.4	30.8	31.2	31.6	32.0	32.5	32.9	33.3
27	27.1	27.5	27.9	28.3	28.7	29.1	29.5	30.0	30.4	30.8	31.2	31.6	32.0	32.4	32.8	33.2	33.7
28	27.5	27.9	28.3	28.7	29.1	29.5	29.9	30.3	30.7	31.1	31.6	32.0	32.4	32.8	33.2	33.6	34.0
29	27.8	28.3	28.7	29.1	29.5	29.9	30.3	30.7	31.1	31.5	31.9	32.4	32.8	33.2	33.6	34.0	34.4
30	28.2	28.6	29.0	29.4	29.9	30.3	30.7	31.1	31.5	31.9	32.3	32.7	33.2	33.6	34.0	34.4	34.8
31	28.6	29.0	29.4	29.8	30.2	30.6	31.1	31.5	31.9	32.3	32.7	33.1	33.5	33.9	34.4	34.8	35.2
32	29.0	29.4	29.8	30.2	30.6	31.0	31.4	31.8	32.3	32.7	33.1	33.5	33.9	34.3	34.7	35.2	35.6
33	29.3	29.8	30.2	30.6	31.0	31.4	31.8	32.2	32.6	33.1	33.5	33.9	34.3	34.7	35.1	35.6	36.0
34	29.7	30.1	30.5	31.0	31.4	31.8	32.2	32.6	33.0	33.4	33.8	34.3	34.7	35.1	35.5	35.9	36.4
35	30.1	30.5	30.9	31.3	31.7	32.2	32.6	33.0	33.4	33.8	34.2	34.7	35.1	35.5	35.9	36.3	36.7
36	30.5	30.9	31.3	31.7	32.1	32.5	33.0	33.4	33.8	34.2	34.6	35.0	35.5	35.9	36.3	36.7	37.1
37	30.9	31.3	31.7	32.1	32.5	32.9	33.3	33.8	34.2	34.6	35.0	35.4	35.8	36.3	36.7	37.1	37.5
38	31.2	31.6	32.1	32.5	32.9	33.3	33.7	34.1	34.6	35.0	35.4	35.8	36.2	36.6	37.1	37.5	37.9
39	31.6	32.0	32.4	32.9	33.3	33.7	34.1	34.5	34.9	35.4	35.8	36.2	36.6	37.0	37.5	37.9	38.3
40	32.0	32.4	32.8	33.2	33.7	34.1	34.5	34.9	35.3	35.7	36.2	36.6	37.0	37.4	37.8	38.3	38.7
41	32.4	32.8	33.2	33.6	34.0	34.5	34.9	35.3	35.7	36.1	36.5	37.0	37.4	37.8	38.2	38.7	39.1
42	32.8	33.2	33.6	34.0	34.4	34.8	35.3	35.7	36.1	36.5	36.9	37.4	37.8	38.2	38.6	39.1	39.5
43	33.1	33.6	34.0	34.4	34.8	35.2	35.6	36.1	36.5	36.9	37.3	37.7	38.2	38.6	39.0	39.4	39.9
44	33.5	33.9	34.4	34.8	35.2	35.6	36.0	36.4	36.9	37.3	37.7	38.1	38.6	39.0	39.4	39.8	40.3
45	33.9	34.3	34.7	35.2	35.6	36.0	36.4	36.8	37.3	37.7	38.1	38.5	38.9	39.4	39.8	40.2	40.7
46	34.3	34.7	35.1	35.5	36.0	36.4	36.8	37.2	37.6	38.1	38.5	38.9	39.3	39.8	40.2	40.6	41.1
47	34.7	35.1	35.5	35.9	36.3	36.8	37.2	37.6	38.0	38.5	38.9	39.3	39.7	40.2	40.6	41.0	41.4
48	35.1	35.5	35.9	36.3	36.7	37.2	37.6	38.0	38.4	38.8	39.3	39.7	40.1	40.6	41.0	41.4	41.8
49	35.4	35.9	36.3	36.7	37.1	37.5	38.0	38.4	38.8	39.2	39.7	40.1	40.5	40.9	41.4	41.8	42.2
50	35.8	36.2	36.7	37.1	37.5	37.9	38.4	38.8	39.2	39.6	40.1	40.5	40.9	41.3	41.8	42.2	42.6

APPENDIX

B RDA'S AND NUTRITIVE VALUES

TABLE B.1. Recommended Daily Dietary Allowances (RDA's)[1]
(Designed for the maintenance of good nutrition of practically all healthy persons in the United States)

Sex-age category	Persons: Age (Years) From	To	Weight: Kilograms	Pounds	Height: Centimeters	Inches	Food energy: Calories	Protein: Grams	Minerals: Calcium, Milligrams	Phosphorus, Milligrams	Iron, Milligrams	Vitamin A: Retinol equivalents[2]	International units[3]	Thiamin: Milligrams	Riboflavin: Milligrams	Niacin: Milligrams	Ascorbic acid: Milligrams
Infants	0	0.5	6	13	60	24	kg × 115 lb × 52.3	kg × 2.2 lb × 1.0	360	240	10	420	1,400	0.3	0.4	6	35
	0.5	1	9	20	71	28	kg × 105 lb × 47.7	kg × 2.0 lb × 0.9	540	360	15	400	2,000	.5	6	8	35
Children	1	3	13	29	90	35	1,300	23	800	800	15	400	2,000	.7	.8	9	45
	4	6	20	44	112	44	1,700	30	800	800	10	500	2,500	.9	1.0	11	45
	7	10	28	62	132	52	2,400	34	800	800	10	700	3,300	1.2	1.4	16	45
Males	11	14	45	99	157	62	2,700	45	1,200	1,200	18	1,000	5,000	1.4	1.6	18	50
	15	18	66	145	176	69	2,800	56	1,200	1,200	18	1,000	5,000	1.4	1.7	18	60
	19	22	70	154	177	70	2,900	56	800	800	10	1,000	5,000	1.5	1.7	19	60
	23	50	70	154	178	70	2,700	56	800	800	10	1,000	5,000	1.4	1.6	18	60
	51+		70	154	178	70	[4]2,400	56	800	800	10	1,000	5,000	1.2	1.4	16	60
Females	11	14	46	101	157	62	2,200	46	1,200	1,200	18	800	4,000	1.1	1.3	15	50
	15	18	55	120	163	64	2,100	46	1,200	1,200	18	800	4,000	1.1	1.3	14	60
	19	22	55	120	163	64	2,100	44	800	800	18	800	4,000	1.1	1.3	14	60
	23	50	55	120	163	64	2,000	44	800	800	18	800	4,000	1.0	1.2	13	60
	51+		55	120	163	64	[4]1,800	44	800	800	10	800	4,000	1.0	1.2	13	60
Pregnant							+300	+30	+400	+400	[5]18+	+200	+1,000	+.4	+.3	+2	+20
Lactating							+500	+20	+400	+400	18	+400	+2,000	+.5	+.5	+5	+40

1. Source: Adapted from Recommended Dietary Allowances, 9th ed., 1980, 185 pp. Washington DC: National Academy of Sciences, National Research Council. Also available in libraries. This publication tabulates the RDA for selected nutrients, discusses the basis for all RDA, and reviews current knowledge of the dietary needs for other nutrients.

2. 1 retinol equivalent = 1 μg retinol or 6 μg beta-carotene.

3. 1 international unit = 0.3 μg retinol or 0.6 μg beta-carotene.

4. After age 75 years, energy requirement is 2,050 calories for males and 1,600 calories for females.

5. The increased requirement cannot be met by ordinary diets; therefore the use of supplemental iron is recommended.

NOTE—The Recommended Daily Dietary Allowances (RDA) should not be confused with the U.S. Recommended Daily Allowances (U.S. RDA). The RDA are amounts of nutrients recommended by the Food and Nutrition Board of the National Research Council and are considered adequate for maintenance of good nutrition in healthy persons in the United States. The allowances are revised from time to time in accordance with newer knowledge of nutritional needs.

The U.S. RDA are the amounts of protein, vitamins, and minerals established by the Food and Drug Administration as standards for nutrition labeling. These allowances were derived from the RDA set by the Food and Nutrition Board. The U.S. RDA for most nutrients approximates the highest RDA of the sex-age categories in this table, excluding the allowances for pregnant and lactating females. Therefore, a diet that furnishes the U.S. RDA for a nutrient will furnish the RDA for most people and more than the RDA for many. U.S. RDA are protein, 45 grams (eggs, fish, meat, milk, poultry), 65 grams (other foods); vitamin A, 5,000 International Units; thiamin, 1.5 milligrams; riboflavin, 1.7 milligrams; niacin, 20 milligrams; ascorbic acid, 60 milligrams; calcium, 1 gram; phosphorus, 1 gram; iron, 18 milligrams. For additional information on U.S. RDA, see the "Federal Register," vol. 38, no. 49 (March 14, 1973), pp. 6959-6960, and Agriculture Information Bulletin 382, "Nutrition Labeling—Tools for Its Use."

TABLE B.2. Nutritive Values of the Edible Part of Foods

(Tr indicates nutrient present in trace amount.)

Item No.	Foods, approximate measures, units, and weight (weight of edible portion only)			Water	Food energy	Protein	Fat	Fatty acids: Saturated	Fatty acids: Monounsaturated	Fatty acids: Polyunsaturated
	Beverages		Grams	Percent	Calories	Grams	Grams	Grams	Grams	Grams
	Alcoholic:									
	Beer:									
1	Regular	12 fl oz	360	92	150	1	0	0.0	0.0	0.0
2	Light	12 fl oz	355	95	95	1	0	0.0	0.0	0.0
	Gin, rum, vodka, whiskey:									
3	80-proof	1-1/2 fl oz	42	67	95	0	0	0.0	0.0	0.0
4	86-proof	1-1/2 fl oz	42	64	105	0	0	0.0	0.0	0.0
5	90-proof	1-1/2 fl oz	42	62	110	0	0	0.0	0.0	0.0
	Wines:									
6	Dessert	3-1/2 fl oz	103	77	140	Tr	0	0.0	0.0	0.0
	Table:									
7	Red	3-1/2 fl oz	102	88	75	Tr	0	0.0	0.0	0.0
8	White	3-1/2 fl oz	102	87	80	Tr	0	0.0	0.0	0.0
	Carbonated:[2]									
9	Club soda	12 fl oz	355	100	0	0	0	0.0	0.0	0.0
	Cola type:									
10	Regular	12 fl oz	369	89	160	0	0	0.0	0.0	0.0
11	Diet, artificially sweetened	12 fl oz	355	100	Tr	0	0	0.0	0.0	0.0
12	Ginger ale	12 fl oz	366	91	125	0	0	0.0	0.0	0.0
13	Grape	12 fl oz	372	88	180	0	0	0.0	0.0	0.0
14	Lemon-lime	12 fl oz	372	89	155	0	0	0.0	0.0	0.0
15	Orange	12 fl oz	372	88	180	0	0	0.0	0.0	0.0
16	Pepper type	12 fl oz	369	89	160	0	0	0.0	0.0	0.0
17	Root beer	12 fl oz	370	89	165	0	0	0.0	0.0	0.0
	Cocoa and chocolate-flavored beverages. See Dairy Products (items 95-98).									
	Coffee:									
18	Brewed	6 fl oz	180	100	Tr	Tr	Tr	Tr	Tr	Tr
19	Instant, prepared (2 tsp powder plus 6 fl oz water)	6 fl oz	182	99	Tr	Tr	Tr	Tr	Tr	Tr
	Fruit drinks, noncarbonated:									
	Canned:									
20	Fruit punch drink	6 fl oz	190	88	85	Tr	0	0.0	0.0	0.0
21	Grape drink	6 fl oz	187	86	100	Tr	0	0.0	0.0	0.0
22	Pineapple-grapefruit juice drink	6 fl oz	187	87	90	Tr	Tr	Tr	Tr	Tr
	Frozen:									
	Lemonade concentrate:									
23	Undiluted	6-fl-oz can	219	49	425	Tr	Tr	Tr	Tr	Tr
24	Diluted with 4-1/3 parts water by volume	6 fl oz	185	89	80	Tr	Tr	Tr	Tr	Tr
	Limeade concentrate:									
25	Undiluted	6-fl-oz can	218	50	410	Tr	Tr	Tr	Tr	Tr
26	Diluted with 4-1/3 parts water by volume	6 fl oz	185	89	75	Tr	Tr	Tr	Tr	Tr
	Fruit juices. See type under Fruits and Fruit Juices.									
	Milk beverages. See Dairy Products (items 92-105).									
	Tea:									
27	Brewed	8 fl oz	240	100	Tr	Tr	Tr	Tr	Tr	Tr
	Instant, powder, prepared:									
28	Unsweetened (1 tsp powder plus 8 fl oz water)	8 fl oz	241	100	Tr	Tr	Tr	Tr	Tr	Tr
29	Sweetened (3 tsp powder plus 8 fl oz water)	8 fl oz	262	91	85	Tr	Tr	Tr	Tr	Tr

[1]Value not determined.
[2]Mineral content varies depending on water source.

Nutrients in Indicated Quantity													
Cholesterol	Carbohydrate	Calcium	Phosphorus	Iron	Potassium	Sodium	Vitamin A value (IU)	Vitamin A value (RE)	Thiamin	Riboflavin	Niacin	Ascorbic acid	Item No.
Milligrams	Grams	Milligrams	Milligrams	Milligrams	Milligrams	Milligrams	International units	Retinol equivalents	Milligrams	Milligrams	Milligrams	Milligrams	
0	13	14	50	0.1	115	18	0	0	0.02	0.09	1.8	0	1
0	5	14	43	0.1	64	11	0	0	0.03	0.11	1.4	0	2
0	Tr	Tr	Tr	Tr	1	Tr	0	0	Tr	Tr	Tr	0	3
0	Tr	Tr	Tr	Tr	1	Tr	0	0	Tr	Tr	Tr	0	4
0	Tr	Tr	Tr	Tr	1	Tr	0	0	Tr	Tr	Tr	0	5
0	8	8	9	0.2	95	9	(1)	(1)	0.01	0.02	0.2	0	6
0	3	8	18	0.4	113	5	(1)	(1)	0.00	0.03	0.1	0	7
0	3	9	14	0.3	83	5	(1)	(1)	0.00	0.01	0.1	0	8
0	0	18	0	Tr	0	78	0	0	0.00	0.00	0.0	0	9
0	41	11	52	0.2	7	18	0	0	0.00	0.00	0.0	0	10
0	Tr	14	39	0.2	7	[3]32	0	0	0.00	0.00	0.0	0	11
0	32	11	0	0.1	4	29	0	0	0.00	0.00	0.0	0	12
0	46	15	0	0.4	4	48	0	0	0.00	0.00	0.0	0	13
0	39	7	0	0.4	4	33	0	0	0.00	0.00	0.0	0	14
0	46	15	4	0.3	7	52	0	0	0.00	0.00	0.0	0	15
0	41	11	41	0.1	4	37	0	0	0.00	0.00	0.0	0	16
0	42	15	0	0.2	4	48	0	0	0.00	0.00	0.0	0	17
0	Tr	4	2	Tr	124	2	0	0	0.00	0.02	0.4	0	18
0	1	2	6	0.1	71	Tr	0	0	0.00	0.03	0.6	0	19
0	22	15	2	0.4	48	15	20	2	0.03	0.04	Tr	[4]61	20
0	26	2	2	0.3	9	11	Tr	Tr	0.01	0.01	Tr	[4]64	21
0	23	13	7	0.9	97	24	60	6	0.06	0.04	0.5	[4]110	22
0	112	9	13	0.4	153	4	40	4	0.04	0.07	0.7	66	23
0	21	2	2	0.1	30	1	10	1	0.01	0.02	0.2	13	24
0	108	11	13	0.2	129	Tr	Tr	Tr	0.02	0.02	0.2	26	25
0	20	2	2	Tr	24	Tr	Tr	Tr	Tr	Tr	Tr	4	26
0	Tr	0	2	Tr	36	1	0	0	0.00	0.03	Tr	0	27
0	1	1	4	Tr	61	1	0	0	0.00	0.02	0.1	0	28
0	22	1	3	Tr	49	Tr	0	0	0.00	0.04	0.1	0	29

[3]Blend of aspartame and saccharin; if only sodium saccharin is used, sodium is 75 mg; if only aspartame is used, sodium is 23 mg.

[4]With added ascorbic acid.

Item No.	Foods, approximate measures, units, and weight (weight of edible portion only)			Water	Food energy	Protein	Fat	Fatty acids: Saturated	Fatty acids: Monounsaturated	Fatty acids: Polyunsaturated
	Dairy Products		Grams	Percent	Calories	Grams	Grams	Grams	Grams	Grams
	Butter. See Fats and Oils (items 128-130).									
	Cheese:									
	Natural:									
30	Blue	1 oz	28	42	100	6	8	5.3	2.2	0.2
31	Camembert (3 wedges per 4-oz container)	1 wedge	38	52	115	8	9	5.8	2.7	0.3
	Cheddar:									
32	Cut pieces	1 oz	28	37	115	7	9	6.0	2.7	0.3
33		1 in³	17	37	70	4	6	3.6	1.6	0.2
34	Shredded	1 cup	113	37	455	28	37	23.8	10.6	1.1
	Cottage (curd not pressed down):									
	Creamed (cottage cheese, 4% fat):									
35	Large curd	1 cup	225	79	235	28	10	6.4	2.9	0.3
36	Small curd	1 cup	210	79	215	26	9	6.0	2.7	0.3
37	With fruit	1 cup	226	72	280	22	8	4.9	2.2	0.2
38	Lowfat (2%)	1 cup	226	79	205	31	4	2.8	1.2	0.1
39	Uncreamed (cottage cheese dry curd, less than 1/2% fat)	1 cup	145	80	125	25	1	0.4	0.2	Tr
40	Cream	1 oz	28	54	100	2	10	6.2	2.8	0.4
41	Feta	1 oz	28	55	75	4	6	4.2	1.3	0.2
	Mozzarella, made with:									
42	Whole milk	1 oz	28	54	80	6	6	3.7	1.9	0.2
43	Part skim milk (low moisture)	1 oz	28	49	80	8	5	3.1	1.4	0.1
44	Muenster	1 oz	28	42	105	7	9	5.4	2.5	0.2
	Parmesan, grated:									
45	Cup, not pressed down	1 cup	100	18	455	42	30	19.1	8.7	0.7
46	Tablespoon	1 tbsp	5	18	25	2	2	1.0	0.4	Tr
47	Ounce	1 oz	28	18	130	12	9	5.4	2.5	0.2
48	Provolone	1 oz	28	41	100	7	8	4.8	2.1	0.2
	Ricotta, made with:									
49	Whole milk	1 cup	246	72	430	28	32	20.4	8.9	0.9
50	Part skim milk	1 cup	246	74	340	28	19	12.1	5.7	0.6
51	Swiss	1 oz	28	37	105	8	8	5.0	2.1	0.3
	Pasteurized process cheese:									
52	American	1 oz	28	39	105	6	9	5.6	2.5	0.3
53	Swiss	1 oz	28	42	95	7	7	4.5	2.0	0.2
54	Pasteurized process cheese food, American	1 oz	28	43	95	6	7	4.4	2.0	0.2
55	Pasteurized process cheese spread, American	1 oz	28	48	80	5	6	3.8	1.8	0.2
	Cream, sweet:									
56	Half-and-half (cream and milk)	1 cup	242	81	315	7	28	17.3	8.0	1.0
57		1 tbsp	15	81	20	Tr	2	1.1	0.5	0.1
58	Light, coffee, or table	1 cup	240	74	470	6	46	28.8	13.4	1.7
59		1 tbsp	15	74	30	Tr	3	1.8	0.8	0.1
	Whipping, unwhipped (volume about double when whipped):									
60	Light	1 cup	239	64	700	5	74	46.2	21.7	2.1
61		1 tbsp	15	64	45	Tr	5	2.9	1.4	0.1
62	Heavy	1 cup	238	58	820	5	88	54.8	25.4	3.3
63		1 tbsp	15	58	50	Tr	6	3.5	1.6	0.2
64	Whipped topping, (pressurized)	1 cup	60	61	155	2	13	8.3	3.9	0.5
65		1 tbsp	3	61	10	Tr	1	0.4	0.2	Tr
66	Cream, sour	1 cup	230	71	495	7	48	30.0	13.9	1.8
67		1 tbsp	12	71	25	Tr	3	1.6	0.7	0.1

Nutrients in Indicated Quantity

Cholesterol	Carbohydrate	Calcium	Phosphorus	Iron	Potassium	Sodium	Vitamin A value (IU)	Vitamin A value (RE)	Thiamin	Riboflavin	Niacin	Ascorbic acid	Item No.
Milligrams	Grams	Milligrams	Milligrams	Milligrams	Milligrams	Milligrams	International units	Retinol equivalents	Milligrams	Milligrams	Milligrams	Milligrams	
21	1	150	110	0.1	73	396	200	65	0.01	0.11	0.3	0	30
27	Tr	147	132	0.1	71	320	350	96	0.01	0.19	0.2	0	31
30	Tr	204	145	0.2	28	176	300	86	0.01	0.11	Tr	0	32
18	Tr	123	87	0.1	17	105	180	52	Tr	0.06	Tr	0	33
119	1	815	579	0.8	111	701	1,200	342	0.03	0.42	0.1	0	34
34	6	135	297	0.3	190	911	370	108	0.05	0.37	0.3	Tr	35
31	6	126	277	0.3	177	850	340	101	0.04	0.34	0.3	Tr	36
25	30	108	236	0.2	151	915	280	81	0.04	0.29	0.2	Tr	37
19	8	155	340	0.4	217	918	160	45	0.05	0.42	0.3	Tr	38
10	3	46	151	0.3	47	19	40	12	0.04	0.21	0.2	0	39
31	1	23	30	0.3	34	84	400	124	Tr	0.06	Tr	0	40
25	1	140	96	0.2	18	316	130	36	0.04	0.24	0.3	0	41
22	1	147	105	0.1	19	106	220	68	Tr	0.07	Tr	0	42
15	1	207	149	0.1	27	150	180	54	0.01	0.10	Tr	0	43
27	Tr	203	133	0.1	38	178	320	90	Tr	0.09	Tr	0	44
79	4	1,376	807	1.0	107	1,861	700	173	0.05	0.39	0.3	0	45
4	Tr	69	40	Tr	5	93	40	9	Tr	0.02	Tr	0	46
22	1	390	229	0.3	30	528	200	49	0.01	0.11	0.1	0	47
20	1	214	141	0.1	39	248	230	75	0.01	0.09	Tr	0	48
124	7	509	389	0.9	257	207	1,210	330	0.03	0.48	0.3	0	49
76	13	669	449	1.1	307	307	1,060	278	0.05	0.46	0.2	0	50
26	1	272	171	Tr	31	74	240	72	0.01	0.10	Tr	0	51
27	Tr	174	211	0.1	46	406	340	82	0.01	0.10	Tr	0	52
24	1	219	216	0.2	61	388	230	65	Tr	0.08	Tr	0	53
18	2	163	130	0.2	79	337	260	62	0.01	0.13	Tr	0	54
16	2	159	202	0.1	69	381	220	54	0.01	0.12	Tr	0	55
89	10	254	230	0.2	314	98	1,050	259	0.08	0.36	0.2	2	56
6	1	16	14	Tr	19	6	70	16	0.01	0.02	Tr	Tr	57
159	9	231	192	0.1	292	95	1,730	437	0.08	0.36	0.1	2	58
10	1	14	12	Tr	18	6	110	27	Tr	0.02	Tr	Tr	59
265	7	166	146	0.1	231	82	2,690	705	0.06	0.30	0.1	1	60
17	Tr	10	9	Tr	15	5	170	44	Tr	0.02	Tr	Tr	61
326	7	154	149	0.1	179	89	3,500	1,002	0.05	0.26	0.1	1	62
21	Tr	10	9	Tr	11	6	220	63	Tr	0.02	Tr	Tr	63
46	7	61	54	Tr	88	78	550	124	0.02	0.04	Tr	0	64
2	Tr	3	3	Tr	4	4	30	6	Tr	Tr	Tr	0	65
102	10	268	195	0.1	331	123	1,820	448	0.08	0.34	0.2	2	66
5	1	14	10	Tr	17	6	90	23	Tr	0.02	Tr	Tr	67

Item No.	Foods, approximate measures, units, and weight (weight of edible portion only)			Water	Food energy	Protein	Fat	Fatty acids: Saturated	Fatty acids: Monounsaturated	Fatty acids: Polyunsaturated
	Dairy Products—Con.		Grams	Percent	Calories	Grams	Grams	Grams	Grams	Grams
	Cream products, imitation (made with vegetable fat):									
	Sweet:									
	Creamers:									
68	Liquid (frozen)	1 tbsp	15	77	20	Tr	1	1.4	Tr	Tr
69	Powdered	1 tsp	2	2	10	Tr	1	0.7	Tr	Tr
	Whipped topping:									
70	Frozen	1 cup	75	50	240	1	19	16.3	1.2	0.4
71		1 tbsp	4	50	15	Tr	1	0.9	0.1	Tr
72	Powdered, made with whole milk	1 cup	80	67	150	3	10	8.5	0.7	0.2
73		1 tbsp	4	67	10	Tr	Tr	0.4	Tr	Tr
74	Pressurized	1 cup	70	60	185	1	16	13.2	1.3	0.2
75		1 tbsp	4	60	10	Tr	1	0.8	0.1	Tr
76	Sour dressing (filled cream type product, nonbutterfat)	1 cup	235	75	415	8	39	31.2	4.6	1.1
77		1 tbsp	12	75	20	Tr	2	1.6	0.2	0.1
	Ice cream. See Milk desserts, frozen (items 106-111).									
	Ice milk. See Milk desserts, frozen (items 112-114).									
	Milk:									
	Fluid:									
78	Whole (3.3% fat)	1 cup	244	88	150	8	8	5.1	2.4	0.3
	Lowfat (2%):									
79	No milk solids added	1 cup	244	89	120	8	5	2.9	1.4	0.2
80	Milk solids added, label claim less than 10 g of protein per cup	1 cup	245	89	125	9	5	2.9	1.4	0.2
	Lowfat (1%):									
81	No milk solids added	1 cup	244	90	100	8	3	1.6	0.7	0.1
82	Milk solids added, label claim less than 10 g of protein per cup	1 cup	245	90	105	9	2	1.5	0.7	0.1
	Nonfat (skim):									
83	No milk solids added	1 cup	245	91	85	8	Tr	0.3	0.1	Tr
84	Milk solids added, label claim less than 10 g of protein per cup	1 cup	245	90	90	9	1	0.4	0.2	Tr
85	Buttermilk	1 cup	245	90	100	8	2	1.3	0.6	0.1
	Canned:									
86	Condensed, sweetened	1 cup	306	27	980	24	27	16.8	7.4	1.0
	Evaporated:									
87	Whole milk	1 cup	252	74	340	17	19	11.6	5.9	0.6
88	Skim milk	1 cup	255	79	200	19	1	0.3	0.2	Tr
	Dried:									
89	Buttermilk	1 cup	120	3	465	41	7	4.3	2.0	0.3
	Nonfat, instantized:									
90	Envelope, 3.2 oz, net wt.[6]	1 envelope	91	4	325	32	1	0.4	0.2	Tr
91	Cup	1 cup	68	4	245	24	Tr	0.3	0.1	Tr
	Milk beverages:									
	Chocolate milk (commercial):									
92	Regular	1 cup	250	82	210	8	8	5.3	2.5	0.3
93	Lowfat (2%)	1 cup	250	84	180	8	5	3.1	1.5	0.2
94	Lowfat (1%)	1 cup	250	85	160	8	3	1.5	0.8	0.1

[5] Vitamin A value is largely from beta-carotene used for coloring.
[6] Yields 1 qt of fluid milk when reconstituted according to package directions.

Nutrients in Indicated Quantity

Cholesterol	Carbohydrate	Calcium	Phosphorus	Iron	Potassium	Sodium	Vitamin A value (IU)	Vitamin A value (RE)	Thiamin	Riboflavin	Niacin	Ascorbic acid	Item No.
Milligrams	Grams	Milligrams	Milligrams	Milligrams	Milligrams	Milligrams	International units	Retinol equivalents	Milligrams	Milligrams	Milligrams	Milligrams	
0	2	1	10	Tr	29	12	[5]10	[5]1	0.00	0.00	0.0	0	68
0	1	Tr	8	Tr	16	4	Tr	Tr	0.00	Tr	0.0	0	69
0	17	5	6	0.1	14	19	[5]650	[5]65	0.00	0.00	0.0	0	70
0	1	Tr	Tr	Tr	1	1	[5]30	[5]3	0.00	0.00	0.0	0	71
8	13	72	69	Tr	121	53	[5]290	[5]39	0.02	0.09	Tr	1	72
Tr	1	4	3	Tr	6	3	[5]10	[5]2	Tr	Tr	Tr	Tr	73
0	11	4	13	Tr	13	43	[5]330	[5]33	0.00	0.00	0.0	0	74
0	1	Tr	1	Tr	1	2	[5]20	[5]2	0.00	0.00	0.0	0	75
13	11	266	205	0.1	380	113	20	5	0.09	0.38	0.2	2	76
1	1	14	10	Tr	19	6	Tr	Tr	Tr	0.02	Tr	Tr	77
33	11	291	228	0.1	370	120	310	76	0.09	0.40	0.2	2	78
18	12	297	232	0.1	377	122	500	139	0.10	0.40	0.2	2	79
18	12	313	245	0.1	397	128	500	140	0.10	0.42	0.2	2	80
10	12	300	235	0.1	381	123	500	144	0.10	0.41	0.2	2	81
10	12	313	245	0.1	397	128	500	145	0.10	0.42	0.2	2	82
4	12	302	247	0.1	406	126	500	149	0.09	0.34	0.2	2	83
5	12	316	255	0.1	418	130	500	149	0.10	0.43	0.2	2	84
9	12	285	219	0.1	371	257	80	20	0.08	0.38	0.1	2	85
104	166	868	775	0.6	1,136	389	1,000	248	0.28	1.27	0.6	8	86
74	25	657	510	0.5	764	267	610	136	0.12	0.80	0.5	5	87
9	29	738	497	0.7	845	293	1,000	298	0.11	0.79	0.4	3	88
83	59	1,421	1,119	0.4	1,910	621	260	65	0.47	1.89	1.1	7	89
17	47	1,120	896	0.3	1,552	499	[7]2,160	[7]646	0.38	1.59	0.8	5	90
12	35	837	670	0.2	1,160	373	[7]1,610	[7]483	0.28	1.19	0.6	4	91
31	26	280	251	0.6	417	149	300	73	0.09	0.41	0.3	2	92
17	26	284	254	0.6	422	151	500	143	0.09	0.41	0.3	2	93
7	26	287	256	0.6	425	152	500	148	0.10	0.42	0.3	2	94

[7]With added vitamin A.

Item No.	Foods, approximate measures, units, and weight (weight of edible portion only)			Water	Food energy	Protein	Fat	Fatty acids		
								Saturated	Monounsaturated	Polyunsaturated
	Dairy Products—Con.		Grams	Percent	Calories	Grams	Grams	Grams	Grams	Grams
	Milk beverages:									
	Cocoa and chocolate-flavored beverages:									
95	Powder containing nonfat dry milk	1 oz	28	1	100	3	1	0.6	0.3	Tr
96	Prepared (6 oz water plus 1 oz powder)	1 serving	206	86	100	3	1	0.6	0.3	Tr
97	Powder without nonfat dry milk	3/4 oz	21	1	75	1	1	0.3	0.2	Tr
98	Prepared (8 oz whole milk plus 3/4 oz powder)	1 serving	265	81	225	9	9	5.4	2.5	0.3
99	Eggnog (commercial)	1 cup	254	74	340	10	19	11.3	5.7	0.9
	Malted milk:									
	Chocolate:									
100	Powder	3/4 oz	21	2	85	1	1	0.5	0.3	0.1
101	Prepared (8 oz whole milk plus 3/4 oz powder)	1 serving	265	81	235	9	9	5.5	2.7	0.4
	Natural:									
102	Powder	3/4 oz	21	3	85	3	2	0.9	0.5	0.3
103	Prepared (8 oz whole milk plus 3/4 oz powder)	1 serving	265	81	235	11	10	6.0	2.9	0.6
	Shakes, thick:									
104	Chocolate	10-oz container	283	72	335	9	8	4.8	2.2	0.3
105	Vanilla	10-oz container	283	74	315	11	9	5.3	2.5	0.3
	Milk desserts, frozen:									
	Ice cream, vanilla:									
	Regular (about 11% fat):									
106	Hardened	1/2 gal	1,064	61	2,155	38	115	71.3	33.1	4.3
107		1 cup	133	61	270	5	14	8.9	4.1	0.5
108		3 fl oz	50	61	100	2	5	3.4	1.6	0.2
109	Soft serve (frozen custard)	1 cup	173	60	375	7	23	13.5	6.7	1.0
110	Rich (about 16% fat), hardened	1/2 gal	1,188	59	2,805	33	190	118.3	54.9	7.1
111		1 cup	148	59	350	4	24	14.7	6.8	0.9
	Ice milk, vanilla:									
112	Hardened (about 4% fat)	1/2 gal	1,048	69	1,470	41	45	28.1	13.0	1.7
113		1 cup	131	69	185	5	6	3.5	1.6	0.2
114	Soft serve (about 3% fat)	1 cup	175	70	225	8	5	2.9	1.3	0.2
115	Sherbet (about 2% fat)	1/2 gal	1,542	66	2,160	17	31	19.0	8.8	1.1
116		1 cup	193	66	270	2	4	2.4	1.1	0.1
	Yogurt:									
	With added milk solids:									
	Made with lowfat milk:									
117	Fruit-flavored[8]	8-oz container	227	74	230	10	2	1.6	0.7	0.1
118	Plain	8-oz container	227	85	145	12	4	2.3	1.0	0.1
119	Made with nonfat milk	8-oz container	227	85	125	13	Tr	0.3	0.1	Tr
	Without added milk solids:									
120	Made with whole milk	8-oz container	227	88	140	8	7	4.8	2.0	0.2
	Eggs									
	Eggs, large (24 oz per dozen):									
	Raw:									
121	Whole, without shell	1 egg	50	75	80	6	6	1.7	2.2	0.7
122	White	1 white	33	88	15	3	Tr	0.0	0.0	0.0
123	Yolk	1 yolk	17	49	65	3	6	1.7	2.2	0.7
	Cooked:									
124	Fried in butter	1 egg	46	68	95	6	7	2.7	2.7	0.8
125	Hard-cooked, shell removed	1 egg	50	75	80	6	6	1.7	2.2	0.7
126	Poached	1 egg	50	74	80	6	6	1.7	2.2	0.7
127	Scrambled (milk added) in butter. Also omelet	1 egg	64	73	110	7	8	3.2	2.9	0.8

[8] Carbohydrate content varies widely because of amount of sugar added and amount and solids content of added flavoring. Consult the label if more precise values for carbohydrate and calories are needed.

Nutrients in Indicated Quantity

Cholesterol	Carbohydrate	Calcium	Phosphorus	Iron	Potassium	Sodium	Vitamin A value (IU)	Vitamin A value (RE)	Thiamin	Riboflavin	Niacin	Ascorbic acid	Item No.
Milligrams	Grams	Milligrams	Milligrams	Milligrams	Milligrams	Milligrams	International units	Retinol equivalents	Milligrams	Milligrams	Milligrams	Milligrams	
1	22	90	88	0.3	223	139	Tr	Tr	0.03	0.17	0.2	Tr	95
1	22	90	88	0.3	223	139	Tr	Tr	0.03	0.17	0.2	Tr	96
0	19	7	26	0.7	136	56	Tr	Tr	Tr	0.03	0.1	Tr	97
33	30	298	254	0.9	508	176	310	76	0.10	0.43	0.3	3	98
149	34	330	278	0.5	420	138	890	203	0.09	0.48	0.3	4	99
1	18	13	37	0.4	130	49	20	5	0.04	0.04	0.4	0	100
34	29	304	265	0.5	500	168	330	80	0.14	0.43	0.7	2	101
4	15	56	79	0.2	159	96	70	17	0.11	0.14	1.1	0	102
37	27	347	307	0.3	529	215	380	93	0.20	0.54	1.3	2	103
30	60	374	357	0.9	634	314	240	59	0.13	0.63	0.4	0	104
33	50	413	326	0.3	517	270	320	79	0.08	0.55	0.4	0	105
476	254	1,406	1,075	1.0	2,052	929	4,340	1,064	0.42	2.63	1.1	6	106
59	32	176	134	0.1	257	116	540	133	0.05	0.33	0.1	1	107
22	12	66	51	Tr	96	44	200	50	0.02	0.12	0.1	Tr	108
153	38	236	199	0.4	338	153	790	199	0.08	0.45	0.2	1	109
703	256	1,213	927	0.8	1,771	868	7,200	1,758	0.36	2.27	0.9	5	110
88	32	151	115	0.1	221	108	900	219	0.04	0.28	0.1	1	111
146	232	1,409	1,035	1.5	2,117	836	1,710	419	0.61	2.78	0.9	6	112
18	29	176	129	0.2	265	105	210	52	0.08	0.35	0.1	1	113
13	38	274	202	0.3	412	163	175	44	0.12	0.54	0.2	1	114
113	469	827	594	2.5	1,585	706	1,480	308	0.26	0.71	1.0	31	115
14	59	103	74	0.3	198	88	190	39	0.03	0.09	0.1	4	116
10	43	345	271	0.2	442	133	100	25	0.08	0.40	0.2	1	117
14	16	415	326	0.2	531	159	150	36	0.10	0.49	0.3	2	118
4	17	452	355	0.2	579	174	20	5	0.11	0.53	0.3	2	119
29	11	274	215	0.1	351	105	280	68	0.07	0.32	0.2	1	120
274	1	28	90	1.0	65	69	260	78	0.04	0.15	Tr	0	121
0	Tr	4	4	Tr	45	50	0	0	Tr	0.09	Tr	0	122
272	Tr	26	86	0.9	15	8	310	94	0.04	0.07	Tr	0	123
278	1	29	91	1.1	66	162	320	94	0.04	0.14	Tr	0	124
274	1	28	90	1.0	65	69	260	78	0.04	0.14	Tr	0	125
273	1	28	90	1.0	65	146	260	78	0.03	0.13	Tr	0	126
282	2	54	109	1.0	97	176	350	102	0.04	0.18	Tr	Tr	127

Item No.	Foods, approximate measures, units, and weight (weight of edible portion only)			Water	Food energy	Protein	Fat	Fatty acids: Saturated	Fatty acids: Monounsaturated	Fatty acids: Polyunsaturated
	Fats and Oils		Grams	Percent	Calories	Grams	Grams	Grams	Grams	Grams
	Butter (4 sticks per lb):									
128	Stick	1/2 cup	113	16	810	1	92	57.1	26.4	3.4
129	Tablespoon (1/8 stick)	1 tbsp	14	16	100	Tr	11	7.1	3.3	0.4
130	Pat (1 in square, 1/3 in high; 90 per lb)	1 pat	5	16	35	Tr	4	2.5	1.2	0.2
131	Fats, cooking (vegetable shortenings)	1 cup	205	0	1,810	0	205	51.3	91.2	53.5
132		1 tbsp	13	0	115	0	13	3.3	5.8	3.4
133	Lard	1 cup	205	0	1,850	0	205	80.4	92.5	23.0
134		1 tbsp	13	0	115	0	13	5.1	5.9	1.5
	Margarine:									
135	Imitation (about 40% fat), soft	8-oz container	227	58	785	1	88	17.5	35.6	31.3
136		1 tbsp	14	58	50	Tr	5	1.1	2.2	1.9
	Regular (about 80% fat):									
	Hard (4 sticks per lb):									
137	Stick	1/2 cup	113	16	810	1	91	17.9	40.5	28.7
138	Tablespoon (1/8 stick)	1 tbsp	14	16	100	Tr	11	2.2	5.0	3.6
139	Pat (1 in square, 1/3 in high; 90 per lb)	1 pat	5	16	35	Tr	4	0.8	1.8	1.3
140	Soft	8-oz container	227	16	1,625	2	183	31.3	64.7	78.5
141		1 tbsp	14	16	100	Tr	11	1.9	4.0	4.8
	Spread (about 60% fat):									
	Hard (4 sticks per lb):									
142	Stick	1/2 cup	113	37	610	1	69	15.9	29.4	20.5
143	Tablespoon (1/8 stick)	1 tbsp	14	37	75	Tr	9	2.0	3.6	2.5
144	Pat (1 in square, 1/3 in high; 90 per lb)	1 pat	5	37	25	Tr	3	0.7	1.3	0.9
145	Soft	8-oz container	227	37	1,225	1	138	29.1	71.5	31.3
146		1 tbsp	14	37	75	Tr	9	1.8	4.4	1.9
	Oils, salad or cooking:									
147	Corn	1 cup	218	0	1,925	0	218	27.7	52.8	128.0
148		1 tbsp	14	0	125	0	14	1.8	3.4	8.2
149	Olive	1 cup	216	0	1,910	0	216	29.2	159.2	18.1
150		1 tbsp	14	0	125	0	14	1.9	10.3	1.2
151	Peanut	1 cup	216	0	1,910	0	216	36.5	99.8	69.1
152		1 tbsp	14	0	125	0	14	2.4	6.5	4.5
153	Safflower	1 cup	218	0	1,925	0	218	19.8	26.4	162.4
154		1 tbsp	14	0	125	0	14	1.3	1.7	10.4
155	Soybean oil, hydrogenated (partially hardened)	1 cup	218	0	1,925	0	218	32.5	93.7	82.0
156		1 tbsp	14	0	125	0	14	2.1	6.0	5.3
157	Soybean-cottonseed oil blend, hydrogenated	1 cup	218	0	1,925	0	218	39.2	64.3	104.9
158		1 tbsp	14	0	125	0	14	2.5	4.1	6.7
159	Sunflower	1 cup	218	0	1,925	0	218	22.5	42.5	143.2
160		1 tbsp	14	0	125	0	14	1.4	2.7	9.2
	Salad dressings:									
	Commercial:									
161	Blue cheese	1 tbsp	15	32	75	1	8	1.5	1.8	4.2
	French:									
162	Regular	1 tbsp	16	35	85	Tr	9	1.4	4.0	3.5
163	Low calorie	1 tbsp	16	75	25	Tr	2	0.2	0.3	1.0
	Italian:									
164	Regular	1 tbsp	15	34	80	Tr	9	1.3	3.7	3.2
165	Low calorie	1 tbsp	15	86	5	Tr	Tr	Tr	Tr	Tr
	Mayonnaise:									
166	Regular	1 tbsp	14	15	100	Tr	11	1.7	3.2	5.8
167	Imitation	1 tbsp	15	63	35	Tr	3	0.5	0.7	1.6
168	Mayonnaise type	1 tbsp	15	40	60	Tr	5	0.7	1.4	2.7
169	Tartar sauce	1 tbsp	14	34	75	Tr	8	1.2	2.6	3.9
	Thousand island:									
170	Regular	1 tbsp	16	46	60	Tr	6	1.0	1.3	3.2
171	Low calorie	1 tbsp	15	69	25	Tr	2	0.2	0.4	0.9

[9] For salted butter; unsalted butter contains 12 mg sodium per stick, 2 mg per tbsp, or 1 mg per pat.
[10] Values for vitamin A are year-round average.

Nutrients in Indicated Quantity

Cholesterol	Carbohydrate	Calcium	Phosphorus	Iron	Potassium	Sodium	Vitamin A value (IU)	Vitamin A value (RE)	Thiamin	Riboflavin	Niacin	Ascorbic acid	Item No.
Milligrams	Grams	Milligrams	Milligrams	Milligrams	Milligrams	Milligrams	International units	Retinol equivalents	Milligrams	Milligrams	Milligrams	Milligrams	
247	Tr	27	26	0.2	29	[9]933	[10]3,460	[10]852	0.01	0.04	Tr	0	128
31	Tr	3	3	Tr	4	[9]116	[10]430	[10]106	Tr	Tr	Tr	0	129
11	Tr	1	1	Tr	1	[9]41	[10]150	[10]38	Tr	Tr	Tr	0	130
0	0	0	0	0.0	0	0	0	0	0.00	0.00	0.0	0	131
0	0	0	0	0.0	0	0	0	0	0.00	0.00	0.0	0	132
195	0	0	0	0.0	0	0	0	0	0.00	0.00	0.0	0	133
12	0	0	0	0.0	0	0	0	0	0.00	0.00	0.0	0	134
0	1	40	31	0.0	57	[11]2,178	[12]7,510	[12]2,254	0.01	0.05	Tr	Tr	135
0	Tr	2	2	0.0	4	[11]134	[12]460	[12]139	Tr	Tr	Tr	Tr	136
0	1	34	26	0.1	48	[11]1,066	[12]3,740	[12]1,122	0.01	0.04	Tr	Tr	137
0	Tr	4	3	Tr	6	[11]132	[12]460	[12]139	Tr	0.01	Tr	Tr	138
0	Tr	1	1	Tr	2	[11]47	[12]170	[12]50	Tr	Tr	Tr	Tr	139
0	1	60	46	0.0	86	[11]2,449	[12]7,510	[12]2,254	0.02	0.07	Tr	Tr	140
0	Tr	4	3	0.0	5	[11]151	[12]460	[12]139	Tr	Tr	Tr	Tr	141
0	0	24	18	0.0	34	[11]1,123	[12]3,740	[12]1,122	0.01	0.03	Tr	Tr	142
0	0	3	2	0.0	4	[11]139	[12]460	[12]139	Tr	Tr	Tr	Tr	143
0	0	1	1	0.0	1	[11]50	[12]170	[12]50	Tr	Tr	Tr	Tr	144
0	0	47	37	0.0	68	[11]2,256	[12]7,510	[12]2,254	0.02	0.06	Tr	Tr	145
0	0	3	2	0.0	4	[11]139	[12]460	[12]139	Tr	Tr	Tr	Tr	146
0	0	0	0	0.0	0	0	0	0	0.00	0.00	0.0	0	147
0	0	0	0	0.0	0	0	0	0	0.00	0.00	0.0	0	148
0	0	0	0	0.0	0	0	0	0	0.00	0.00	0.0	0	149
0	0	0	0	0.0	0	0	0	0	0.00	0.00	0.0	0	150
0	0	0	0	0.0	0	0	0	0	0.00	0.00	0.0	0	151
0	0	0	0	0.0	0	0	0	0	0.00	0.00	0.0	0	152
0	0	0	0	0.0	0	0	0	0	0.00	0.00	0.0	0	153
0	0	0	0	0.0	0	0	0	0	0.00	0.00	0.0	0	154
0	0	0	0	0.0	0	0	0	0	0.00	0.00	0.0	0	155
0	0	0	0	0.0	0	0	0	0	0.00	0.00	0.0	0	156
0	0	0	0	0.0	0	0	0	0	0.00	0.00	0.0	0	157
0	0	0	0	0.0	0	0	0	0	0.00	0.00	0.0	0	158
0	0	0	0	0.0	0	0	0	0	0.00	0.00	0.0	0	159
0	0	0	0	0.0	0	0	0	0	0.00	0.00	0.0	0	160
3	1	12	11	Tr	6	164	30	10	Tr	0.02	Tr	Tr	161
0	1	2	1	Tr	2	188	Tr	Tr	Tr	Tr	Tr	Tr	162
0	2	6	5	Tr	3	306	Tr	Tr	Tr	Tr	Tr	Tr	163
0	1	1	1	Tr	5	162	30	3	Tr	Tr	Tr	Tr	164
0	2	1	1	Tr	4	136	Tr	Tr	Tr	Tr	Tr	Tr	165
8	Tr	3	4	0.1	5	80	40	12	0.00	0.00	Tr	0	166
4	2	Tr	Tr	0.0	2	75	0	0	0.00	0.00	0.0	0	167
4	4	2	4	Tr	1	107	30	13	Tr	Tr	Tr	0	168
4	1	3	4	0.1	11	182	30	9	Tr	Tr	0.0	Tr	169
4	2	2	3	0.1	18	112	50	15	Tr	Tr	Tr	0	170
2	2	2	3	0.1	17	150	50	14	Tr	Tr	Tr	0	171

[11]For salted margarine.

[12]Based on average vitamin A content of fortified margarine. Federal specifications for fortified margarine require a minimum of 15,000 IU per pound.

Item No.	Foods, approximate measures, units, and weight (weight of edible portion only)			Water	Food energy	Protein	Fat	Fatty acids: Saturated	Fatty acids: Monounsaturated	Fatty acids: Polyunsaturated
	Fats and Oils—Con.		Grams	Percent	Calories	Grams	Grams	Grams	Grams	Grams
	Salad dressings:									
	Prepared from home recipe:									
172	Cooked type[13]	1 tbsp	16	69	25	1	2	0.5	0.6	0.3
173	Vinegar and oil	1 tbsp	16	47	70	0	8	1.5	2.4	3.9
	Fish and Shellfish									
	Clams:									
174	Raw, meat only	3 oz	85	82	65	11	1	0.3	0.3	0.3
175	Canned, drained solids	3 oz	85	77	85	13	2	0.5	0.5	0.4
176	Crabmeat, canned	1 cup	135	77	135	23	3	0.5	0.8	1.4
177	Fish sticks, frozen, reheated, (stick, 4 by 1 by 1/2 in)	1 fish stick	28	52	70	6	3	0.8	1.4	0.8
	Flounder or Sole, baked, with lemon juice:									
178	With butter	3 oz	85	73	120	16	6	3.2	1.5	0.5
179	With margarine	3 oz	85	73	120	16	6	1.2	2.3	1.9
180	Without added fat	3 oz	85	78	80	17	1	0.3	0.2	0.4
181	Haddock, breaded, fried[14]	3 oz	85	61	175	17	9	2.4	3.9	2.4
182	Halibut, broiled, with butter and lemon juice	3 oz	85	67	140	20	6	3.3	1.6	0.7
183	Herring, pickled	3 oz	85	59	190	17	13	4.3	4.6	3.1
184	Ocean perch, breaded, fried[14]	1 fillet	85	59	185	16	11	2.6	4.6	2.8
	Oysters:									
185	Raw, meat only (13-19 medium Selects)	1 cup	240	85	160	20	4	1.4	0.5	1.4
186	Breaded, fried[14]	1 oyster	45	65	90	5	5	1.4	2.1	1.4
	Salmon:									
187	Canned (pink), solids and liquid	3 oz	85	71	120	17	5	0.9	1.5	2.1
188	Baked (red)	3 oz	85	67	140	21	5	1.2	2.4	1.4
189	Smoked	3 oz	85	59	150	18	8	2.6	3.9	0.7
190	Sardines, Atlantic, canned in oil, drained solids	3 oz	85	62	175	20	9	2.1	3.7	2.9
191	Scallops, breaded, frozen, reheated	6 scallops	90	59	195	15	10	2.5	4.1	2.5
	Shrimp:									
192	Canned, drained solids	3 oz	85	70	100	21	1	0.2	0.2	0.4
193	French fried (7 medium)[16]	3 oz	85	55	200	16	10	2.5	4.1	2.6
194	Trout, broiled, with butter and lemon juice	3 oz	85	63	175	21	9	4.1	2.9	1.6
	Tuna, canned, drained solids:									
195	Oil pack, chunk light	3 oz	85	61	165	24	7	1.4	1.9	3.1
196	Water pack, solid white	3 oz	85	63	135	30	1	0.3	0.2	0.3
197	Tuna salad[17]	1 cup	205	63	375	33	19	3.3	4.9	9.2
	Fruits and Fruit Juices									
	Apples:									
	Raw:									
	Unpeeled, without cores:									
198	2-3/4-in diam. (about 3 per lb with cores)	1 apple	138	84	80	Tr	Tr	0.1	Tr	0.1
199	3-1/4-in diam. (about 2 per lb with cores)	1 apple	212	84	125	Tr	1	0.1	Tr	0.2
200	Peeled, sliced	1 cup	110	84	65	Tr	Tr	0.1	Tr	0.1
201	Dried, sulfured	10 rings	64	32	155	1	Tr	Tr	Tr	0.1
202	Apple juice, bottled or canned[19]	1 cup	248	88	115	Tr	Tr	Tr	Tr	0.1
	Applesauce, canned:									
203	Sweetened	1 cup	255	80	195	Tr	Tr	0.1	Tr	0.1
204	Unsweetened	1 cup	244	88	105	Tr	Tr	Tr	Tr	Tr

[13] Fatty acid values apply to product made with regular margarine.
[14] Dipped in egg, milk, and breadcrumbs; fried in vegetable shortening.
[15] If bones are discarded, value for calcium will be greatly reduced.
[16] Dipped in egg, breadcrumbs, and flour; fried in vegetable shortening.

Nutrients in Indicated Quantity

Cholesterol	Carbohydrate	Calcium	Phosphorus	Iron	Potassium	Sodium	Vitamin A value (IU)	Vitamin A value (RE)	Thiamin	Riboflavin	Niacin	Ascorbic acid	Item No.
Milligrams	Grams	Milligrams	Milligrams	Milligrams	Milligrams	Milligrams	International units	Retinol equivalents	Milligrams	Milligrams	Milligrams	Milligrams	
9	2	13	14	0.1	19	117	70	20	0.01	0.02	Tr	Tr	172
0	Tr	0	0	0.0	1	Tr	0	0	0.00	0.00	0.0	0	173
43	2	59	138	2.6	154	102	90	26	0.09	0.15	1.1	9	174
54	2	47	116	3.5	119	102	90	26	0.01	0.09	0.9	3	175
135	1	61	246	1.1	149	1,350	50	14	0.11	0.11	2.6	0	176
26	4	11	58	0.3	94	53	20	5	0.03	0.05	0.6	0	177
68	Tr	13	187	0.3	272	145	210	54	0.05	0.08	1.6	1	178
55	Tr	14	187	0.3	273	151	230	69	0.05	0.08	1.6	1	179
59	Tr	13	197	0.3	286	101	30	10	0.05	0.08	1.7	1	180
75	7	34	183	1.0	270	123	70	20	0.06	0.10	2.9	0	181
62	Tr	14	206	0.7	441	103	610	174	0.06	0.07	7.7	1	182
85	0	29	128	0.9	85	850	110	33	0.04	0.18	2.8	0	183
66	7	31	191	1.2	241	138	70	20	0.10	0.11	2.0	0	184
120	8	226	343	15.6	290	175	740	223	0.34	0.43	6.0	24	185
35	5	49	73	3.0	64	70	150	44	0.07	0.10	1.3	4	186
34	0	[15]167	243	0.7	307	443	60	18	0.03	0.15	6.8	0	187
60	0	26	269	0.5	305	55	290	87	0.18	0.14	5.5	0	188
51	0	12	208	0.8	327	1,700	260	77	0.17	0.17	6.8	0	189
85	0	[15]371	424	2.6	349	425	190	56	0.03	0.17	4.6	0	190
70	10	39	203	2.0	369	298	70	21	0.11	0.11	1.6	0	191
128	1	98	224	1.4	104	1,955	50	15	0.01	0.03	1.5	0	192
168	11	61	154	2.0	189	384	90	26	0.06	0.09	2.8	0	193
71	Tr	26	259	1.0	297	122	230	60	0.07	0.07	2.3	1	194
55	0	7	199	1.6	298	303	70	20	0.04	0.09	10.1	0	195
48	0	17	202	0.6	255	468	110	32	0.03	0.10	13.4	0	196
80	19	31	281	2.5	531	877	230	53	0.06	0.14	13.3	6	197
0	21	10	10	0.2	159	Tr	70	7	0.02	0.02	0.1	8	198
0	32	15	15	0.4	244	Tr	110	11	0.04	0.03	0.2	12	199
0	16	4	8	0.1	124	Tr	50	5	0.02	0.01	0.1	4	200
0	42	9	24	0.9	288	[18]56	0	0	0.00	0.10	0.6	2	201
0	29	17	17	0.9	295	7	Tr	Tr	0.05	0.04	0.2	[20]2	202
0	51	10	18	0.9	156	8	30	3	0.03	0.07	0.5	[20]4	203
0	28	7	17	0.3	183	5	70	7	0.03	0.06	0.5	[20]3	204

[17] Made with drained chunk light tuna, celery, onion, pickle relish, and mayonnaise-type salad dressing.
[18] Sodium bisulfite used to preserve color; unsulfited product would contain less sodium.
[19] Also applies to pasteurized apple cider.
[20] Without added ascorbic acid. For value with added ascorbic acid, refer to label.

Item No.	Foods, approximate measures, units, and weight (weight of edible portion only)			Water	Food energy	Pro-tein	Fat	Fatty acids		
								Satu-rated	Mono-unsatu-rated	Poly-unsatu-rated
	Fruits and Fruit Juices—Con.		Grams	Per-cent	Cal-ories	Grams	Grams	Grams	Grams	Grams
	Apricots:									
205	Raw, without pits (about 12 per lb with pits)	3 apricots	106	86	50	1	Tr	Tr	0.2	0.1
	Canned (fruit and liquid):									
206	Heavy syrup pack	1 cup	258	78	215	1	Tr	Tr	0.1	Tr
207		3 halves	85	78	70	Tr	Tr	Tr	Tr	Tr
208	Juice pack	1 cup	248	87	120	2	Tr	Tr	Tr	Tr
209		3 halves	84	87	40	1	Tr	Tr	Tr	Tr
	Dried:									
210	Uncooked (28 large or 37 medium halves per cup)	1 cup	130	31	310	5	1	Tr	0.3	0.1
211	Cooked, unsweetened, fruit and liquid	1 cup	250	76	210	3	Tr	Tr	0.2	0.1
212	Apricot nectar, canned	1 cup	251	85	140	1	Tr	Tr	0.1	Tr
	Avocados, raw, whole, without skin and seed:									
213	California (about 2 per lb with skin and seed)	1 avocado	173	73	305	4	30	4.5	19.4	3.5
214	Florida (about 1 per lb with skin and seed)	1 avocado	304	80	340	5	27	5.3	14.8	4.5
	Bananas, raw, without peel:									
215	Whole (about 2-1/2 per lb with peel)	1 banana	114	74	105	1	1	0.2	Tr	0.1
216	Sliced	1 cup	150	74	140	2	1	0.3	0.1	0.1
217	Blackberries, raw	1 cup	144	86	75	1	1	0.2	0.1	0.1
	Blueberries:									
218	Raw	1 cup	145	85	80	1	1	Tr	0.1	0.3
219	Frozen, sweetened	10-oz container	284	77	230	1	Tr	Tr	0.1	0.2
220		1 cup	230	77	185	1	Tr	Tr	Tr	0.1
	Cantaloup. See Melons (item 251).									
	Cherries:									
221	Sour, red, pitted, canned, water pack	1 cup	244	90	90	2	Tr	0.1	0.1	0.1
222	Sweet, raw, without pits and stems	10 cherries	68	81	50	1	1	0.1	0.2	0.2
223	Cranberry juice cocktail, bottled, sweetened	1 cup	253	85	145	Tr	Tr	Tr	Tr	0.1
224	Cranberry sauce, sweetened, canned, strained	1 cup	277	61	420	1	Tr	Tr	0.1	0.2
	Dates:									
225	Whole, without pits	10 dates	83	23	230	2	Tr	0.1	0.1	Tr
226	Chopped	1 cup	178	23	490	4	1	0.3	0.2	Tr
227	Figs, dried	10 figs	187	28	475	6	2	0.4	0.5	1.0
	Fruit cocktail, canned, fruit and liquid:									
228	Heavy syrup pack	1 cup	255	80	185	1	Tr	Tr	Tr	0.1
229	Juice pack	1 cup	248	87	115	1	Tr	Tr	Tr	Tr
	Grapefruit:									
230	Raw, without peel, membrane and seeds (3-3/4-in diam., 1 lb 1 oz, whole, with refuse)	1/2 grapefruit	120	91	40	1	Tr	Tr	Tr	Tr
231	Canned, sections with syrup	1 cup	254	84	150	1	Tr	Tr	Tr	0.1
	Grapefruit juice:									
232	Raw	1 cup	247	90	95	1	Tr	Tr	Tr	0.1
	Canned:									
233	Unsweetened	1 cup	247	90	95	1	Tr	Tr	Tr	0.1
234	Sweetened	1 cup	250	87	115	1	Tr	Tr	Tr	0.1
	Frozen concentrate, unsweetened									
235	Undiluted	6-fl-oz can	207	62	300	4	1	0.1	0.1	0.2
236	Diluted with 3 parts water by volume	1 cup	247	89	100	1	Tr	Tr	Tr	0.1

[20] Without added ascorbic acid. For value with added ascorbic acid, refer to label.
[21] With added ascorbic acid.

Nutrients in Indicated Quantity													
Cholesterol	Carbohydrate	Calcium	Phosphorus	Iron	Potassium	Sodium	Vitamin A value (IU)	Vitamin A value (RE)	Thiamin	Riboflavin	Niacin	Ascorbic acid	Item No.
Milligrams	Grams	Milligrams	Milligrams	Milligrams	Milligrams	Milligrams	International units	Retinol equivalents	Milligrams	Milligrams	Milligrams	Milligrams	
0	12	15	20	0.6	314	1	2,770	277	0.03	0.04	0.6	11	205
0	55	23	31	0.8	361	10	3,170	317	0.05	0.06	1.0	8	206
0	18	8	10	0.3	119	3	1,050	105	0.02	0.02	0.3	3	207
0	31	30	50	0.7	409	10	4,190	419	0.04	0.05	0.9	12	208
0	10	10	17	0.3	139	3	1,420	142	0.02	0.02	0.3	4	209
0	80	59	152	6.1	1,791	13	9,410	941	0.01	0.20	3.9	3	210
0	55	40	103	4.2	1,222	8	5,910	591	0.02	0.08	2.4	4	211
0	36	18	23	1.0	286	8	3,300	330	0.02	0.04	0.7	[20]2	212
0	12	19	73	2.0	1,097	21	1,060	106	0.19	0.21	3.3	14	213
0	27	33	119	1.6	1,484	15	1,860	186	0.33	0.37	5.8	24	214
0	27	7	23	0.4	451	1	90	9	0.05	0.11	0.6	10	215
0	35	9	30	0.5	594	2	120	12	0.07	0.15	0.8	14	216
0	18	46	30	0.8	282	Tr	240	24	0.04	0.06	0.6	30	217
0	20	9	15	0.2	129	9	150	15	0.07	0.07	0.5	19	218
0	62	17	20	1.1	170	3	120	12	0.06	0.15	0.7	3	219
0	50	14	16	0.9	138	2	100	10	0.05	0.12	0.6	2	220
0	22	27	24	3.3	239	17	1,840	184	0.04	0.10	0.4	5	221
0	11	10	13	0.3	152	Tr	150	15	0.03	0.04	0.3	5	222
0	38	8	3	0.4	61	10	10	1	0.01	0.04	0.1	[21]108	223
0	108	11	17	0.6	72	80	60	6	0.04	0.06	0.3	6	224
0	61	27	33	1.0	541	2	40	4	0.07	0.08	1.8	0	225
0	131	57	71	2.0	1,161	5	90	9	0.16	0.18	3.9	0	226
0	122	269	127	4.2	1,331	21	250	25	0.13	0.16	1.3	1	227
0	48	15	28	0.7	224	15	520	52	0.05	0.05	1.0	5	228
0	29	20	35	0.5	236	10	760	76	0.03	0.04	1.0	7	229
0	10	14	10	0.1	167	Tr	[22]10	[22]1	0.04	0.02	0.3	41	230
0	39	36	25	1.0	328	5	Tr	Tr	0.10	0.05	0.6	54	231
0	23	22	37	0.5	400	2	20	2	0.10	0.05	0.5	94	232
0	22	17	27	0.5	378	2	20	2	0.10	0.05	0.6	72	233
0	28	20	28	0.9	405	5	20	2	0.10	0.06	0.8	67	234
0	72	56	101	1.0	1,002	6	60	6	0.30	0.16	1.6	248	235
0	24	20	35	0.3	336	2	20	2	0.10	0.05	0.5	83	236

[22]For white grapefruit; pink grapefruit have about 310 IU or 31 RE.

Item No.	Foods, approximate measures, units, and weight (weight of edible portion only)			Water	Food energy	Protein	Fat	Fatty acids Saturated	Fatty acids Monounsaturated	Fatty acids Polyunsaturated
	Fruits and Fruit Juices—Con.		Grams	Percent	Calories	Grams	Grams	Grams	Grams	Grams
	Grapes, European type (adherent skin), raw:									
237	Thompson Seedless	10 grapes	50	81	35	Tr	Tr	0.1	Tr	0.1
238	Tokay and Emperor, seeded types	10 grapes	57	81	40	Tr	Tr	0.1	Tr	0.1
	Grape juice:									
239	Canned or bottled	1 cup	253	84	155	1	Tr	0.1	Tr	0.1
	Frozen concentrate, sweetened:									
240	Undiluted	6-fl-oz can	216	54	385	1	1	0.2	Tr	0.2
241	Diluted with 3 parts water by volume	1 cup	250	87	125	Tr	Tr	0.1	Tr	0.1
242	Kiwifruit, raw, without skin (about 5 per lb with skin)	1 kiwifruit	76	83	45	1	Tr	Tr	0.1	0.1
243	Lemons, raw, without peel and seeds (about 4 per lb with peel and seeds)	1 lemon	58	89	15	1	Tr	Tr	Tr	0.1
	Lemon juice:									
244	Raw	1 cup	244	91	60	1	Tr	Tr	Tr	Tr
245	Canned or bottled, unsweetened	1 cup	244	92	50	1	1	0.1	Tr	0.2
246		1 tbsp	15	92	5	Tr	Tr	Tr	Tr	Tr
247	Frozen, single-strength, unsweetened	6-fl-oz can	244	92	55	1	1	0.1	Tr	0.2
	Lime juice:									
248	Raw	1 cup	246	90	65	1	Tr	Tr	Tr	0.1
249	Canned, unsweetened	1 cup	246	93	50	1	1	0.1	0.1	0.2
250	Mangos, raw, without skin and seed (about 1-1/2 per lb with skin and seed)	1 mango	207	82	135	1	1	0.1	0.2	0.1
	Melons, raw, without rind and cavity contents:									
251	Cantaloup, orange-fleshed (5-in diam., 2-1/3 lb, whole, with rind and cavity contents)	1/2 melon	267	90	95	2	1	0.1	0.1	0.3
252	Honeydew (6-1/2-in diam., 5-1/4 lb, whole, with rind and cavity contents)	1/10 melon	129	90	45	1	Tr	Tr	Tr	0.1
253	Nectarines, raw, without pits (about 3 per lb with pits)	1 nectarine	136	86	65	1	1	0.1	0.2	0.3
	Oranges, raw:									
254	Whole, without peel and seeds (2-5/8-in diam., about 2-1/2 per lb, with peel and seeds)	1 orange	131	87	60	1	Tr	Tr	Tr	Tr
255	Sections without membranes	1 cup	180	87	85	2	Tr	Tr	Tr	Tr
	Orange juice:									
256	Raw, all varieties	1 cup	248	88	110	2	Tr	0.1	0.1	0.1
257	Canned, unsweetened	1 cup	249	89	105	1	Tr	Tr	0.1	0.1
258	Chilled	1 cup	249	88	110	2	1	0.1	0.1	0.2
	Frozen concentrate:									
259	Undiluted	6-fl-oz can	213	58	340	5	Tr	0.1	0.1	0.1
260	Diluted with 3 parts water by volume	1 cup	249	88	110	2	Tr	Tr	Tr	Tr
261	Orange and grapefruit juice, canned	1 cup	247	89	105	1	Tr	Tr	Tr	Tr
262	Papayas, raw, 1/2-in cubes	1 cup	140	86	65	1	Tr	0.1	0.1	Tr
	Peaches:									
	Raw:									
263	Whole, 2-1/2-in diam., peeled, pitted (about 4 per lb with peels and pits)	1 peach	87	88	35	1	Tr	Tr	Tr	Tr
264	Sliced	1 cup	170	88	75	1	Tr	Tr	0.1	0.1
	Canned, fruit and liquid:									
265	Heavy syrup pack	1 cup	256	79	190	1	Tr	Tr	0.1	0.1
266		1 half	81	79	60	Tr	Tr	Tr	Tr	Tr
267	Juice pack	1 cup	248	87	110	2	Tr	Tr	Tr	Tr
268		1 half	77	87	35	Tr	Tr	Tr	Tr	Tr

[20] Without added ascorbic acid. For value with added ascorbic acid, refer to label.
[21] With added ascorbic acid.

Nutrients in Indicated Quantity

Cholesterol	Carbohydrate	Calcium	Phosphorus	Iron	Potassium	Sodium	Vitamin A value (IU)	Vitamin A value (RE)	Thiamin	Riboflavin	Niacin	Ascorbic acid	Item No.
Milligrams	Grams	Milligrams	Milligrams	Milligrams	Milligrams	Milligrams	International units	Retinol equivalents	Milligrams	Milligrams	Milligrams	Milligrams	
0	9	6	7	0.1	93	1	40	4	0.05	0.03	0.2	5	237
0	10	6	7	0.1	105	1	40	4	0.05	0.03	0.2	6	238
0	38	23	28	0.6	334	8	20	2	0.07	0.09	0.7	[20]Tr	239
0	96	28	32	0.8	160	15	60	6	0.11	0.20	0.9	[21]179	240
0	32	10	10	0.3	53	5	20	2	0.04	0.07	0.3	[21]60	241
0	11	20	30	0.3	252	4	130	13	0.02	0.04	0.4	74	242
0	5	15	9	0.3	80	1	20	2	0.02	0.01	0.1	31	243
0	21	17	15	0.1	303	2	50	5	0.07	0.02	0.2	112	244
0	16	27	22	0.3	249	[23]51	40	4	0.10	0.02	0.5	61	245
0	1	2	1	Tr	15	[23]3	Tr	Tr	0.01	Tr	Tr	4	246
0	16	20	20	0.3	217	2	30	3	0.14	0.03	0.3	77	247
0	22	22	17	0.1	268	2	20	2	0.05	0.02	0.2	72	248
0	16	30	25	0.6	185	[23]39	40	4	0.08	0.01	0.4	16	249
0	35	21	23	0.3	323	4	8,060	806	0.12	0.12	1.2	57	250
0	22	29	45	0.6	825	24	8,610	861	0.10	0.06	1.5	113	251
0	12	8	13	0.1	350	13	50	5	0.10	0.02	0.8	32	252
0	16	7	22	0.2	288	Tr	1,000	100	0.02	0.06	1.3	7	253
0	15	52	18	0.1	237	Tr	270	27	0.11	0.05	0.4	70	254
0	21	72	25	0.2	326	Tr	370	37	0.16	0.07	0.5	96	255
0	26	27	42	0.5	496	2	500	50	0.22	0.07	1.0	124	256
0	25	20	35	1.1	436	5	440	44	0.15	0.07	0.8	86	257
0	25	25	27	0.4	473	2	190	19	0.28	0.05	0.7	82	258
0	81	68	121	0.7	1,436	6	590	59	0.60	0.14	1.5	294	259
0	27	22	40	0.2	473	2	190	19	0.20	0.04	0.5	97	260
0	25	20	35	1.1	390	7	290	29	0.14	0.07	0.8	72	261
0	17	35	12	0.3	247	9	400	40	0.04	0.04	0.5	92	262
0	10	4	10	0.1	171	Tr	470	47	0.01	0.04	0.9	6	263
0	19	9	20	0.2	335	Tr	910	91	0.03	0.07	1.7	11	264
0	51	8	28	0.7	236	15	850	85	0.03	0.06	1.6	7	265
0	16	2	9	0.2	75	5	270	27	0.01	0.02	0.5	2	266
0	29	15	42	0.7	317	10	940	94	0.02	0.04	1.4	9	267
0	9	5	13	0.2	99	3	290	29	0.01	0.01	0.4	3	268

[23]Sodium benzoate and sodium bisulfite added as preservatives.

Item No.	Foods, approximate measures, units, and weight (weight of edible portion only)			Water	Food energy	Protein	Fat	Fatty acids		
								Saturated	Monounsaturated	Polyunsaturated
	Fruits and Fruit Juices—Con.		Grams	Percent	Calories	Grams	Grams	Grams	Grams	Grams
	Peaches:									
	Dried:									
269	Uncooked	1 cup	160	32	380	6	1	0.1	0.4	0.6
270	Cooked, unsweetened, fruit and liquid	1 cup	258	78	200	3	1	0.1	0.2	0.3
271	Frozen, sliced, sweetened	10-oz container	284	75	265	2	Tr	Tr	0.1	0.2
272		1 cup	250	75	235	2	Tr	Tr	0.1	0.2
	Pears:									
	Raw, with skin, cored:									
273	Bartlett, 2-1/2-in diam. (about 2-1/2 per lb with cores and stems)	1 pear	166	84	100	1	1	Tr	0.1	0.2
274	Bosc, 2-1/2-in diam. (about 3 per lb with cores and stems)	1 pear	141	84	85	1	1	Tr	0.1	0.1
275	D'Anjou, 3-in diam. (about 2 per lb with cores and stems)	1 pear	200	84	120	1	1	Tr	0.2	0.2
	Canned, fruit and liquid:									
276	Heavy syrup pack	1 cup	255	80	190	1	Tr	Tr	0.1	0.1
277		1 half	79	80	60	Tr	Tr	Tr	Tr	Tr
278	Juice pack	1 cup	248	86	125	1	Tr	Tr	Tr	Tr
279		1 half	77	86	40	Tr	Tr	Tr	Tr	Tr
	Pineapple:									
280	Raw, diced	1 cup	155	87	75	1	1	Tr	0.1	0.2
	Canned, fruit and liquid:									
	Heavy syrup pack:									
281	Crushed, chunks, tidbits	1 cup	255	79	200	1	Tr	Tr	Tr	0.1
282	Slices	1 slice	58	79	45	Tr	Tr	Tr	Tr	Tr
	Juice pack:									
283	Chunks or tidbits	1 cup	250	84	150	1	Tr	Tr	Tr	0.1
284	Slices	1 slice	58	84	35	Tr	Tr	Tr	Tr	Tr
285	Pineapple juice, unsweetened, canned	1 cup	250	86	140	1	Tr	Tr	Tr	0.1
	Plantains, without peel:									
286	Raw	1 plantain	179	65	220	2	1	0.3	0.1	0.1
287	Cooked, boiled, sliced	1 cup	154	67	180	1	Tr	0.1	Tr	0.1
	Plums, without pits:									
	Raw:									
288	2-1/8-in diam. (about 6-1/2 per lb with pits)	1 plum	66	85	35	1	Tr	Tr	0.3	0.1
289	1-1/2-in diam. (about 15 per lb with pits)	1 plum	28	85	15	Tr	Tr	Tr	0.1	Tr
	Canned, purple, fruit and liquid:									
290	Heavy syrup pack	1 cup	258	76	230	1	Tr	Tr	0.2	0.1
291		3 plums	133	76	120	Tr	Tr	Tr	0.1	Tr
292	Juice pack	1 cup	252	84	145	1	Tr	Tr	Tr	Tr
293		3 plums	95	84	55	Tr	Tr	Tr	Tr	Tr
	Prunes, dried:									
294	Uncooked	4 extra large or 5 large prunes	49	32	115	1	Tr	Tr	0.2	0.1
295	Cooked, unsweetened, fruit and liquid	1 cup	212	70	225	2	Tr	Tr	0.3	0.1
296	Prune juice, canned or bottled	1 cup	256	81	180	2	Tr	Tr	0.1	Tr
	Raisins, seedless:									
297	Cup, not pressed down	1 cup	145	15	435	5	1	0.2	Tr	0.2
298	Packet, 1/2 oz (1-1/2 tbsp)	1 packet	14	15	40	Tr	Tr	Tr	Tr	Tr
	Raspberries:									
299	Raw	1 cup	123	87	60	1	1	Tr	0.1	0.4
300	Frozen, sweetened	10-oz container	284	73	295	2	Tr	Tr	Tr	0.3
301		1 cup	250	73	255	2	Tr	Tr	Tr	0.2

[21] With added ascorbic acid.

Nutrients in Indicated Quantity

Cholesterol	Carbohydrate	Calcium	Phosphorus	Iron	Potassium	Sodium	Vitamin A value (IU)	Vitamin A value (RE)	Thiamin	Riboflavin	Niacin	Ascorbic acid	Item No.
Milligrams	Grams	Milligrams	Milligrams	Milligrams	Milligrams	Milligrams	International units	Retinol equivalents	Milligrams	Milligrams	Milligrams	Milligrams	
0	98	45	190	6.5	1,594	11	3,460	346	Tr	0.34	7.0	8	269
0	51	23	98	3.4	826	5	510	51	0.01	0.05	3.9	10	270
0	68	9	31	1.1	369	17	810	81	0.04	0.10	1.9	[21]268	271
0	60	8	28	0.9	325	15	710	71	0.03	0.09	1.6	[21]236	272
0	25	18	18	0.4	208	Tr	30	3	0.03	0.07	0.2	7	273
0	21	16	16	0.4	176	Tr	30	3	0.03	0.06	0.1	6	274
0	30	22	22	0.5	250	Tr	40	4	0.04	0.08	0.2	8	275
0	49	13	18	0.6	166	13	10	1	0.03	0.06	0.6	3	276
0	15	4	6	0.2	51	4	Tr	Tr	0.01	0.02	0.2	1	277
0	32	22	30	0.7	238	10	10	1	0.03	0.03	0.5	4	278
0	10	7	9	0.2	74	3	Tr	Tr	0.01	0.01	0.2	1	279
0	19	11	11	0.6	175	2	40	4	0.14	0.06	0.7	24	280
0	52	36	18	1.0	265	3	40	4	0.23	0.06	0.7	19	281
0	12	8	4	0.2	60	1	10	1	0.05	0.01	0.2	4	282
0	39	35	15	0.7	305	3	100	10	0.24	0.05	0.7	24	283
0	9	8	3	0.2	71	1	20	2	0.06	0.01	0.2	6	284
0	34	43	20	0.7	335	3	10	1	0.14	0.06	0.6	27	285
0	57	5	61	1.1	893	7	2,020	202	0.09	0.10	1.2	33	286
0	48	3	43	0.9	716	8	1,400	140	0.07	0.08	1.2	17	287
0	9	3	7	0.1	114	Tr	210	21	0.03	0.06	0.3	6	288
0	4	1	3	Tr	48	Tr	90	9	0.01	0.03	0.1	3	289
0	60	23	34	2.2	235	49	670	67	0.04	0.10	0.8	1	290
0	31	12	17	1.1	121	25	340	34	0.02	0.05	0.4	1	291
0	38	25	38	0.9	388	3	2,540	254	0.06	0.15	1.2	7	292
0	14	10	14	0.3	146	1	960	96	0.02	0.06	0.4	3	293
0	31	25	39	1.2	365	2	970	97	0.04	0.08	1.0	2	294
0	60	49	74	2.4	708	4	650	65	0.05	0.21	1.5	6	295
0	45	31	64	3.0	707	10	10	1	0.04	0.18	2.0	10	296
0	115	71	141	3.0	1,089	17	10	1	0.23	0.13	1.2	5	297
0	11	7	14	0.3	105	2	Tr	Tr	0.02	0.01	0.1	Tr	298
0	14	27	15	0.7	187	Tr	160	16	0.04	0.11	1.1	31	299
0	74	43	48	1.8	324	3	170	17	0.05	0.13	0.7	47	300
0	65	38	43	1.6	285	3	150	15	0.05	0.11	0.6	41	301

Item No.	Foods, approximate measures, units, and weight (weight of edible portion only)			Water	Food energy	Protein	Fat	Fatty acids: Saturated	Fatty acids: Monounsaturated	Fatty acids: Polyunsaturated
	Fruits and Fruit Juices—Con.		Grams	Percent	Calories	Grams	Grams	Grams	Grams	Grams
302	Rhubarb, cooked, added sugar-----	1 cup----------	240	68	280	1	Tr	Tr	Tr	0.1
	Strawberries:									
303	Raw, capped, whole------------	1 cup----------	149	92	45	1	1	Tr	0.1	0.3
304	Frozen, sweetened, sliced------	10-oz container	284	73	275	2	Tr	Tr	0.1	0.2
305		1 cup----------	255	73	245	1	Tr	Tr	Tr	0.2
	Tangerines:									
306	Raw, without peel and seeds (2-3/8-in diam., about 4 per lb, with peel and seeds)-----	1 tangerine-----	84	88	35	1	Tr	Tr	Tr	Tr
307	Canned, light syrup, fruit and liquid----------------------	1 cup----------	252	83	155	1	Tr	Tr	Tr	0.1
308	Tangerine juice, canned, sweetened------------------------	1 cup----------	249	87	125	1	Tr	Tr	Tr	0.1
	Watermelon, raw, without rind and seeds:									
309	Piece (4 by 8 in wedge with rind and seeds; 1/16 of 32-2/3-lb melon, 10 by 16 in)	1 piece---------	482	92	155	3	2	0.3	0.2	1.0
310	Diced------------------------	1 cup----------	160	92	50	1	1	0.1	0.1	0.3
	Grain Products									
311	Bagels, plain or water, enriched, 3-1/2-in diam.[24] ---------------	1 bagel---------	68	29	200	7	2	0.3	0.5	0.7
312	Barley, pearled, light, uncooked	1 cup----------	200	11	700	16	2	0.3	0.2	0.9
	Biscuits, baking powder, 2-in diam. (enriched flour, vegetable shortening):									
313	From home recipe---------------	1 biscuit-------	28	28	100	2	5	1.2	2.0	1.3
314	From mix----------------------	1 biscuit-------	28	29	95	2	3	0.8	1.4	0.9
315	From refrigerated dough--------	1 biscuit-------	20	30	65	1	2	0.6	0.9	0.6
	Breadcrumbs, enriched:									
316	Dry, grated--------------------	1 cup----------	100	7	390	13	5	1.5	1.6	1.0
	Soft. See White bread (item 351).									
	Breads:									
317	Boston brown bread, canned, slice, 3-1/4 in by 1/2 in[25]--	1 slice---------	45	45	95	2	1	0.3	0.1	0.1
	Cracked-wheat bread (3/4 enriched wheat flour, 1/4 cracked wheat flour):[25]									
318	Loaf, 1 lb-------------------	1 loaf----------	454	35	1,190	42	16	3.1	4.3	5.7
319	Slice (18 per loaf)----------	1 slice---------	25	35	65	2	1	0.2	0.2	0.3
320	Toasted--------------------	1 slice---------	21	26	65	2	1	0.2	0.2	0.3
	French or vienna bread, enriched:[25]									
321	Loaf, 1 lb-------------------	1 loaf----------	454	34	1,270	43	18	3.8	5.7	5.9
	Slice:									
322	French, 5 by 2-1/2 by 1 in	1 slice---------	35	34	100	3	1	0.3	0.4	0.5
323	Vienna, 4-3/4 by 4 by 1/2 in----------------------	1 slice---------	25	34	70	2	1	0.2	0.3	0.3
	Italian bread, enriched:									
324	Loaf, 1 lb-------------------	1 loaf----------	454	32	1,255	41	4	0.6	0.3	1.6
325	Slice, 4-1/2 by 3-1/4 by 3/4 in------------------------	1 slice---------	30	32	85	3	Tr	Tr	Tr	0.1
	Mixed grain bread, enriched:[25]									
326	Loaf, 1 lb-------------------	1 loaf----------	454	37	1,165	45	17	3.2	4.1	6.5
327	Slice (18 per loaf)----------	1 slice---------	25	37	65	2	1	0.2	0.2	0.4
328	Toasted--------------------	1 slice---------	23	27	65	2	1	0.2	0.2	0.4

[24] Egg bagels have 44 mg cholesterol and 22 IU or 7 RE vitamin A per bagel.
[25] Made with vegetable shortening.

Nutrients in Indicated Quantity

Cholesterol	Carbohydrate	Calcium	Phosphorus	Iron	Potassium	Sodium	Vitamin A value (IU)	Vitamin A value (RE)	Thiamin	Riboflavin	Niacin	Ascorbic acid	Item No.
Milligrams	Grams	Milligrams	Milligrams	Milligrams	Milligrams	Milligrams	International units	Retinol equivalents	Milligrams	Milligrams	Milligrams	Milligrams	
0	75	348	19	0.5	230	2	170	17	0.04	0.06	0.5	8	302
0	10	21	28	0.6	247	1	40	4	0.03	0.10	0.3	84	303
0	74	31	37	1.7	278	9	70	7	0.05	0.14	1.1	118	304
0	66	28	33	1.5	250	8	60	6	0.04	0.13	1.0	106	305
0	9	12	8	0.1	132	1	770	77	0.09	0.02	0.1	26	306
0	41	18	25	0.9	197	15	2,120	212	0.13	0.11	1.1	50	307
0	30	45	35	0.5	443	2	1,050	105	0.15	0.05	0.2	55	308
0	35	39	43	0.8	559	10	1,760	176	0.39	0.10	1.0	46	309
0	11	13	14	0.3	186	3	590	59	0.13	0.03	0.3	15	310
0	38	29	46	1.8	50	245	0	0	0.26	0.20	2.4	0	311
0	158	32	378	4.2	320	6	0	0	0.24	0.10	6.2	0	312
Tr	13	47	36	0.7	32	195	10	3	0.08	0.08	0.8	Tr	313
Tr	14	58	128	0.7	56	262	20	4	0.12	0.11	0.8	Tr	314
1	10	4	79	0.5	18	249	0	0	0.08	0.05	0.7	0	315
5	73	122	141	4.1	152	736	0	0	0.35	0.35	4.8	0	316
3	21	41	72	0.9	131	113	[26]0	[26]0	0.06	0.04	0.7	0	317
0	227	295	581	12.1	608	1,966	Tr	Tr	1.73	1.73	15.3	Tr	318
0	12	16	32	0.7	34	106	Tr	Tr	0.10	0.09	0.8	Tr	319
0	12	16	32	0.7	34	106	Tr	Tr	0.07	0.09	0.8	Tr	320
0	230	499	386	14.0	409	2,633	Tr	Tr	2.09	1.59	18.2	Tr	321
0	18	39	30	1.1	32	203	Tr	Tr	0.16	0.12	1.4	Tr	322
0	13	28	21	0.8	23	145	Tr	Tr	0.12	0.09	1.0	Tr	323
0	256	77	350	12.7	336	2,656	0	0	1.80	1.10	15.0	0	324
0	17	5	23	0.8	22	176	0	0	0.12	0.07	1.0	0	325
0	212	472	962	14.8	990	1,870	Tr	Tr	1.77	1.73	18.9	Tr	326
0	12	27	55	0.8	56	106	Tr	Tr	0.10	0.10	1.1	Tr	327
0	12	27	55	0.8	56	106	Tr	Tr	0.08	0.10	1.1	Tr	328

[26] Made with white cornmeal. If made with yellow cornmeal, value is 32 IU or 3 RE.

Item No.	Foods, approximate measures, units, and weight (weight of edible portion only)			Water	Food energy	Protein	Fat	Fatty acids: Saturated	Fatty acids: Monounsaturated	Fatty acids: Polyunsaturated
	Grain Products—Con.		Grams	Percent	Calories	Grams	Grams	Grams	Grams	Grams
	Breads:									
	Oatmeal bread, enriched:[25]									
329	Loaf, 1 lb	1 loaf	454	37	1,145	38	20	3.7	7.1	8.2
330	Slice (18 per loaf)	1 slice	25	37	65	2	1	0.2	0.4	0.5
331	Toasted	1 slice	23	30	65	2	1	0.2	0.4	0.5
332	Pita bread, enriched, white, 6-1/2-in diam.	1 pita	60	31	165	6	1	0.1	0.1	0.4
	Pumpernickel (2/3 rye flour, 1/3 enriched wheat flour):[25]									
333	Loaf, 1 lb	1 loaf	454	37	1,160	42	16	2.6	3.6	6.4
334	Slice, 5 by 4 by 3/8 in	1 slice	32	37	80	3	1	0.2	0.3	0.5
335	Toasted	1 slice	29	28	80	3	1	0.2	0.3	0.5
	Raisin bread, enriched:[25]									
336	Loaf, 1 lb	1 loaf	454	33	1,260	37	18	4.1	6.5	6.7
337	Slice (18 per loaf)	1 slice	25	33	65	2	1	0.2	0.3	0.4
338	Toasted	1 slice	21	24	65	2	1	0.2	0.3	0.4
	Rye bread, light (2/3 enriched wheat flour, 1/3 rye flour):[25]									
339	Loaf, 1 lb	1 loaf	454	37	1,190	38	17	3.3	5.2	5.5
340	Slice, 4-3/4 by 3-3/4 by 7/16 in	1 slice	25	37	65	2	1	0.2	0.3	0.3
341	Toasted	1 slice	22	28	65	2	1	0.2	0.3	0.3
	Wheat bread, enriched:[25]									
342	Loaf, 1 lb	1 loaf	454	37	1,160	43	19	3.9	7.3	4.5
343	Slice (18 per loaf)	1 slice	25	37	65	2	1	0.2	0.4	0.3
344	Toasted	1 slice	23	28	65	3	1	0.2	0.4	0.3
	White bread, enriched:[25]									
345	Loaf, 1 lb	1 loaf	454	37	1,210	38	18	5.6	6.5	4.2
346	Slice (18 per loaf)	1 slice	25	37	65	2	1	0.3	0.4	0.2
347	Toasted	1 slice	22	28	65	2	1	0.3	0.4	0.2
348	Slice (22 per loaf)	1 slice	20	37	55	2	1	0.2	0.3	0.2
349	Toasted	1 slice	17	28	55	2	1	0.2	0.3	0.2
350	Cubes	1 cup	30	37	80	2	1	0.4	0.4	0.3
351	Crumbs, soft	1 cup	45	37	120	4	2	0.6	0.6	0.4
	Whole-wheat bread:[25]									
352	Loaf, 1 lb	1 loaf	454	38	1,110	44	20	5.8	6.8	5.2
353	Slice (16 per loaf)	1 slice	28	38	70	3	1	0.4	0.4	0.3
354	Toasted	1 slice	25	29	70	3	1	0.4	0.4	0.3
	Bread stuffing (from enriched bread), prepared from mix:									
355	Dry type	1 cup	140	33	500	9	31	6.1	13.3	9.6
356	Moist type	1 cup	203	61	420	9	26	5.3	11.3	8.0
	Breakfast cereals:									
	Hot type, cooked:									
	Corn (hominy) grits:									
357	Regular and quick, enriched	1 cup	242	85	145	3	Tr	Tr	0.1	0.2
358	Instant, plain	1 pkt	137	85	80	2	Tr	Tr	Tr	0.1
	Cream of Wheat®:									
359	Regular, quick, instant	1 cup	244	86	140	4	Tr	0.1	Tr	0.2
360	Mix'n Eat, plain	1 pkt	142	82	100	3	Tr	Tr	Tr	0.1
361	Malt-O-Meal®	1 cup	240	88	120	4	Tr	Tr	Tr	0.1
	Oatmeal or rolled oats:									
362	Regular, quick, instant, nonfortified	1 cup	234	85	145	6	2	0.4	0.8	1.0
	Instant, fortified:									
363	Plain	1 pkt	177	86	105	4	2	0.3	0.6	0.7
364	Flavored	1 pkt	164	76	160	5	2	0.3	0.7	0.8

[25] Made with vegetable shortening.
[27] Nutrient added.
[28] Cooked without salt. If salt is added according to label recommendations, sodium content is 540 mg.
[29] For white corn grits. Cooked yellow grits contain 145 IU or 14 RE.
[30] Value based on label declaration for added nutrients.

Nutrients in Indicated Quantity													
Cholesterol	Carbohydrate	Calcium	Phosphorus	Iron	Potassium	Sodium	Vitamin A value (IU)	Vitamin A value (RE)	Thiamin	Riboflavin	Niacin	Ascorbic acid	Item No.
Milligrams	Grams	Milligrams	Milligrams	Milligrams	Milligrams	Milligrams	International units	Retinol equivalents	Milligrams	Milligrams	Milligrams	Milligrams	
0	212	267	563	12.0	707	2,231	0	0	2.09	1.20	15.4	0	329
0	12	15	31	0.7	39	124	0	0	0.12	0.07	0.9	0	330
0	12	15	31	0.7	39	124	0	0	0.09	0.07	0.9	0	331
0	33	49	60	1.4	71	339	0	0	0.27	0.12	2.2	0	332
0	218	322	990	12.4	1,966	2,461	0	0	1.54	2.36	15.0	0	333
0	16	23	71	0.9	141	177	0	0	0.11	0.17	1.1	0	334
0	16	23	71	0.9	141	177	0	0	0.09	0.17	1.1	0	335
0	239	463	395	14.1	1,058	1,657	Tr	Tr	1.50	2.81	18.6	Tr	336
0	13	25	22	0.8	59	92	Tr	Tr	0.08	0.15	1.0	Tr	337
0	13	25	22	0.8	59	92	Tr	Tr	0.06	0.15	1.0	Tr	338
0	218	363	658	12.3	926	3,164	0	0	1.86	1.45	15.0	0	339
0	12	20	36	0.7	51	175	0	0	0.10	0.08	0.8	0	340
0	12	20	36	0.7	51	175	0	0	0.08	0.08	0.8	0	341
0	213	572	835	15.8	627	2,447	Tr	Tr	2.09	1.45	20.5	Tr	342
0	12	32	47	0.9	35	138	Tr	Tr	0.12	0.08	1.2	Tr	343
0	12	32	47	0.9	35	138	Tr	Tr	0.10	0.08	1.2	Tr	344
0	222	572	490	12.9	508	2,334	Tr	Tr	2.13	1.41	17.0	Tr	345
0	12	32	27	0.7	28	129	Tr	Tr	0.12	0.08	0.9	Tr	346
0	12	32	27	0.7	28	129	Tr	Tr	0.09	0.08	0.9	Tr	347
0	10	25	21	0.6	22	101	Tr	Tr	0.09	0.06	0.7	Tr	348
0	10	25	21	0.6	22	101	Tr	Tr	0.07	0.06	0.7	Tr	349
0	15	38	32	0.9	34	154	Tr	Tr	0.14	0.09	1.1	Tr	350
0	22	57	49	1.3	50	231	Tr	Tr	0.21	0.14	1.7	Tr	351
0	206	327	1,180	15.5	799	2,887	Tr	Tr	1.59	0.95	17.4	Tr	352
0	13	20	74	1.0	50	180	Tr	Tr	0.10	0.06	1.1	Tr	353
0	13	20	74	1.0	50	180	Tr	Tr	0.08	0.06	1.1	Tr	354
0	50	92	136	2.2	126	1,254	910	273	0.17	0.20	2.5	0	355
67	40	81	134	2.0	118	1,023	850	256	0.10	0.18	1.6	0	356
0	31	0	29	[27]1.5	53	[28]0	[29]0	[29]0	[27]0.24	[27]0.15	[27]2.0	0	357
0	18	7	16	[27]1.0	29	343	0	0	[27]0.18	[27]0.08	[27]1.3	0	358
0	29	[30]54	[31]43	[30]10.9	46	[31,32]5	0	0	[30]0.24	[30]0.07	[30]1.5	0	359
0	21	[30]20	[30]20	[30]8.1	38	241	[30]1,250	[30]376	[30]0.43	[30]0.28	[30]5.0	0	360
0	26	5	[30]24	[30]9.6	31	[33]2	0	0	[30]0.48	[30]0.24	[30]5.8	0	361
0	25	19	178	1.6	131	[34]2	40	4	0.26	0.05	0.3	0	362
0	18	[27]163	133	[27]6.3	99	[27]285	[27]1,510	[27]453	[27]0.53	[27]0.28	[27]5.5	0	363
0	31	[27]168	148	[27]6.7	137	[27]254	[27]1,530	[27]460	[27]0.53	[27]0.38	[27]5.9	Tr	364

[31] For regular and instant cereal. For quick cereal, phosphorus is 102 mg and sodium is 142 mg.
[32] Cooked without salt. If salt is added according to label recommendations, sodium content is 390 mg.
[33] Cooked without salt. If salt is added according to label recommendations, sodium content is 324 mg.
[34] Cooked without salt. If salt is added according to label recommendations, sodium content is 374 mg.

Item No.	Foods, approximate measures, units, and weight (weight of edible portion only)			Water	Food energy	Protein	Fat	Fatty acids: Saturated	Fatty acids: Monounsaturated	Fatty acids: Polyunsaturated
	Grain Products—Con.		Grams	Percent	Calories	Grams	Grams	Grams	Grams	Grams
	Breakfast cereals:									
	Ready to eat:									
365	All-Bran® (about 1/3 cup)	1 oz	28	3	70	4	1	0.1	0.1	0.3
366	Cap'n Crunch® (about 3/4 cup)	1 oz	28	3	120	1	3	1.7	0.3	0.4
367	Cheerios® (about 1-1/4 cup)	1 oz	28	5	110	4	2	0.3	0.6	0.7
	Corn Flakes (about 1-1/4 cup):									
368	Kellogg's®	1 oz	28	3	110	2	Tr	Tr	Tr	Tr
369	Toasties®	1 oz	28	3	110	2	Tr	Tr	Tr	Tr
	40% Bran Flakes:									
370	Kellogg's® (about 3/4 cup)	1 oz	28	3	90	4	1	0.1	0.1	0.3
371	Post® (about 2/3 cup)	1 oz	28	3	90	3	Tr	0.1	0.1	0.2
372	Froot Loops® (about 1 cup)	1 oz	28	3	110	2	1	0.2	0.1	0.1
373	Golden Grahams® (about 3/4 cup)	1 oz	28	2	110	2	1	0.7	0.1	0.2
374	Grape-Nuts® (about 1/4 cup)	1 oz	28	3	100	3	Tr	Tr	Tr	0.1
375	Honey Nut Cheerios® (about 3/4 cup)	1 oz	28	3	105	3	1	0.1	0.3	0.3
376	Lucky Charms® (about 1 cup)	1 oz	28	3	110	3	1	0.2	0.4	0.4
377	Nature Valley® Granola (about 1/3 cup)	1 oz	28	4	125	3	5	3.3	0.7	0.7
378	100% Natural Cereal (about 1/4 cup)	1 oz	28	2	135	3	6	4.1	1.2	0.5
379	Product 19® (about 3/4 cup)	1 oz	28	3	110	3	Tr	Tr	Tr	0.1
	Raisin Bran:									
380	Kellogg's® (about 3/4 cup)	1 oz	28	8	90	3	1	0.1	0.1	0.3
381	Post® (about 1/2 cup)	1 oz	28	9	85	3	1	0.1	0.1	0.3
382	Rice Krispies® (about 1 cup)	1 oz	28	2	110	2	Tr	Tr	Tr	0.1
383	Shredded Wheat (about 2/3 cup)	1 oz	28	5	100	3	1	0.1	0.1	0.3
384	Special K® (about 1-1/3 cup)	1 oz	28	2	110	6	Tr	Tr	Tr	Tr
385	Super Sugar Crisp® (about 7/8 cup)	1 oz	28	2	105	2	Tr	Tr	Tr	0.1
386	Sugar Frosted Flakes, Kellogg's® (about 3/4 cup)	1 oz	28	3	110	1	Tr	Tr	Tr	Tr
387	Sugar Smacks® (about 3/4 cup)	1 oz	28	3	105	2	1	0.1	0.1	0.2
388	Total® (about 1 cup)	1 oz	28	4	100	3	1	0.1	0.1	0.3
389	Trix® (about 1 cup)	1 oz	28	3	110	2	Tr	0.2	0.1	0.1
390	Wheaties® (about 1 cup)	1 oz	28	5	100	3	Tr	0.1	Tr	0.2
391	Buckwheat flour, light, sifted	1 cup	98	12	340	6	1	0.2	0.4	0.4
392	Bulgur, uncooked	1 cup	170	10	600	19	3	1.2	0.3	1.2
	Cakes prepared from cake mixes with enriched flour:[35]									
	Angelfood:									
393	Whole cake, 9-3/4-in diam. tube cake	1 cake	635	38	1,510	38	2	0.4	0.2	1.0
394	Piece, 1/12 of cake	1 piece	53	38	125	3	Tr	Tr	Tr	0.1
	Coffeecake, crumb:									
395	Whole cake, 7-3/4 by 5-5/8 by 1-1/4 in	1 cake	430	30	1,385	27	41	11.8	16.7	9.6
396	Piece, 1/6 of cake	1 piece	72	30	230	5	7	2.0	2.8	1.6
	Devil's food with chocolate frosting:									
397	Whole, 2-layer cake, 8- or 9-in diam.	1 cake	1,107	24	3,755	49	136	55.6	51.4	19.7
398	Piece, 1/16 of cake	1 piece	69	24	235	3	8	3.5	3.2	1.2
399	Cupcake, 2-1/2-in diam.	1 cupcake	35	24	120	2	4	1.8	1.6	0.6
	Gingerbread:									
400	Whole cake, 8 in square	1 cake	570	37	1,575	18	39	9.6	16.4	10.5
401	Piece, 1/9 of cake	1 piece	63	37	175	2	4	1.1	1.8	1.2

[27] Nutrient added.
[30] Value based on label declaration for added nutrients.

Nutrients in Indicated Quantity													
Cholesterol	Carbohydrate	Calcium	Phosphorus	Iron	Potassium	Sodium	Vitamin A value (IU)	Vitamin A value (RE)	Thiamin	Riboflavin	Niacin	Ascorbic acid	Item No.
Milligrams	Grams	Milligrams	Milligrams	Milligrams	Milligrams	Milligrams	International units	Retinol equivalents	Milligrams	Milligrams	Milligrams	Milligrams	
0	21	23	264	[30]4.5	350	320	[30]1,250	[30]375	[30]0.37	[30]0.43	[30]5.0	[30]15	365
0	23	5	36	[27]7.5	37	213	40	4	[27]0.50	[27]0.55	[27]6.6	0	366
0	20	48	134	[30]4.5	101	307	[30]1,250	[30]375	[30]0.37	[30]0.43	[30]5.0	[30]15	367
0	24	1	18	[30]1.8	26	351	[30]1,250	[30]375	[30]0.37	[30]0.43	[30]5.0	[30]15	368
0	24	1	12	[27]0.7	33	297	[30]1,250	[30]375	[30]0.37	[30]0.43	[30]5.0	0	369
0	22	14	139	[30]8.1	180	264	[30]1,250	[30]375	[30]0.37	[30]0.43	[30]5.0	0	370
0	22	12	179	[30]4.5	151	260	[30]1,250	[30]375	[30]0.37	[30]0.43	[30]5.0	0	371
0	25	3	24	[30]4.5	26	145	[30]1,250	[30]375	[30]0.37	[30]0.43	[30]5.0	[30]15	372
Tr	24	17	41	[30]4.5	63	346	[30]1,250	[30]375	[30]0.37	[30]0.43	[30]5.0	[30]15	373
0	23	11	71	1.2	95	197	[30]1,250	[30]375	[30]0.37	[30]0.43	[30]5.0	0	374
0	23	20	105	[30]4.5	99	257	[30]1,250	[30]375	[30]0.37	[30]0.43	[30]5.0	[30]15	375
0	23	32	79	[30]4.5	59	201	[30]1,250	[30]375	[30]0.37	[30]0.43	[30]5.0	[30]15	376
0	19	18	89	0.9	98	58	20	2	0.10	0.05	0.2	0	377
Tr	18	49	104	0.8	140	12	20	2	0.09	0.15	0.6	0	378
0	24	3	40	[30]18.0	44	325	[30]5,000	[30]1,501	[30]1.50	[30]1.70	[30]20.0	[30]60	379
0	21	10	105	[30]3.5	147	207	[30]960	[30]288	[30]0.28	[30]0.34	[30]3.9	0	380
0	21	13	119	[30]4.5	175	185	[30]1,250	[30]375	[30]0.37	[30]0.43	[30]5.0	0	381
0	25	4	34	[30]1.8	29	340	[30]1,250	[30]375	[30]0.37	[30]0.43	[30]5.0	[30]15	382
0	23	11	100	1.2	102	3	0	0	0.07	0.08	1.5	0	383
Tr	21	8	55	[30]4.5	49	265	[30]1,250	[30]375	[30]0.37	[30]0.43	[30]5.0	[30]15	384
0	26	6	52	[30]1.8	105	25	[30]1,250	[30]375	[30]0.37	[30]0.43	[30]5.0	0	385
0	26	1	21	[30]1.8	18	230	[30]1,250	[30]375	[30]0.37	[30]0.43	[30]5.0	[30]15	386
0	25	3	31	[30]1.8	42	75	[30]1,250	[30]375	[30]0.37	[30]0.43	[30]5.0	[30]15	387
0	22	48	118	[30]18.0	106	352	[30]5,000	[30]1,501	[30]1.50	[30]1.70	[30]20.0	[30]60	388
0	25	6	19	[30]4.5	27	181	[30]1,250	[30]375	[30]0.37	[30]0.43	[30]5.0	[30]15	389
0	23	43	98	[30]4.5	106	354	[30]1,250	[30]375	[30]0.37	[30]0.43	[30]5.0	[30]15	390
0	78	11	86	1.0	314	2	0	0	0.08	0.04	0.4	0	391
0	129	49	575	9.5	389	7	0	0	0.48	0.24	7.7	0	392
0	342	527	1,086	2.7	845	3,226	0	0	0.32	1.27	1.6	0	393
0	29	44	91	0.2	71	269	0	0	0.03	0.11	0.1	0	394
279	225	262	748	7.3	469	1,853	690	194	0.82	0.90	7.7	1	395
47	38	44	125	1.2	78	310	120	32	0.14	0.15	1.3	Tr	396
598	645	653	1,162	22.1	1,439	2,900	1,660	498	1.11	1.66	10.0	1	397
37	40	41	72	1.4	90	181	100	31	0.07	0.10	0.6	Tr	398
19	20	21	37	0.7	46	92	50	16	0.04	0.05	0.3	Tr	399
6	291	513	570	10.8	1,562	1,733	0	0	0.86	1.03	7.4	1	400
1	32	57	63	1.2	173	192	0	0	0.09	0.11	0.8	Tr	401

[35] Excepting angelfood cake, cakes were made from mixes containing vegetable shortening and frostings were made with margarine.

Item No.	Foods, approximate measures, units, and weight (weight of edible portion only)			Water	Food energy	Protein	Fat	Fatty acids		
								Saturated	Monounsaturated	Polyunsaturated
	Grain Products—Con.		Grams	Percent	Calories	Grams	Grams	Grams	Grams	Grams
	Cakes prepared from cake mixes with enriched flour:[35]									
	Yellow with chocolate frosting:									
402	Whole, 2-layer cake, 8- or 9-in diam.	1 cake	1,108	26	3,735	45	125	47.8	48.8	21.8
403	Piece, 1/16 of cake	1 piece	69	26	235	3	8	3.0	3.0	1.4
	Cakes prepared from home recipes using enriched flour:									
	Carrot, with cream cheese frosting:[36]									
404	Whole cake, 10-in diam. tube cake	1 cake	1,536	23	6,175	63	328	66.0	135.2	107.5
405	Piece, 1/16 of cake	1 piece	96	23	385	4	21	4.1	8.4	6.7
	Fruitcake, dark:[36]									
406	Whole cake, 7-1/2-in diam., 2-1/4-in high tube cake	1 cake	1,361	18	5,185	74	228	47.6	113.0	51.7
407	Piece, 1/32 of cake, 2/3-in arc	1 piece	43	18	165	2	7	1.5	3.6	1.6
	Plain sheet cake:[37]									
	Without frosting:									
408	Whole cake, 9-in square	1 cake	777	25	2,830	35	108	29.5	45.1	25.6
409	Piece, 1/9 of cake	1 piece	86	25	315	4	12	3.3	5.0	2.8
	With uncooked white frosting:									
410	Whole cake, 9-in square	1 cake	1,096	21	4,020	37	129	41.6	50.4	26.3
411	Piece, 1/9 of cake	1 piece	121	21	445	4	14	4.6	5.6	2.9
	Pound:[38]									
412	Loaf, 8-1/2 by 3-1/2 by 3-1/4 in	1 loaf	514	22	2,025	33	94	21.1	40.9	26.7
413	Slice, 1/17 of loaf	1 slice	30	22	120	2	5	1.2	2.4	1.6
	Cakes, commercial, made with enriched flour:									
	Pound:									
414	Loaf, 8-1/2 by 3-1/2 by 3 in	1 loaf	500	24	1,935	26	94	52.0	30.0	4.0
415	Slice, 1/17 of loaf	1 slice	29	24	110	2	5	3.0	1.7	0.2
	Snack cakes:									
416	Devil's food with creme filling (2 small cakes per pkg)	1 small cake	28	20	105	1	4	1.7	1.5	0.6
417	Sponge with creme filling (2 small cakes per pkg)	1 small cake	42	19	155	1	5	2.3	2.1	0.5
	White with white frosting:									
418	Whole, 2-layer cake, 8- or 9-in diam.	1 cake	1,140	24	4,170	43	148	33.1	61.6	42.2
419	Piece, 1/16 of cake	1 piece	71	24	260	3	9	2.1	3.8	2.6
	Yellow with chocolate frosting:									
420	Whole, 2-layer cake, 8- or 9-in diam.	1 cake	1,108	23	3,895	40	175	92.0	58.7	10.0
421	Piece, 1/16 of cake	1 piece	69	23	245	2	11	5.7	3.7	0.6
	Cheesecake:									
422	Whole cake, 9-in diam.	1 cake	1,110	46	3,350	60	213	119.9	65.5	14.4
423	Piece, 1/12 of cake	1 piece	92	46	280	5	18	9.9	5.4	1.2
	Cookies made with enriched flour:									
	Brownies with nuts:									
424	Commercial, with frosting, 1-1/2 by 1-3/4 by 7/8 in	1 brownie	25	13	100	1	4	1.6	2.0	0.6
425	From home recipe, 1-3/4 by 1-3/4 by 7/8 in[36]	1 brownie	20	10	95	1	6	1.4	2.8	1.2
	Chocolate chip:									
426	Commercial, 2-1/4-in diam., 3/8 in thick	4 cookies	42	4	180	2	9	2.9	3.1	2.6

[35] Excepting angelfood cake, cakes were made from mixes containing vegetable shortening and frostings were made with margarine.
[36] Made with vegetable oil.

Nutrients in Indicated Quantity

Cholesterol	Carbohydrate	Calcium	Phosphorus	Iron	Potassium	Sodium	Vitamin A value (IU)	Vitamin A value (RE)	Thiamin	Riboflavin	Niacin	Ascorbic acid	Item No.
Milligrams	Grams	Milligrams	Milligrams	Milligrams	Milligrams	Milligrams	International units	Retinol equivalents	Milligrams	Milligrams	Milligrams	Milligrams	
576	638	1,008	2,017	15.5	1,208	2,515	1,550	465	1.22	1.66	11.1	1	402
36	40	63	126	1.0	75	157	100	29	0.08	0.10	0.7	Tr	403
1183	775	707	998	21.0	1,720	4,470	2,240	246	1.83	1.97	14.7	23	404
74	48	44	62	1.3	108	279	140	15	0.11	0.12	0.9	1	405
640	783	1,293	1,592	37.6	6,138	2,123	1,720	422	2.41	2.55	17.0	504	406
20	25	41	50	1.2	194	67	50	13	0.08	0.08	0.5	16	407
552	434	497	793	11.7	614	2,331	1,320	373	1.24	1.40	10.1	2	408
61	48	55	88	1.3	68	258	150	41	0.14	0.15	1.1	Tr	409
636	694	548	822	11.0	669	2,488	2,190	647	1.21	1.42	9.9	2	410
70	77	61	91	1.2	74	275	240	71	0.13	0.16	1.1	Tr	411
555	265	339	473	9.3	483	1,645	3,470	1,033	0.93	1.08	7.8	1	412
32	15	20	28	0.5	28	96	200	60	0.05	0.06	0.5	Tr	413
1100	257	146	517	8.0	443	1,857	2,820	715	0.96	1.12	8.1	0	414
64	15	8	30	0.5	26	108	160	41	0.06	0.06	0.5	0	415
15	17	21	26	1.0	34	105	20	4	0.06	0.09	0.7	0	416
7	27	14	44	0.6	37	155	30	9	0.07	0.06	0.6	0	417
46	670	536	1,585	15.5	832	2,827	640	194	3.19	2.05	27.6	0	418
3	42	33	99	1.0	52	176	40	12	0.20	0.13	1.7	0	419
609	620	366	1,884	19.9	1,972	3,080	1,850	488	0.78	2.22	10.0	0	420
38	39	23	117	1.2	123	192	120	30	0.05	0.14	0.6	0	421
2053	317	622	977	5.3	1,088	2,464	2,820	833	0.33	1.44	5.1	56	422
170	26	52	81	0.4	90	204	230	69	0.03	0.12	0.4	5	423
14	16	13	26	0.6	50	59	70	18	0.08	0.07	0.3	Tr	424
18	11	9	26	0.4	35	51	20	6	0.05	0.05	0.3	Tr	425
5	28	13	41	0.8	68	140	50	15	0.10	0.23	1.0	Tr	426

[37]Cake made with vegetable shortening; frosting with margarine.
[38]Made with margarine.

Item No.	Foods, approximate measures, units, and weight (weight of edible portion only)			Water	Food energy	Protein	Fat	Fatty acids: Saturated	Fatty acids: Monounsaturated	Fatty acids: Polyunsaturated
	Grain Products—Con.		Grams	Percent	Calories	Grams	Grams	Grams	Grams	Grams
	Cookies made with enriched flour:									
	Chocolate chip:									
427	From home recipe, 2-1/3-in diam.[25]	4 cookies	40	3	185	2	11	3.9	4.3	2.0
428	From refrigerated dough, 2-1/4-in diam., 3/8 in thick	4 cookies	48	5	225	2	11	4.0	4.4	2.0
429	Fig bars, square, 1-5/8 by 1-5/8 by 3/8 in or rectangular, 1-1/2 by 1-3/4 by 1/2 in	4 cookies	56	12	210	2	4	1.0	1.5	1.0
430	Oatmeal with raisins, 2-5/8-in diam., 1/4 in thick	4 cookies	52	4	245	3	10	2.5	4.5	2.8
431	Peanut butter cookie, from home recipe, 2-5/8-in diam.[25]	4 cookies	48	3	245	4	14	4.0	5.8	2.8
432	Sandwich type (chocolate or vanilla), 1-3/4-in diam., 3/8 in thick	4 cookies	40	2	195	2	8	2.0	3.6	2.2
	Shortbread:									
433	Commercial	4 small cookies	32	6	155	2	8	2.9	3.0	1.1
434	From home recipe[38]	2 large cookies	28	3	145	2	8	1.3	2.7	3.4
435	Sugar cookie, from refrigerated dough, 2-1/2-in diam., 1/4 in thick	4 cookies	48	4	235	2	12	2.3	5.0	3.6
436	Vanilla wafers, 1-3/4-in diam., 1/4 in thick	10 cookies	40	4	185	2	7	1.8	3.0	1.8
437	Corn chips	1-oz package	28	1	155	2	9	1.4	2.4	3.7
	Cornmeal:									
438	Whole-ground, unbolted, dry form	1 cup	122	12	435	11	5	0.5	1.1	2.5
439	Bolted (nearly whole-grain), dry form	1 cup	122	12	440	11	4	0.5	0.9	2.2
	Degermed, enriched:									
440	Dry form	1 cup	138	12	500	11	2	0.2	0.4	0.9
441	Cooked	1 cup	240	88	120	3	Tr	Tr	0.1	0.2
	Crackers:[39]									
	Cheese:									
442	Plain, 1 in square	10 crackers	10	4	50	1	3	0.9	1.2	0.3
443	Sandwich type (peanut butter)	1 sandwich	8	3	40	1	2	0.4	0.8	0.3
444	Graham, plain, 2-1/2 in square	2 crackers	14	5	60	1	1	0.4	0.6	0.4
445	Melba toast, plain	1 piece	5	4	20	1	Tr	0.1	0.1	0.1
446	Rye wafers, whole-grain, 1-7/8 by 3-1/2 in	2 wafers	14	5	55	1	1	0.3	0.4	0.3
447	Saltines[40]	4 crackers	12	4	50	1	1	0.5	0.4	0.2
448	Snack-type, standard	1 round cracker	3	3	15	Tr	1	0.2	0.4	0.1
449	Wheat, thin	4 crackers	8	3	35	1	1	0.5	0.5	0.4
450	Whole-wheat wafers	2 crackers	8	4	35	1	2	0.5	0.6	0.4
451	Croissants, made with enriched flour, 4-1/2 by 4 by 1-3/4 in	1 croissant	57	22	235	5	12	3.5	6.7	1.4
	Danish pastry, made with enriched flour:									
	Plain without fruit or nuts:									
452	Packaged ring, 12 oz	1 ring	340	27	1,305	21	71	21.8	28.6	15.6
453	Round piece, about 4-1/4-in diam., 1 in high	1 pastry	57	27	220	4	12	3.6	4.8	2.6
454	Ounce	1 oz	28	27	110	2	6	1.8	2.4	1.3
455	Fruit, round piece	1 pastry	65	30	235	4	13	3.9	5.2	2.9
	Doughnuts, made with enriched flour:									
456	Cake type, plain, 3-1/4-in diam., 1 in high	1 doughnut	50	21	210	3	12	2.8	5.0	3.0
457	Yeast-leavened, glazed, 3-3/4-in diam., 1-1/4 in high	1 doughnut	60	27	235	4	13	5.2	5.5	0.9
458	English muffins, plain, enriched	1 muffin	57	42	140	5	1	0.3	0.2	0.3
459	Toasted	1 muffin	50	29	140	5	1	0.3	0.2	0.3

[25]Made with vegetable shortening.
[38]Made with margarine.

Nutrients in Indicated Quantity

Cholesterol	Carbohydrate	Calcium	Phosphorus	Iron	Potassium	Sodium	Vitamin A value (IU)	Vitamin A value (RE)	Thiamin	Riboflavin	Niacin	Ascorbic acid	Item No.
Milligrams	Grams	Milligrams	Milligrams	Milligrams	Milligrams	Milligrams	International units	Retinol equivalents	Milligrams	Milligrams	Milligrams	Milligrams	
18	26	13	34	1.0	82	82	20	5	0.06	0.06	0.6	0	427
22	32	13	34	1.0	62	173	30	8	0.06	0.10	0.9	0	428
27	42	40	34	1.4	162	180	60	6	0.08	0.07	0.7	Tr	429
2	36	18	58	1.1	90	148	40	12	0.09	0.08	1.0	0	430
22	28	21	60	1.1	110	142	20	5	0.07	0.07	1.9	0	431
0	29	12	40	1.4	66	189	0	0	0.09	0.07	0.8	0	432
27	20	13	39	0.8	38	123	30	8	0.10	0.09	0.9	0	433
0	17	6	31	0.6	18	125	300	89	0.08	0.06	0.7	Tr	434
29	31	50	91	0.9	33	261	40	11	0.09	0.06	1.1	0	435
25	29	16	36	0.8	50	150	50	14	0.07	0.10	1.0	0	436
0	16	35	52	0.5	52	233	110	11	0.04	0.05	0.4	1	437
0	90	24	312	2.2	346	1	620	62	0.46	0.13	2.4	0	438
0	91	21	272	2.2	303	1	590	59	0.37	0.10	2.3	0	439
0	108	8	137	5.9	166	1	610	61	0.61	0.36	4.8	0	440
0	26	2	34	1.4	38	0	140	14	0.14	0.10	1.2	0	441
6	6	11	17	0.3	17	112	20	5	0.05	0.04	0.4	0	442
1	5	7	25	0.3	17	90	Tr	Tr	0.04	0.03	0.6	0	443
0	11	6	20	0.4	36	86	0	0	0.02	0.03	0.6	0	444
0	4	6	10	0.1	11	44	0	0	0.01	0.01	0.1	0	445
0	10	7	44	0.5	65	115	0	0	0.06	0.03	0.5	0	446
4	9	3	12	0.5	17	165	0	0	0.06	0.05	0.6	0	447
0	2	3	6	0.1	4	30	Tr	Tr	0.01	0.01	0.1	0	448
0	5	3	15	0.3	17	69	Tr	Tr	0.04	0.03	0.4	0	449
0	5	3	22	0.2	31	59	0	0	0.02	0.03	0.4	0	450
13	27	20	64	2.1	68	452	50	13	0.17	0.13	1.3	0	451
292	152	360	347	6.5	316	1,302	360	99	0.95	1.02	8.5	Tr	452
49	26	60	58	1.1	53	218	60	17	0.16	0.17	1.4	Tr	453
24	13	30	29	0.5	26	109	30	8	0.08	0.09	0.7	Tr	454
56	28	17	80	1.3	57	233	40	11	0.16	0.14	1.4	Tr	455
20	24	22	111	1.0	58	192	20	5	0.12	0.12	1.1	Tr	456
21	26	17	55	1.4	64	222	Tr	Tr	0.28	0.12	1.8	0	457
0	27	96	67	1.7	331	378	0	0	0.26	0.19	2.2	0	458
0	27	96	67	1.7	331	378	0	0	0.23	0.19	2.2	0	459

[39]Crackers made with enriched flour except for rye wafers and whole-wheat wafers.
[40]Made with lard.

Item No.	Foods, approximate measures, units, and weight (weight of edible portion only)			Water	Food energy	Protein	Fat	Fatty acids: Saturated	Fatty acids: Monounsaturated	Fatty acids: Polyunsaturated
	Grain Products—Con.		Grams	Percent	Calories	Grams	Grams	Grams	Grams	Grams
460	French toast, from home recipe	1 slice	65	53	155	6	7	1.6	2.0	1.6
	Macaroni, enriched, cooked (cut lengths, elbows, shells):									
461	Firm stage (hot)	1 cup	130	64	190	7	1	0.1	0.1	0.3
	Tender stage:									
462	Cold	1 cup	105	72	115	4	Tr	0.1	0.1	0.2
463	Hot	1 cup	140	72	155	5	1	0.1	0.1	0.2
	Muffins made with enriched flour, 2-1/2-in diam., 1-1/2 in high:									
	From home recipe:									
464	Blueberry[25]	1 muffin	45	37	135	3	5	1.5	2.1	1.2
465	Bran[36]	1 muffin	45	35	125	3	6	1.4	1.6	2.3
466	Corn (enriched, degermed cornmeal and flour)[25]	1 muffin	45	33	145	3	5	1.5	2.2	1.4
	From commercial mix (egg and water added):									
467	Blueberry	1 muffin	45	33	140	3	5	1.4	2.0	1.2
468	Bran	1 muffin	45	28	140	3	4	1.3	1.6	1.0
469	Corn	1 muffin	45	30	145	3	6	1.7	2.3	1.4
470	Noodles (egg noodles), enriched, cooked	1 cup	160	70	200	7	2	0.5	0.6	0.6
471	Noodles, chow mein, canned	1 cup	45	11	220	6	11	2.1	7.3	0.4
	Pancakes, 4-in diam.:									
472	Buckwheat, from mix (with buckwheat and enriched flours), egg and milk added	1 pancake	27	58	55	2	2	0.9	0.9	0.5
	Plain:									
473	From home recipe using enriched flour	1 pancake	27	50	60	2	2	0.5	0.8	0.5
474	From mix (with enriched flour), egg, milk, and oil added	1 pancake	27	54	60	2	2	0.5	0.9	0.5
	Piecrust, made with enriched flour and vegetable shortening, baked:									
475	From home recipe, 9-in diam.	1 pie shell	180	15	900	11	60	14.8	25.9	15.7
476	From mix, 9-in diam.	Piecrust for 2-crust pie	320	19	1,485	20	93	22.7	41.0	25.0
	Pies, piecrust made with enriched flour, vegetable shortening, 9-in diam.:									
	Apple:									
477	Whole	1 pie	945	48	2,420	21	105	27.4	44.4	26.5
478	Piece, 1/6 of pie	1 piece	158	48	405	3	18	4.6	7.4	4.4
	Blueberry:									
479	Whole	1 pie	945	51	2,285	23	102	25.5	44.4	27.4
480	Piece, 1/6 of pie	1 piece	158	51	380	4	17	4.3	7.4	4.6
	Cherry:									
481	Whole	1 pie	945	47	2,465	25	107	28.4	46.3	27.4
482	Piece, 1/6 of pie	1 piece	158	47	410	4	18	4.7	7.7	4.6
	Creme:									
483	Whole	1 pie	910	43	2,710	20	139	90.1	23.7	6.4
484	Piece, 1/6 of pie	1 piece	152	43	455	3	23	15.0	4.0	1.1
	Custard:									
485	Whole	1 pie	910	58	1,985	56	101	33.7	40.0	19.1
486	Piece, 1/6 of pie	1 piece	152	58	330	9	17	5.6	6.7	3.2
	Lemon meringue:									
487	Whole	1 pie	840	47	2,140	31	86	26.0	34.4	17.6
488	Piece, 1/6 of pie	1 piece	140	47	355	5	14	4.3	5.7	2.9
	Peach:									
489	Whole	1 pie	945	48	2,410	24	101	24.6	43.5	26.5
490	Piece, 1/6 of pie	1 piece	158	48	405	4	17	4.1	7.3	4.4

[25] Made with vegetable shortening.

Nutrients in Indicated Quantity

Cho-les-terol	Carbo-hydrate	Calcium	Phos-phorus	Iron	Potas-sium	Sodium	Vitamin A value (IU)	Vitamin A value (RE)	Thiamin	Ribo-flavin	Niacin	Ascorbic acid	Item No.
Milli-grams	Grams	Milli-grams	Milli-grams	Milli-grams	Milli-grams	Milli-grams	Inter-national units	Retinol equiva-lents	Milli-grams	Milli-grams	Milli-grams	Milli-grams	
112	17	72	85	1.3	86	257	110	32	0.12	0.16	1.0	Tr	460
0	39	14	85	2.1	103	1	0	0	0.23	0.13	1.8	0	461
0	24	8	53	1.3	64	1	0	0	0.15	0.08	1.2	0	462
0	32	11	70	1.7	85	1	0	0	0.20	0.11	1.5	0	463
19	20	54	46	0.9	47	198	40	9	0.10	0.11	0.9	1	464
24	19	60	125	1.4	99	189	230	30	0.11	0.13	1.3	3	465
23	21	66	59	0.9	57	169	80	15	0.11	0.11	0.9	Tr	466
45	22	15	90	0.9	54	225	50	11	0.10	0.17	1.1	Tr	467
28	24	27	182	1.7	50	385	100	14	0.08	0.12	1.9	0	468
42	22	30	128	1.3	31	291	90	16	0.09	0.09	0.8	Tr	469
50	37	16	94	2.6	70	3	110	34	0.22	0.13	1.9	0	470
5	26	14	41	0.4	33	450	0	0	0.05	0.03	0.6	0	471
20	.6	59	91	0.4	66	125	60	17	0.04	0.05	0.2	Tr	472
16	9	27	38	0.5	33	115	30	10	0.06	0.07	0.5	Tr	473
16	8	36	71	0.7	43	160	30	7	0.09	0.12	0.8	Tr	474
0	79	25	90	4.5	90	1,100	0	0	0.54	0.40	5.0	0	475
0	141	131	272	9.3	179	2,602	0	0	1.06	0.80	9.9	0	476
0	360	76	208	9.5	756	2,844	280	28	1.04	0.76	9.5	9	477
0	60	13	35	1.6	126	476	50	5	0.17	0.13	1.6	2	478
0	330	104	217	12.3	945	2,533	850	85	1.04	0.85	10.4	38	479
0	55	17	36	2.1	158	423	140	14	0.17	0.14	1.7	6	480
0	363	132	236	9.5	992	2,873	4,160	416	1.13	0.85	9.5	0	481
0	61	22	40	1.6	166	480	700	70	0.19	0.14	1.6	0	482
46	351	273	919	6.8	796	2,207	1,250	391	0.36	0.89	6.4	0	483
8	59	46	154	1.1	133	369	210	65	0.06	0.15	1.1	0	484
1010	213	874	1,028	9.1	1,247	2,612	2,090	573	0.82	1.91	5.5	0	485
169	36	146	172	1.5	208	436	350	96	0.14	0.32	0.9	0	486
857	317	118	412	8.4	420	2,369	1,430	395	0.59	0.84	5.0	25	487
143	53	20	69	1.4	70	395	240	66	0.10	0.14	0.8	4	488
0	361	95	274	11.3	1,408	2,533	6,900	690	1.04	0.95	14.2	28	489
0	60	16	46	1.9	235	423	1,150	115	0.17	0.16	2.4	5	490

[36] Made with vegetable oil.

Item No.	Foods, approximate measures, units, and weight (weight of edible portion only)			Water	Food energy	Protein	Fat	Fatty acids: Saturated	Fatty acids: Monounsaturated	Fatty acids: Polyunsaturated
	Grain Products—Con.		Grams	Percent	Calories	Grams	Grams	Grams	Grams	Grams
	Pies, piecrust made with enriched flour, vegetable shortening, 9-inch diam.:									
	Pecan:									
491	Whole	1 pie	825	20	3,450	42	189	28.1	101.5	47.0
492	Piece, 1/6 of pie	1 piece	138	20	575	7	32	4.7	17.0	7.9
	Pumpkin:									
493	Whole	1 pie	910	59	1,920	36	102	38.2	40.0	18.2
494	Piece, 1/6 of pie	1 piece	152	59	320	6	17	6.4	6.7	3.0
	Pies, fried:									
495	Apple	1 pie	85	43	255	2	14	5.8	6.6	0.6
496	Cherry	1 pie	85	42	250	2	14	5.8	6.7	0.6
	Popcorn, popped:									
497	Air-popped, unsalted	1 cup	8	4	30	1	Tr	Tr	0.1	0.2
498	Popped in vegetable oil, salted	1 cup	11	3	55	1	3	0.5	1.4	1.2
499	Sugar syrup coated	1 cup	35	4	135	2	1	0.1	0.3	0.6
	Pretzels, made with enriched flour:									
500	Stick, 2-1/4 in long	10 pretzels	3	3	10	Tr	Tr	Tr	Tr	Tr
501	Twisted, dutch, 2-3/4 by 2-5/8 in	1 pretzel	16	3	65	2	1	0.1	0.2	0.2
502	Twisted, thin, 3-1/4 by 2-1/4 by 1/4 in	10 pretzels	60	3	240	6	2	0.4	0.8	0.6
	Rice:									
503	Brown, cooked, served hot	1 cup	195	70	230	5	1	0.3	0.3	0.4
	White, enriched:									
	Commercial varieties, all types:									
504	Raw	1 cup	185	12	670	12	1	0.2	0.2	0.3
505	Cooked, served hot	1 cup	205	73	225	4	Tr	0.1	0.1	0.1
506	Instant, ready-to-serve, hot	1 cup	165	73	180	4	0	0.1	0.1	0.1
	Parboiled:									
507	Raw	1 cup	185	10	685	14	1	0.1	0.1	0.2
508	Cooked, served hot	1 cup	175	73	185	4	Tr	Tr	Tr	0.1
	Rolls, enriched:									
	Commercial:									
509	Dinner, 2-1/2-in diam., 2 in high	1 roll	28	32	85	2	2	0.5	0.8	0.6
510	Frankfurter and hamburger (8 per 11-1/2-oz pkg.)	1 roll	40	34	115	3	2	0.5	0.8	0.6
511	Hard, 3-3/4-in diam., 2 in high	1 roll	50	25	155	5	2	0.4	0.5	0.6
512	Hoagie or submarine, 11-1/2 by 3 by 2-1/2 in	1 roll	135	31	400	11	8	1.8	3.0	2.2
	From home recipe:									
513	Dinner, 2-1/2-in diam., 2 in high	1 roll	35	26	120	3	3	0.8	1.2	0.9
	Spaghetti, enriched, cooked:									
514	Firm stage, "al dente," served hot	1 cup	130	64	190	7	1	0.1	0.1	0.3
515	Tender stage, served hot	1 cup	140	73	155	5	1	0.1	0.1	0.2
516	Toaster pastries	1 pastry	54	13	210	2	6	1.7	3.6	0.4
517	Tortillas, corn	1 tortilla	30	45	65	2	1	0.1	0.3	0.6
	Waffles, made with enriched flour, 7-in diam.:									
518	From home recipe	1 waffle	75	37	245	7	13	4.0	4.9	2.6
519	From mix, egg and milk added	1 waffle	75	42	205	7	8	2.7	2.9	1.5
	Wheat flours:									
	All-purpose or family flour, enriched:									
520	Sifted, spooned	1 cup	115	12	420	12	1	0.2	0.1	0.5
521	Unsifted, spooned	1 cup	125	12	455	13	1	0.2	0.1	0.5
522	Cake or pastry flour, enriched, sifted, spooned	1 cup	96	12	350	7	1	0.1	0.1	0.3
523	Self-rising, enriched, unsifted, spooned	1 cup	125	12	440	12	1	0.2	0.1	0.5
524	Whole-wheat, from hard wheats, stirred	1 cup	120	12	400	16	2	0.3	0.3	1.1

Nutrients in Indicated Quantity

Cholesterol	Carbohydrate	Calcium	Phosphorus	Iron	Potassium	Sodium	Vitamin A value (IU)	Vitamin A value (RE)	Thiamin	Riboflavin	Niacin	Ascorbic acid	Item No
Milligrams	Grams	Milligrams	Milligrams	Milligrams	Milligrams	Milligrams	International units	Retinol equivalents	Milligrams	Milligrams	Milligrams	Milligrams	
569	423	388	850	27.2	1,015	1,823	1,320	322	1.82	0.99	6.6	0	491
95	71	65	142	4.6	170	305	220	54	0.30	0.17	1.1	0	492
655	223	464	628	8.2	1,456	1,947	22,480	2,493	0.82	1.27	7.3	0	493
109	37	78	105	1.4	243	325	3,750	416	0.14	0.21	1.2	0	494
14	31	12	34	0.9	42	326	30	3	0.09	0.06	1.0	1	495
13	32	11	41	0.7	61	371	190	19	0.06	0.06	0.6	1	496
0	6	1	22	0.2	20	Tr	10	1	0.03	0.01	0.2	0	497
0	6	3	31	0.3	19	86	20	2	0.01	0.02	0.1	0	498
0	30	2	47	0.5	90	Tr	30	3	0.13	0.02	0.4	0	499
0	2	1	3	0.1	3	48	0	0	0.01	0.01	0.1	0	500
0	13	4	15	0.3	16	258	0	0	0.05	0.04	0.7	0	501
0	48	16	55	1.2	61	966	0	0	0.19	0.15	2.6	0	502
0	50	23	142	1.0	137	0	0	0	0.18	0.04	2.7	0	503
0	149	44	174	5.4	170	9	0	0	0.81	0.06	6.5	0	504
0	50	21	57	1.8	57	0	0	0	0.23	0.02	2.1	0	505
0	40	5	31	1.3	0	0	0	0	0.21	0.02	1.7	0	506
0	150	111	370	5.4	278	17	0	0	0.81	0.07	6.5	0	507
0	41	33	100	1.4	75	0	0	0	0.19	0.02	2.1	0	508
Tr	14	33	44	0.8	36	155	Tr	Tr	0.14	0.09	1.1	Tr	509
Tr	20	54	44	1.2	56	241	Tr	Tr	0.20	0.13	1.6	Tr	510
Tr	30	24	46	1.4	49	313	0	0	0.20	0.12	1.7	0	511
Tr	72	100	115	3.8	128	683	0	0	0.54	0.33	4.5	0	512
12	20	16	36	1.1	41	98	30	8	0.12	0.12	1.2	0	513
0	39	14	85	2.0	103	1	0	0	0.23	0.13	1.8	0	514
0	32	11	70	1.7	85	1	0	0	0.20	0.11	1.5	0	515
0	38	104	104	2.2	91	248	520	52	0.17	0.18	2.3	4	516
0	13	42	55	0.6	43	1	80	8	0.05	0.03	0.4	0	517
102	26	154	135	1.5	129	445	140	39	0.18	0.24	1.5	Tr	518
59	27	179	257	1.2	146	515	170	49	0.14	0.23	0.9	Tr	519
0	88	18	100	5.1	109	2	0	0	0.73	0.46	6.1	0	520
0	95	20	109	5.5	119	3	0	0	0.80	0.50	6.6	0	521
0	76	16	70	4.2	91	2	0	0	0.58	0.38	5.1	0	522
0	93	331	583	5.5	113	1,349	0	0	0.80	0.50	6.6	0	523
0	85	49	446	5.2	444	4	0	0	0.66	0.14	5.2	0	524

Legumes, Nuts, and Seeds

Item No.	Foods, approximate measures, units, and weight (weight of edible portion only)		Grams	Water Per-cent	Food energy Cal-ories	Pro-tein Grams	Fat Grams	Fatty acids: Satu-rated Grams	Fatty acids: Mono-unsatu-rated Grams	Fatty acids: Poly-unsatu-rated Grams
	Almonds, shelled:									
525	Slivered, packed	1 cup	135	4	795	27	70	6.7	45.8	14.8
526	Whole	1 oz	28	4	165	6	15	1.4	9.6	3.1
	Beans, dry:									
	Cooked, drained:									
527	Black	1 cup	171	66	225	15	1	0.1	0.1	0.5
528	Great Northern	1 cup	180	69	210	14	1	0.1	0.1	0.6
529	Lima	1 cup	190	64	260	16	1	0.2	0.1	0.5
530	Pea (navy)	1 cup	190	69	225	15	1	0.1	0.1	0.7
531	Pinto	1 cup	180	65	265	15	1	0.1	0.1	0.5
	Canned, solids and liquid:									
	White with:									
532	Frankfurters (sliced)	1 cup	255	71	365	19	18	7.4	8.8	0.7
533	Pork and tomato sauce	1 cup	255	71	310	16	7	2.4	2.7	0.7
534	Pork and sweet sauce	1 cup	255	66	385	16	12	4.3	4.9	1.2
535	Red kidney	1 cup	255	76	230	15	1	0.1	0.1	0.6
536	Black-eyed peas, dry, cooked (with residual cooking liquid)	1 cup	250	80	190	13	1	0.2	Tr	0.3
537	Brazil nuts, shelled	1 oz	28	3	185	4	19	4.6	6.5	6.8
538	Carob flour	1 cup	140	3	255	6	Tr	Tr	0.1	0.1
	Cashew nuts, salted:									
539	Dry roasted	1 cup	137	2	785	21	63	12.5	37.4	10.7
540		1 oz	28	2	165	4	13	2.6	7.7	2.2
541	Roasted in oil	1 cup	130	4	750	21	63	12.4	36.9	10.6
542		1 oz	28	4	165	5	14	2.7	8.1	2.3
543	Chestnuts, European (Italian), roasted, shelled	1 cup	143	40	350	5	3	0.6	1.1	1.2
544	Chickpeas, cooked, drained	1 cup	163	60	270	15	4	0.4	0.9	1.9
	Coconut:									
	Raw:									
545	Piece, about 2 by 2 by 1/2 in	1 piece	45	47	160	1	15	13.4	0.6	0.2
546	Shredded or grated	1 cup	80	47	285	3	27	23.8	1.1	0.3
547	Dried, sweetened, shredded	1 cup	93	13	470	3	33	29.3	1.4	0.4
548	Filberts (hazelnuts), chopped	1 cup	115	5	725	15	72	5.3	56.5	6.9
549		1 oz	28	5	180	4	18	1.3	13.9	1.7
550	Lentils, dry, cooked	1 cup	200	72	215	16	1	0.1	0.2	0.5
551	Macadamia nuts, roasted in oil, salted	1 cup	134	2	960	10	103	15.4	80.9	1.8
552		1 oz	28	2	205	2	22	3.2	17.1	0.4
	Mixed nuts, with peanuts, salted:									
553	Dry roasted	1 oz	28	2	170	5	15	2.0	8.9	3.1
554	Roasted in oil	1 oz	28	2	175	5	16	2.5	9.0	3.8
555	Peanuts, roasted in oil, salted	1 cup	145	2	840	39	71	9.9	35.5	22.6
556		1 oz	28	2	165	8	14	1.9	6.9	4.4
557	Peanut butter	1 tbsp	16	1	95	5	8	1.4	4.0	2.5
558	Peas, split, dry, cooked	1 cup	200	70	230	16	1	0.1	0.1	0.3
559	Pecans, halves	1 cup	108	5	720	8	73	5.9	45.5	18.1
560		1 oz	28	5	190	2	19	1.5	12.0	4.7
561	Pine nuts (pinyons), shelled	1 oz	28	6	160	3	17	2.7	6.5	7.3
562	Pistachio nuts, dried, shelled	1 oz	28	4	165	6	14	1.7	9.3	2.1
563	Pumpkin and squash kernels, dry, hulled	1 oz	28	7	155	7	13	2.5	4.0	5.9
564	Refried beans, canned	1 cup	290	72	295	18	3	0.4	0.6	1.4
565	Sesame seeds, dry, hulled	1 tbsp	8	5	45	2	4	0.6	1.7	1.9
566	Soybeans, dry, cooked, drained	1 cup	180	71	235	20	10	1.3	1.9	5.3
	Soy products:									
567	Miso	1 cup	276	53	470	29	13	1.8	2.6	7.3
568	Tofu, piece 2-1/2 by 2-3/4 by 1 in	1 piece	120	85	85	9	5	0.7	1.0	2.9
569	Sunflower seeds, dry, hulled	1 oz	28	5	160	6	14	1.5	2.7	9.3
570	Tahini	1 tbsp	15	3	90	3	8	1.1	3.0	3.5

[41] Cashews without salt contain 21 mg sodium per cup or 4 mg per oz.
[42] Cashews without salt contain 22 mg sodium per cup or 5 mg per oz.
[43] Macadamia nuts without salt contain 9 mg sodium per cup or 2 mg per oz.

Nutrients in Indicated Quantity													
Cholesterol	Carbohydrate	Calcium	Phosphorus	Iron	Potassium	Sodium	Vitamin A value (IU)	Vitamin A value (RE)	Thiamin	Riboflavin	Niacin	Ascorbic acid	Item No.
Milligrams	Grams	Milligrams	Milligrams	Milligrams	Milligrams	Milligrams	International units	Retinol equivalents	Milligrams	Milligrams	Milligrams	Milligrams	
0	28	359	702	4.9	988	15	0	0	0.28	1.05	4.5	1	525
0	6	75	147	1.0	208	3	0	0	0.06	0.22	1.0	Tr	526
0	41	47	239	2.9	608	1	Tr	Tr	0.43	0.05	0.9	0	527
0	38	90	266	4.9	749	13	0	0	0.25	0.13	1.3	0	528
0	49	55	293	5.9	1,163	4	0	0	0.25	0.11	1.3	0	529
0	40	95	281	5.1	790	13	0	0	0.27	0.13	1.3	0	530
0	49	86	296	5.4	882	3	Tr	Tr	0.33	0.16	0.7	0	531
30	32	94	303	4.8	668	1,374	330	33	0.18	0.15	3.3	Tr	532
10	48	138	235	4.6	536	1,181	330	33	0.20	0.08	1.5	5	533
10	54	161	291	5.9	536	969	330	33	0.15	0.10	1.3	5	534
0	42	74	278	4.6	673	968	10	1	0.13	0.10	1.5	0	535
0	35	43	238	3.3	573	20	30	3	0.40	0.10	1.0	0	536
0	4	50	170	1.0	170	1	Tr	Tr	0.28	0.03	0.5	Tr	537
0	126	390	102	5.7	1,275	24	Tr	Tr	0.07	0.07	2.2	Tr	538
0	45	62	671	8.2	774	[41]877	0	0	0.27	0.27	1.9	0	539
0	9	13	139	1.7	160	[41]181	0	0	0.06	0.06	0.4	0	540
0	37	53	554	5.3	689	[42]814	0	0	0.55	0.23	2.3	0	541
0	8	12	121	1.2	150	[42]177	0	0	0.12	0.05	0.5	0	542
0	76	41	153	1.3	847	3	30	3	0.35	0.25	1.9	37	543
0	45	80	273	4.9	475	11	Tr	Tr	0.18	0.09	0.9	0	544
0	7	6	51	1.1	160	9	0	0	0.03	0.01	0.2	1	545
0	12	11	90	1.9	285	16	0	0	0.05	0.02	0.4	3	546
0	44	14	99	1.8	313	244	0	0	0.03	0.02	0.4	1	547
0	18	216	359	3.8	512	3	80	8	0.58	0.13	1.3	1	548
0	4	53	88	0.9	126	1	20	2	0.14	0.03	0.3	Tr	549
0	38	50	238	4.2	498	26	40	4	0.14	0.12	1.2	0	550
0	17	60	268	2.4	441	[43]348	10	1	0.29	0.15	2.7	0	551
0	4	13	57	0.5	93	[43]74	Tr	Tr	0.06	0.03	0.6	0	552
0	7	20	123	1.0	169	[44]190	Tr	Tr	0.06	0.06	1.3	0	553
0	6	31	131	0.9	165	[44]185	10	1	0.14	0.06	1.4	Tr	554
0	27	125	734	2.8	1,019	[45]626	0	0	0.42	0.15	21.5	0	555
0	5	24	143	0.5	199	[45]122	0	0	0.08	0.03	4.2	0	556
0	3	5	60	0.3	110	75	0	0	0.02	0.02	2.2	0	557
0	42	22	178	3.4	592	26	80	8	0.30	0.18	1.8	0	558
0	20	39	314	2.3	423	1	140	14	0.92	0.14	1.0	2	559
0	5	10	83	0.6	111	Tr	40	4	0.24	0.04	0.3	1	560
0	5	2	10	0.9	178	20	10	1	0.35	0.06	1.2	1	561
0	7	38	143	1.9	310	2	70	7	0.23	0.05	0.3	Tr	562
0	5	12	333	4.2	229	5	110	11	0.06	0.09	0.5	Tr	563
0	51	141	245	5.1	1,141	1,228	0	0	0.14	0.16	1.4	17	564
0	1	11	62	0.6	33	3	10	1	0.06	0.01	0.4	0	565
0	19	131	322	4.9	972	4	50	5	0.38	0.16	1.1	0	566
0	65	188	853	4.7	922	8,142	110	11	0.17	0.28	0.8	0	567
0	3	108	151	2.3	50	8	0	0	0.07	0.04	0.1	0	568
0	5	33	200	1.9	195	1	10	1	0.65	0.07	1.3	Tr	569
0	3	21	119	0.7	69	5	10	1	0.24	0.02	0.8	1	570

[44]Mixed nuts without salt contain 3 mg sodium per oz.
[45]Peanuts without salt contain 22 mg sodium per cup or 4 mg per oz.

Item No.	Foods, approximate measures, units, and weight (weight of edible portion only)			Water	Food energy	Protein	Fat	Fatty acids: Saturated	Fatty acids: Monounsaturated	Fatty acids: Polyunsaturated
			Grams	Percent	Calories	Grams	Grams	Grams	Grams	Grams
	Legumes, Nuts, and Seeds—Con.									
	Walnuts:									
571	Black, chopped	1 cup	125	4	760	30	71	4.5	15.9	46.9
572		1 oz	28	4	170	7	16	1.0	3.6	10.6
573	English or Persian, pieces or chips	1 cup	120	4	770	17	74	6.7	17.0	47.0
574		1 oz	28	4	180	4	18	1.6	4.0	11.1
	Meat and Meat Products									
	Beef, cooked:[46]									
	Cuts braised, simmered, or pot roasted:									
	Relatively fat such as chuck blade:									
575	Lean and fat, piece, 2-1/2 by 2-1/2 by 3/4 in	3 oz	85	43	325	22	26	10.8	11.7	0.9
576	Lean only from item 575	2.2 oz	62	53	170	19	9	3.9	4.2	0.3
	Relatively lean, such as bottom round:									
577	Lean and fat, piece, 4-1/8 by 2-1/4 by 1/2 in	3 oz	85	54	220	25	13	4.8	5.7	0.5
578	Lean only from item 577	2.8 oz	78	57	175	25	8	2.7	3.4	0.3
	Ground beef, broiled, patty, 3 by 5/8 in:									
579	Lean	3 oz	85	56	230	21	16	6.2	6.9	0.6
580	Regular	3 oz	85	54	245	20	18	6.9	7.7	0.7
581	Heart, lean, braised	3 oz	85	65	150	24	5	1.2	0.8	1.6
582	Liver, fried, slice, 6-1/2 by 2-3/8 by 3/8 in[47]	3 oz	85	56	185	23	7	2.5	3.6	1.3
	Roast, oven cooked, no liquid added:									
	Relatively fat, such as rib:									
583	Lean and fat, 2 pieces, 4-1/8 by 2-1/4 by 1/4 in	3 oz	85	46	315	19	26	10.8	11.4	0.9
584	Lean only from item 583	2.2 oz	61	57	150	17	9	3.6	3.7	0.3
	Relatively lean, such as eye of round:									
585	Lean and fat, 2 pieces, 2-1/2 by 2-1/2 by 3/8 in	3 oz	85	57	205	23	12	4.9	5.4	0.5
586	Lean only from item 585	2.6 oz	75	63	135	22	5	1.9	2.1	0.2
	Steak:									
	Sirloin, broiled:									
587	Lean and fat, piece, 2-1/2 by 2-1/2 by 3/4 in	3 oz	85	53	240	23	15	6.4	6.9	0.6
588	Lean only from item 587	2.5 oz	72	59	150	22	6	2.6	2.8	0.3
589	Beef, canned, corned	3 oz	85	59	185	22	10	4.2	4.9	0.4
590	Beef, dried, chipped	2.5 oz	72	48	145	24	4	1.8	2.0	0.2
	Lamb, cooked:									
	Chops, (3 per lb with bone):									
	Arm, braised:									
591	Lean and fat	2.2 oz	63	44	220	20	15	6.9	6.0	0.9
592	Lean only from item 591	1.7 oz	48	49	135	17	7	2.9	2.6	0.4
	Loin, broiled:									
593	Lean and fat	2.8 oz	80	54	235	22	16	7.3	6.4	1.0
594	Lean only from item 593	2.3 oz	64	61	140	19	6	2.6	2.4	0.4
	Leg, roasted:									
595	Lean and fat, 2 pieces, 4-1/8 by 2-1/4 by 1/4 in	3 oz	85	59	205	22	13	5.6	4.9	0.8
596	Lean only from item 595	2.6 oz	73	64	140	20	6	2.4	2.2	0.4
	Rib, roasted:									
597	Lean and fat, 3 pieces, 2-1/2 by 2-1/2 by 1/4 in	3 oz	85	47	315	18	26	12.1	10.6	1.5
598	Lean only from item 597	2 oz	57	60	130	15	7	3.2	3.0	0.5

[46]Outer layer of fat was removed to within approximately 1/2 inch of the lean. Deposits of fat within the cut were not removed.
[47]Fried in vegetable shortening.

Nutrients in Indicated Quantity

Cholesterol	Carbohydrate	Calcium	Phosphorus	Iron	Potassium	Sodium	Vitamin A value (IU)	Vitamin A value (RE)	Thiamin	Riboflavin	Niacin	Ascorbic acid	Item No.
Milligrams	Grams	Milligrams	Milligrams	Milligrams	Milligrams	Milligrams	International units	Retinol equivalents	Milligrams	Milligrams	Milligrams	Milligrams	
0	15	73	580	3.8	655	1	370	37	0.27	0.14	0.9	Tr	571
0	3	16	132	0.9	149	Tr	80	8	0.06	0.03	0.2	Tr	572
0	22	113	380	2.9	602	12	150	15	0.46	0.18	1.3	4	573
0	5	27	90	0.7	142	3	40	4	0.11	0.04	0.3	1	574
87	0	11	163	2.5	163	53	Tr	Tr	0.06	0.19	2.0	0	575
66	0	8	146	2.3	163	44	Tr	Tr	0.05	0.17	1.7	0	576
81	0	5	217	2.8	248	43	Tr	Tr	0.06	0.21	3.3	0	577
75	0	4	212	2.7	240	40	Tr	Tr	0.06	0.20	3.0	0	578
74	0	9	134	1.8	256	65	Tr	Tr	0.04	0.18	4.4	0	579
76	0	9	144	2.1	248	70	Tr	Tr	0.03	0.16	4.9	0	580
164	0	5	213	6.4	198	54	Tr	Tr	0.12	1.31	3.4	5	581
410	7	9	392	5.3	309	90	[48]30,690	[48]9,120	0.18	3.52	12.3	23	582
72	0	8	145	2.0	246	54	Tr	Tr	0.06	0.16	3.1	0	583
49	0	5	127	1.7	218	45	Tr	Tr	0.05	0.13	2.7	0	584
62	0	5	177	1.6	308	50	Tr	Tr	0.07	0.14	3.0	0	585
52	0	3	170	1.5	297	46	Tr	Tr	0.07	0.13	2.8	0	586
77	0	9	186	2.6	306	53	Tr	Tr	0.10	0.23	3.3	0	587
64	0	8	176	2.4	290	48	Tr	Tr	0.09	0.22	3.1	0	588
80	0	17	90	3.7	51	802	Tr	Tr	0.02	0.20	2.9	0	589
46	0	14	287	2.3	142	3,053	Tr	Tr	0.05	0.23	2.7	0	590
77	0	16	132	1.5	195	46	Tr	Tr	0.04	0.16	4.4	0	591
59	0	12	111	1.3	162	36	Tr	Tr	0.03	0.13	3.0	0	592
78	0	16	162	1.4	272	62	Tr	Tr	0.09	0.21	5.5	0	593
60	0	12	145	1.3	241	54	Tr	Tr	0.08	0.18	4.4	0	594
78	0	8	162	1.7	273	57	Tr	Tr	0.09	0.24	5.5	0	595
65	0	6	150	1.5	247	50	Tr	Tr	0.08	0.20	4.6	0	596
77	0	19	139	1.4	224	60	Tr	Tr	0.08	0.18	5.5	0	597
50	0	12	111	1.0	179	46	Tr	Tr	0.05	0.13	3.5	0	598

[48] Value varies widely.

Item No.	Foods, approximate measures, units, and weight (weight of edible portion only)			Water	Food energy	Protein	Fat	Fatty acids Saturated	Monounsaturated	Polyunsaturated
	Meat and Meat Products—Con.		Grams	Percent	Calories	Grams	Grams	Grams	Grams	Grams
	Pork, cured, cooked:									
	Bacon:									
599	Regular	3 medium slices	19	13	110	6	9	3.3	4.5	1.1
600	Canadian-style	2 slices	46	62	85	11	4	1.3	1.9	0.4
	Ham, light cure, roasted:									
601	Lean and fat, 2 pieces, 4-1/8 by 2-1/4 by 1/4 in	3 oz	85	58	205	18	14	5.1	6.7	1.5
602	Lean only from item 601	2.4 oz	68	66	105	17	4	1.3	1.7	0.4
603	Ham, canned, roasted, 2 pieces, 4-1/8 by 2-1/4 by 1/4 in	3 oz	85	67	140	18	7	2.4	3.5	0.8
	Luncheon meat:									
604	Canned, spiced or unspiced, slice, 3 by 2 by 1/2 in	2 slices	42	52	140	5	13	4.5	6.0	1.5
605	Chopped ham (8 slices per 6 oz pkg)	2 slices	42	64	95	7	7	2.4	3.4	0.9
	Cooked ham (8 slices per 8-oz pkg):									
606	Regular	2 slices	57	65	105	10	6	1.9	2.8	0.7
607	Extra lean	2 slices	57	71	75	11	3	0.9	1.3	0.3
	Pork, fresh, cooked:									
	Chop, loin (cut 3 per lb with bone):									
	Broiled:									
608	Lean and fat	3.1 oz	87	50	275	24	19	7.0	8.8	2.2
609	Lean only from item 608	2.5 oz	72	57	165	23	8	2.6	3.4	0.9
	Pan fried:									
610	Lean and fat	3.1 oz	89	45	335	21	27	9.8	12.5	3.1
611	Lean only from item 610	2.4 oz	67	54	180	19	11	3.7	4.8	1.3
	Ham (leg), roasted:									
612	Lean and fat, piece, 2-1/2 by 2-1/2 by 3/4 in	3 oz	85	53	250	21	18	6.4	8.1	2.0
613	Lean only from item 612	2.5 oz	72	60	160	20	8	2.7	3.6	1.0
	Rib, roasted:									
614	Lean and fat, piece, 2-1/2 by 3/4 in	3 oz	85	51	270	21	20	7.2	9.2	2.3
615	Lean only from item 614	2.5 oz	71	57	175	20	10	3.4	4.4	1.2
	Shoulder cut, braised:									
616	Lean and fat, 3 pieces, 2-1/2 by 2-1/2 by 1/4 in	3 oz	85	47	295	23	22	7.9	10.0	2.4
617	Lean only from item 616	2.4 oz	67	54	165	22	8	2.8	3.7	1.0
	Sausages (See also Luncheon meats, items 604-607):									
618	Bologna, slice (8 per 8-oz pkg)	2 slices	57	54	180	7	16	6.1	7.6	1.4
619	Braunschweiger, slice (6 per 6-oz pkg)	2 slices	57	48	205	8	18	6.2	8.5	2.1
620	Brown and serve (10-11 per 8-oz pkg), browned	1 link	13	45	50	2	5	1.7	2.2	0.5
621	Frankfurter (10 per 1-lb pkg), cooked (reheated)	1 frankfurter	45	54	145	5	13	4.8	6.2	1.2
622	Pork link (16 per 1-lb pkg), cooked[50]	1 link	13	45	50	3	4	1.4	1.8	0.5
	Salami:									
623	Cooked type, slice (8 per 8-oz pkg)	2 slices	57	60	145	8	11	4.6	5.2	1.2
624	Dry type, slice (12 per 4-oz pkg)	2 slices	20	35	85	5	7	2.4	3.4	0.6
625	Sandwich spread (pork, beef)	1 tbsp	15	60	35	1	3	0.9	1.1	0.4
626	Vienna sausage (7 per 4-oz can)	1 sausage	16	60	45	2	4	1.5	2.0	0.3
	Veal, medium fat, cooked, bone removed:									
627	Cutlet, 4-1/8 by 2-1/4 by 1/2 in, braised or broiled	3 oz	85	60	185	23	9	4.1	4.1	0.6
628	Rib, 2 pieces, 4-1/8 by 2-1/4 by 1/4 in, roasted	3 oz	85	55	230	23	14	6.0	6.0	1.0

[49] Contains added sodium ascorbate. If sodium ascorbate is not added, ascorbic acid content is negligible.

Nutrients in Indicated Quantity

Cholesterol	Carbohydrate	Calcium	Phosphorus	Iron	Potassium	Sodium	Vitamin A value (IU)	Vitamin A value (RE)	Thiamin	Riboflavin	Niacin	Ascorbic acid	Item No.
Milligrams	Grams	Milligrams	Milligrams	Milligrams	Milligrams	Milligrams	International units	Retinol equivalents	Milligrams	Milligrams	Milligrams	Milligrams	
16	Tr	2	64	0.3	92	303	0	0	0.13	0.05	1.4	6	599
27	1	5	136	0.4	179	711	0	0	0.38	0.09	3.2	10	600
53	0	6	182	0.7	243	1,009	0	0	0.51	0.19	3.8	0	601
37	0	5	154	0.6	215	902	0	0	0.46	0.17	3.4	0	602
35	Tr	6	188	0.9	298	908	0	0	0.82	0.21	4.3	[49]19	603
26	1	3	34	0.3	90	541	0	0	0.15	0.08	1.3	Tr	604
21	0	3	65	0.3	134	576	0	0	0.27	0.09	1.6	[49]8	605
32	2	4	141	0.6	189	751	0	0	0.49	0.14	3.0	[49]16	606
27	1	4	124	0.4	200	815	0	0	0.53	0.13	2.8	[49]15	607
84	0	3	184	0.7	312	61	10	3	0.87	0.24	4.3	Tr	608
71	0	4	176	0.7	302	56	10	1	0.83	0.22	4.0	Tr	609
92	0	4	190	0.7	323	64	10	3	0.91	0.24	4.6	Tr	610
72	0	3	178	0.7	305	57	10	1	0.84	0.22	4.0	Tr	611
79	0	5	210	0.9	280	50	10	2	0.54	0.27	3.9	Tr	612
68	0	5	202	0.8	269	46	10	1	0.50	0.25	3.6	Tr	613
69	0	9	190	0.8	313	37	10	3	0.50	0.24	4.2	Tr	614
56	0	8	182	0.7	300	33	10	2	0.45	0.22	3.8	Tr	615
93	0	6	162	1.4	286	75	10	3	0.46	0.26	4.4	Tr	616
76	0	5	151	1.3	271	68	10	1	0.40	0.24	4.0	Tr	617
31	2	7	52	0.9	103	581	0	0	0.10	0.08	1.5	[49]12	618
89	2	5	96	5.3	113	652	8,010	2,405	0.14	0.87	4.8	[49]6	619
9	Tr	1	14	0.1	25	105	0	0	0.05	0.02	0.4	0	620
23	1	5	39	0.5	75	504	0	0	0.09	0.05	1.2	[49]12	621
11	Tr	4	24	0.2	47	168	0	0	0.10	0.03	0.6	Tr	622
37	1	7	66	1.5	113	607	0	0	0.14	0.21	2.0	[49]7	623
16	1	2	28	0.3	76	372	0	0	0.12	0.06	1.0	[49]5	624
6	2	2	9	0.1	17	152	10	1	0.03	0.02	0.3	0	625
8	Tr	2	8	0.1	16	152	0	0	0.01	0.02	0.3	0	626
109	0	9	196	0.8	258	56	Tr	Tr	0.06	0.21	4.6	0	627
109	0	10	211	0.7	259	57	Tr	Tr	0.11	0.26	6.6	0	628

[50] One patty (8 per pound) of bulk sausage is equivalent to 2 links.

Item No.	Foods, approximate measures, units, and weight (weight of edible portion only)			Water	Food energy	Protein	Fat	Fatty acids: Saturated	Fatty acids: Monounsaturated	Fatty acids: Polyunsaturated
	Mixed Dishes and Fast Foods		Grams	Percent	Calories	Grams	Grams	Grams	Grams	Grams
	Mixed dishes:									
629	Beef and vegetable stew, from home recipe	1 cup	245	82	220	16	11	4.4	4.5	0.5
630	Beef potpie, from home recipe, baked, piece, 1/3 of 9-in diam. pie[51]	1 piece	210	55	515	21	30	7.9	12.9	7.4
631	Chicken a la king, cooked, from home recipe	1 cup	245	68	470	27	34	12.9	13.4	6.2
632	Chicken and noodles, cooked, from home recipe	1 cup	240	71	365	22	18	5.1	7.1	3.9
	Chicken chow mein:									
633	Canned	1 cup	250	89	95	7	Tr	0.1	0.1	0.8
634	From home recipe	1 cup	250	78	255	31	10	4.1	4.9	3.5
635	Chicken potpie, from home recipe, baked, piece, 1/3 of 9-in diam. pie[51]	1 piece	232	57	545	23	31	10.3	15.5	6.6
636	Chili con carne with beans, canned	1 cup	255	72	340	19	16	5.8	7.2	1.0
637	Chop suey with beef and pork, from home recipe	1 cup	250	75	300	26	17	4.3	7.4	4.2
	Macaroni (enriched) and cheese:									
638	Canned[52]	1 cup	240	80	230	9	10	4.7	2.9	1.3
639	From home recipe[38]	1 cup	200	58	430	17	22	9.8	7.4	3.6
640	Quiche Lorraine, 1/8 of 8-in diam. quiche[51]	1 slice	176	47	600	13	48	23.2	17.8	4.1
	Spaghetti (enriched) in tomato sauce with cheese:									
641	Canned	1 cup	250	80	190	6	2	0.4	0.4	0.5
642	From home recipe	1 cup	250	77	260	9	9	3.0	3.6	1.2
	Spaghetti (enriched) with meatballs and tomato sauce:									
643	Canned	1 cup	250	78	260	12	10	2.4	3.9	3.1
644	From home recipe	1 cup	248	70	330	19	12	3.9	4.4	2.2
	Fast food entrees:									
	Cheeseburger:									
645	Regular	1 sandwich	112	46	300	15	15	7.3	5.6	1.0
646	4 oz patty	1 sandwich	194	46	525	30	31	15.1	12.2	1.4
	Chicken, fried. See Poultry and Poultry Products (items 656-659).									
647	Enchilada	1 enchilada	230	72	235	20	16	7.7	6.7	0.6
648	English muffin, egg, cheese, and bacon	1 sandwich	138	49	360	18	18	8.0	8.0	0.7
	Fish sandwich:									
649	Regular, with cheese	1 sandwich	140	43	420	16	23	6.3	6.9	7.7
650	Large, without cheese	1 sandwich	170	48	470	18	27	6.3	8.7	9.5
	Hamburger:									
651	Regular	1 sandwich	98	46	245	12	11	4.4	5.3	0.5
652	4 oz patty	1 sandwich	174	50	445	25	21	7.1	11.7	0.6
653	Pizza, cheese, 1/8 of 15-in diam. pizza[51]	1 slice	120	46	290	15	9	4.1	2.6	1.3
654	Roast beef sandwich	1 sandwich	150	52	345	22	13	3.5	6.9	1.8
655	Taco	1 taco	81	55	195	9	11	4.1	5.5	0.8

[38] Made with margarine.
[51] Crust made with vegetable shortening and enriched flour.

Nutrients in Indicated Quantity

Cholesterol	Carbohydrate	Calcium	Phosphorus	Iron	Potassium	Sodium	Vitamin A value (IU)	Vitamin A value (RE)	Thiamin	Riboflavin	Niacin	Ascorbic acid	Item No.
Milligrams	Grams	Milligrams	Milligrams	Milligrams	Milligrams	Milligrams	International units	Retinol equivalents	Milligrams	Milligrams	Milligrams	Milligrams	
71	15	29	184	2.9	613	292	5,690	568	0.15	0.17	4.7	17	629
42	39	29	149	3.8	334	596	4,220	517	0.29	0.29	4.8	6	630
221	12	127	358	2.5	404	760	1,130	272	0.10	0.42	5.4	12	631
103	26	26	247	2.2	149	600	430	130	0.05	0.17	4.3	Tr	632
8	18	45	85	1.3	418	725	150	28	0.05	0.10	1.0	13	633
75	10	58	293	2.5	473	718	280	50	0.08	0.23	4.3	10	634
56	42	70	232	3.0	343	594	7,220	735	0.32	0.32	4.9	5	635
28	31	82	321	4.3	594	1,354	150	15	0.08	0.18	3.3	8	636
68	13	60	248	4.8	425	1,053	600	60	0.28	0.38	5.0	33	637
24	26	199	182	1.0	139	730	260	72	0.12	0.24	1.0	Tr	638
44	40	362	322	1.8	240	1,086	860	232	0.20	0.40	1.8	1	639
285	29	211	276	1.0	283	653	1,640	454	0.11	0.32	Tr	Tr	640
3	39	40	88	2.8	303	955	930	120	0.35	0.28	4.5	10	641
8	37	80	135	2.3	408	955	1,080	140	0.25	0.18	2.3	13	642
23	29	53	113	3.3	245	1,220	1,000	100	0.15	0.18	2.3	5	643
89	39	124	236	3.7	665	1,009	1,590	159	0.25	0.30	4.0	22	644
44	28	135	174	2.3	219	672	340	65	0.26	0.24	3.7	1	645
104	40	236	320	4.5	407	1,224	670	128	0.33	0.48	7.4	3	646
19	24	97	198	3.3	653	1,332	2,720	352	0.18	0.26	Tr	Tr	647
213	31	197	290	3.1	201	832	650	160	0.46	0.50	3.7	1	648
56	39	132	223	1.8	274	667	160	25	0.32	0.26	3.3	2	649
91	41	61	246	2.2	375	621	110	15	0.35	0.23	3.5	1	650
32	28	56	107	2.2	202	463	80	14	0.23	0.24	3.8	1	651
71	38	75	225	4.8	404	763	160	28	0.38	0.38	7.8	1	652
56	39	220	216	1.6	230	699	750	106	0.34	0.29	4.2	2	653
55	34	60	222	4.0	338	757	240	32	0.40	0.33	6.0	2	654
21	15	109	134	1.2	263	456	420	57	0.09	0.07	1.4	1	655

[52] Made with corn oil.

Item No.	Foods, approximate measures, units, and weight (weight of edible portion only)			Water	Food energy	Protein	Fat	Fatty acids: Saturated	Fatty acids: Monounsaturated	Fatty acids: Polyunsaturated
	Poultry and Poultry Products		Grams	Percent	Calories	Grams	Grams	Grams	Grams	Grams
	Chicken:									
	Fried, flesh, with skin:[53]									
	Batter dipped:									
656	Breast, 1/2 breast (5.6 oz with bones)	4.9 oz	140	52	365	35	18	4.9	7.6	4.3
657	Drumstick (3.4 oz with bones)	2.5 oz	72	53	195	16	11	3.0	4.6	2.7
	Flour coated:									
658	Breast, 1/2 breast (4.2 oz with bones)	3.5 oz	98	57	220	31	9	2.4	3.4	1.9
659	Drumstick (2.6 oz with bones)	1.7 oz	49	57	120	13	7	1.8	2.7	1.6
	Roasted, flesh only:									
660	Breast, 1/2 breast (4.2 oz with bones and skin)	3.0 oz	86	65	140	27	3	0.9	1.1	0.7
661	Drumstick, (2.9 oz with bones and skin)	1.6 oz	44	67	75	12	2	0.7	0.8	0.6
662	Stewed, flesh only, light and dark meat, chopped or diced	1 cup	140	67	250	38	9	2.6	3.3	2.2
663	Chicken liver, cooked	1 liver	20	68	30	5	1	0.4	0.3	0.2
664	Duck, roasted, flesh only	1/2 duck	221	64	445	52	25	9.2	8.2	3.2
	Turkey, roasted, flesh only:									
665	Dark meat, piece, 2-1/2 by 1-5/8 by 1/4 in	4 pieces	85	63	160	24	6	2.1	1.4	1.8
666	Light meat, piece, 4 by 2 by 1/4 in	2 pieces	85	66	135	25	3	0.9	0.5	0.7
	Light and dark meat:									
667	Chopped or diced	1 cup	140	65	240	41	7	2.3	1.4	2.0
668	Pieces (1 slice white meat, 4 by 2 by 1/4 in and 2 slices dark meat, 2-1/2 by 1-5/8 by 1/4 in)	3 pieces	85	65	145	25	4	1.4	0.9	1.2
	Poultry food products:									
	Chicken:									
669	Canned, boneless	5 oz	142	69	235	31	11	3.1	4.5	2.5
670	Frankfurter (10 per 1-lb pkg)	1 frankfurter	45	58	115	6	9	2.5	3.8	1.8
671	Roll, light (6 slices per 6 oz pkg)	2 slices	57	69	90	11	4	1.1	1.7	0.9
	Turkey:									
672	Gravy and turkey, frozen	5-oz package	142	85	95	8	4	1.2	1.4	0.7
673	Ham, cured turkey thigh meat (8 slices per 8-oz pkg)	2 slices	57	71	75	11	3	1.0	0.7	0.9
674	Loaf, breast meat (8 slices per 6-oz pkg)	2 slices	42	72	45	10	1	0.2	0.2	0.1
675	Patties, breaded, battered, fried (2.25 oz)	1 patty	64	50	180	9	12	3.0	4.8	3.0
676	Roast, boneless, frozen, seasoned, light and dark meat, cooked	3 oz	85	68	130	18	5	1.6	1.0	1.4
	Soups, Sauces, and Gravies									
	Soups:									
	Canned, condensed:									
	Prepared with equal volume of milk:									
677	Clam chowder, New England	1 cup	248	85	165	9	7	3.0	2.3	1.1
678	Cream of chicken	1 cup	248	85	190	7	11	4.6	4.5	1.6
679	Cream of mushroom	1 cup	248	85	205	6	14	5.1	3.0	4.6
680	Tomato	1 cup	248	85	160	6	6	2.9	1.6	1.1

[53] Fried in vegetable shortening.

Nutrients in Indicated Quantity													
Cho-les-terol	Carbo-hydrate	Calcium	Phos-phorus	Iron	Potas-sium	Sodium	Vitamin A value (IU)	Vitamin A value (RE)	Thiamin	Ribo-flavin	Niacin	Ascorbic acid	Item No.
Milli-grams	Grams	Milli-grams	Milli-grams	Milli-grams	Milli-grams	Milli-grams	Inter-national units	Retinol equiva-lents	Milli-grams	Milli-grams	Milli-grams	Milli-grams	
119	13	28	259	1.8	281	385	90	28	0.16	0.20	14.7	0	656
62	6	12	106	1.0	134	194	60	19	0.08	0.15	3.7	0	657
87	2	16	228	1.2	254	74	50	15	0.08	0.13	13.5	0	658
44	1	6	86	0.7	112	44	40	12	0.04	0.11	3.0	0	659
73	0	13	196	0.9	220	64	20	5	0.06	0.10	11.8	0	660
41	0	5	81	0.6	108	42	30	8	0.03	0.10	2.7	0	661
116	0	20	210	1.6	252	98	70	21	0.07	0.23	8.6	0	662
126	Tr	3	62	1.7	28	10	3,270	983	0.03	0.35	0.9	3	663
197	0	27	449	6.0	557	144	170	51	0.57	1.04	11.3	0	664
72	0	27	173	2.0	246	67	0	0	0.05	0.21	3.1	0	665
59	0	16	186	1.1	259	54	0	0	0.05	0.11	5.8	0	666
106	0	35	298	2.5	417	98	0	0	0.09	0.25	7.6	0	667
65	0	21	181	1.5	253	60	0	0	0.05	0.15	4.6	0	668
88	0	20	158	2.2	196	714	170	48	0.02	0.18	9.0	3	669
45	3	43	48	0.9	38	616	60	17	0.03	0.05	1.4	0	670
28	1	24	89	0.6	129	331	50	14	0.04	0.07	3.0	0	671
26	7	20	115	1.3	87	787	60	18	0.03	0.18	2.6	0	672
32	Tr	6	108	1.6	184	565	0	0	0.03	0.14	2.0	0	673
17	0	3	97	0.2	118	608	0	0	0.02	0.05	3.5	[54]0	674
40	10	9	173	1.4	176	512	20	7	0.06	0.12	1.5	0	675
45	3	4	207	1.4	253	578	0	0	0.04	0.14	5.3	0	676
22	17	186	156	1.5	300	992	160	40	0.07	0.24	1.0	3	677
27	15	181	151	0.7	273	1,047	710	94	0.07	0.26	0.9	1	678
20	15	179	156	0.6	270	1,076	150	37	0.08	0.28	0.9	2	679
17	22	159	149	1.8	449	932	850	109	0.13	0.25	1.5	68	680

[54] If sodium ascorbate is added, product contains 11 mg ascorbic acid.

Item No.	Foods, approximate measures, units, and weight (weight of edible portion only)			Water	Food energy	Protein	Fat	Fatty acids: Saturated	Fatty acids: Monounsaturated	Fatty acids: Polyunsaturated
	Soups, Sauces, and Gravies—Con.		Grams	Percent	Calories	Grams	Grams	Grams	Grams	Grams
	Soups:									
	Canned, condensed:									
	Prepared with equal volume of water:									
681	Bean with bacon	1 cup	253	84	170	8	6	1.5	2.2	1.8
682	Beef broth, bouillon, consomme	1 cup	240	98	15	3	1	0.3	0.2	Tr
683	Beef noodle	1 cup	244	92	85	5	3	1.1	1.2	0.5
684	Chicken noodle	1 cup	241	92	75	4	2	0.7	1.1	0.6
685	Chicken rice	1 cup	241	94	60	4	2	0.5	0.9	0.4
686	Clam chowder, Manhattan	1 cup	244	90	80	4	2	0.4	0.4	1.3
687	Cream of chicken	1 cup	244	91	115	3	7	2.1	3.3	1.5
688	Cream of mushroom	1 cup	244	90	130	2	9	2.4	1.7	4.2
689	Minestrone	1 cup	241	91	80	4	3	0.6	0.7	1.1
690	Pea, green	1 cup	250	83	165	9	3	1.4	1.0	0.4
691	Tomato	1 cup	244	90	85	2	2	0.4	0.4	1.0
692	Vegetable beef	1 cup	244	92	80	6	2	0.9	0.8	0.1
693	Vegetarian	1 cup	241	92	70	2	2	0.3	0.8	0.7
	Dehydrated:									
	Unprepared:									
694	Bouillon	1 pkt	6	3	15	1	1	0.3	0.2	Tr
695	Onion	1 pkt	7	4	20	1	Tr	0.1	0.2	Tr
	Prepared with water:									
696	Chicken noodle	1 pkt (6-fl-oz)	188	94	40	2	1	0.2	0.4	0.3
697	Onion	1 pkt (6-fl-oz)	184	96	20	1	Tr	0.1	0.2	0.1
698	Tomato vegetable	1 pkt (6-fl-oz)	189	94	40	1	1	0.3	0.2	0.1
	Sauces:									
	From dry mix:									
699	Cheese, prepared with milk	1 cup	279	77	305	16	17	9.3	5.3	1.6
700	Hollandaise, prepared with water	1 cup	259	84	240	5	20	11.6	5.9	0.9
701	White sauce, prepared with milk	1 cup	264	81	240	10	13	6.4	4.7	1.7
	From home recipe:									
702	White sauce, medium[55]	1 cup	250	73	395	10	30	9.1	11.9	7.2
	Ready to serve:									
703	Barbecue	1 tbsp	16	81	10	Tr	Tr	Tr	0.1	0.1
704	Soy	1 tbsp	18	68	10	2	0	0.0	0.0	0.0
	Gravies:									
	Canned:									
705	Beef	1 cup	233	87	125	9	5	2.7	2.3	0.2
706	Chicken	1 cup	238	85	190	5	14	3.4	6.1	3.6
707	Mushroom	1 cup	238	89	120	3	6	1.0	2.8	2.4
	From dry mix:									
708	Brown	1 cup	261	91	80	3	2	0.9	0.8	0.1
709	Chicken	1 cup	260	91	85	3	2	0.5	0.9	0.4
	Sugars and Sweets									
	Candy:									
710	Caramels, plain or chocolate	1 oz	28	8	115	1	3	2.2	0.3	0.1
	Chocolate:									
711	Milk, plain	1 oz	28	1	145	2	9	5.4	3.0	0.3
712	Milk, with almonds	1 oz	28	2	150	3	10	4.8	4.1	0.7
713	Milk, with peanuts	1 oz	28	1	155	4	11	4.2	3.5	1.5
714	Milk, with rice cereal	1 oz	28	2	140	2	7	4.4	2.5	0.2
715	Semisweet, small pieces (60 per oz)	1 cup or 6 oz	170	1	860	7	61	36.2	19.9	1.9
716	Sweet (dark)	1 oz	28	1	150	1	10	5.9	3.3	0.3
717	Fondant, uncoated (mints, candy corn, other)	1 oz	28	3	105	Tr	0	0.0	0.0	0.0
718	Fudge, chocolate, plain	1 oz	28	8	115	1	3	2.1	1.0	0.1
719	Gum drops	1 oz	28	12	100	Tr	Tr	Tr	Tr	0.1

[55] Made with enriched flour, margarine, and whole milk.

Nutrients in Indicated Quantity

Cholesterol	Carbohydrate	Calcium	Phosphorus	Iron	Potassium	Sodium	Vitamin A value (IU)	Vitamin A value (RE)	Thiamin	Riboflavin	Niacin	Ascorbic acid	Item No.
Milligrams	Grams	Milligrams	Milligrams	Milligrams	Milligrams	Milligrams	International units	Retinol equivalents	Milligrams	Milligrams	Milligrams	Milligrams	
3	23	81	132	2.0	402	951	890	89	0.09	0.03.	0.6	2	681
Tr	Tr	14	31	0.4	130	782	0	0	Tr	0.05	1.9	0	682
5	9	15	46	1.1	100	952	630	63	0.07	0.06	1.1	Tr	683
7	9	17	36	0.8	55	1,106	710	71	0.05	0.06	1.4	Tr	684
7	7	17	22	0.7	101	815	660	66	0.02	0.02	1.1	Tr	685
2	12	34	59	1.9	261	1,808	920	92	0.06	0.05	1.3	3	686
10	9	34	37	0.6	88	986	560	56	0.03	0.06	0.8	Tr	687
2	9	46	49	0.5	100	1,032	0	0	0.05	0.09	0.7	1	688
2	11	34	55	0.9	313	911	2,340	234	0.05	0.04	0.9	1	689
0	27	28	125	2.0	190	988	200	20	0.11	0.07	1.2	2	690
0	17	12	34	1.8	264	871	690	69	0.09	0.05	1.4	66	691
5	10	17	41	1.1	173	956	1,890	189	0.04	0.05	1.0	2	692
0	12	22	34	1.1	210	822	3,010	301	0.05	0.05	0.9	1	693
1	1	4	19	0.1	27	1,019	Tr	Tr	Tr	0.01	0.3	0	694
Tr	4	10	23	0.1	47	627	Tr	Tr	0.02	0.04	0.4	Tr	695
2	6	24	24	0.4	23	957	50	5	0.05	0.04	0.7	Tr	696
0	4	9	22	0.1	48	635	Tr	Tr	0.02	0.04	0.4	Tr	697
0	8	6	23	0.5	78	856	140	14	0.04	0.03	0.6	5	698
53	23	569	438	0.3	552	1,565	390	117	0.15	0.56	0.3	2	699
52	14	124	127	0.9	124	1,564	730	220	0.05	0.18	0.1	Tr	700
34	21	425	256	0.3	444	797	310	92	0.08	0.45	0.5	3	701
32	24	292	238	0.9	381	888	1,190	340	0.15	0.43	0.8	2	702
0	2	3	3	0.1	28	130	140	14	Tr	Tr	0.1	1	703
0	2	3	38	0.5	64	1,029	0	0	0.01	0.02	0.6	0	704
7	11	14	70	1.6	189	117	0	0	0.07	0.08	1.5	0	705
5	13	48	69	1.1	259	1,373	880	264	0.04	0.10	1.1	0	706
0	13	17	36	1.6	252	1,357	0	0	0.08	0.15	1.6	0	707
2	14	66	47	0.2	61	1,147	0	0	0.04	0.09	0.9	0	708
3	14	39	47	0.3	62	1,134	0	0	0.05	0.15	0.8	3	709
1	22	42	35	0.4	54	64	Tr	Tr	0.01	0.05	0.1	Tr	710
6	16	50	61	0.4	96	23	30	10	0.02	0.10	0.1	Tr	711
5	15	65	77	0.5	125	23	30	8	0.02	0.12	0.2	Tr	712
5	13	49	83	0.4	138	19	30	8	0.07	0.07	1.4	Tr	713
6	18	48	57	0.2	100	46	30	8	0.01	0.08	0.1	Tr	714
0	97	51	178	5.8	593	24	30	3	0.10	0.14	0.9	Tr	715
0	16	7	41	0.6	86	5	10	1	0.01	0.04	0.1	Tr	716
0	27	2	Tr	0.1	1	57	0	0	Tr	Tr	Tr	0	717
1	21	22	24	0.3	42	54	Tr	Tr	0.01	0.03	0.1	Tr	718
0	25	2	Tr	0.1	1	10	0	0	0.00	Tr	Tr	0	719

Item No.	Foods, approximate measures, units, and weight (weight of edible portion only)			Water	Food energy	Protein	Fat	Fatty acids: Saturated	Fatty acids: Monounsaturated	Fatty acids: Polyunsaturated
	Sugars and Sweets—Con.		Grams	Percent	Calories	Grams	Grams	Grams	Grams	Grams
	Candy:									
720	Hard	1 oz	28	1	110	0	0	0.0	0.0	0.0
721	Jelly beans	1 oz	28	6	105	Tr	Tr	Tr	Tr	0.1
722	Marshmallows	1 oz	28	17	90	1	0	0.0	0.0	0.0
723	Custard, baked	1 cup	265	77	305	14	15	6.8	5.4	0.7
724	Gelatin dessert prepared with gelatin dessert powder and water	1/2 cup	120	84	70	2	0	0.0	0.0	0.0
725	Honey, strained or extracted	1 cup	339	17	1,030	1	0	0.0	0.0	0.0
726		1 tbsp	21	17	65	Tr	0	0.0	0.0	0.0
727	Jams and preserves	1 tbsp	20	29	55	Tr	Tr	0.0	Tr	Tr
728		1 packet	14	29	40	Tr	Tr	0.0	Tr	Tr
729	Jellies	1 tbsp	18	28	50	Tr	Tr	Tr	Tr	Tr
730		1 packet	14	28	40	Tr	Tr	Tr	Tr	Tr
731	Popsicle, 3-fl-oz size	1 popsicle	95	80	70	0	0	0.0	0.0	0.0
	Puddings:									
	Canned:									
732	Chocolate	5-oz can	142	68	205	3	11	9.5	0.5	0.1
733	Tapioca	5-oz can	142	74	160	3	5	4.8	Tr	Tr
734	Vanilla	5-oz can	142	69	220	2	10	9.5	0.2	0.1
	Dry mix, prepared with whole milk:									
	Chocolate:									
735	Instant	1/2 cup	130	71	155	4	4	2.3	1.1	0.2
736	Regular (cooked)	1/2 cup	130	73	150	4	4	2.4	1.1	0.1
737	Rice	1/2 cup	132	73	155	4	4	2.3	1.1	0.1
738	Tapioca	1/2 cup	130	75	145	4	4	2.3	1.1	0.1
	Vanilla:									
739	Instant	1/2 cup	130	73	150	4	4	2.2	1.1	0.2
740	Regular (cooked)	1/2 cup	130	74	145	4	4	2.3	1.0	0.1
	Sugars:									
741	Brown, pressed down	1 cup	220	2	820	0	0	0.0	0.0	0.0
	White:									
742	Granulated	1 cup	200	1	770	0	0	0.0	0.0	0.0
743		1 tbsp	12	1	45	0	0	0.0	0.0	0.0
744		1 packet	6	1	25	0	0	0.0	0.0	0.0
745	Powdered, sifted, spooned into cup	1 cup	100	1	385	0	0	0.0	0.0	0.0
	Syrups:									
	Chocolate-flavored syrup or topping:									
746	Thin type	2 tbsp	38	37	85	1	Tr	0.2	0.1	0.1
747	Fudge type	2 tbsp	38	25	125	2	5	3.1	1.7	0.2
748	Molasses, cane, blackstrap	2 tbsp	40	24	85	0	0	0.0	0.0	0.0
749	Table syrup (corn and maple)	2 tbsp	42	25	122	0	0	0.0	0.0	0.0
	Vegetables and Vegetable Products									
750	Alfalfa seeds, sprouted, raw	1 cup	33	91	10	1	Tr	Tr	Tr	0.1
751	Artichokes, globe or French, cooked, drained	1 artichoke	120	87	55	3	Tr	Tr	Tr	0.1
	Asparagus, green:									
	Cooked, drained:									
	From raw:									
752	Cuts and tips	1 cup	180	92	45	5	1	0.1	Tr	0.2
753	Spears, 1/2-in diam. at base	4 spears	60	92	15	2	Tr	Tr	Tr	0.1
	From frozen:									
754	Cuts and tips	1 cup	180	91	50	5	1	0.2	Tr	0.3
755	Spears, 1/2-in diam. at base	4 spears	60	91	15	2	Tr	0.1	Tr	0.1
756	Canned, spears, 1/2-in diam. at base	4 spears	80	95	10	1	Tr	Tr	Tr	0.1
757	Bamboo shoots, canned, drained	1 cup	131	94	25	2	1	0.1	Tr	0.2

[56] For regular pack; special dietary pack contains 3 mg sodium.

Nutrients in Indicated Quantity

Cho-les-terol	Carbo-hydrate	Calcium	Phos-phorus	Iron	Potas-sium	Sodium	Vitamin A value (IU)	Vitamin A value (RE)	Thiamin	Ribo-flavin	Niacin	Ascorbic acid	Item No.
Milli-grams	Grams	Milli-grams	Milli-grams	Milli-grams	Milli-grams	Milli-grams	Inter-national units	Retinol equiva-lents	Milli-grams	Milli-grams	Milli-grams	Milli-grams	
0	28	Tr	2	0.1	1	7	0	0	0.10	0.00	0.0	0	720
0	26	1	1	0.3	11	7	0	0	0.00	Tr	Tr	0	721
0	23	1	2	0.5	2	25	0	0	0.00	Tr	Tr	0	722
278	29	297	310	1.1	387	209	530	146	0.11	0.50	0.3	1	723
0	17	2	23	Tr	Tr	55	0	0	0.00	0.00	0.0	0	724
0	279	17	20	1.7	173	17	0	0	0.02	0.14	1.0	3	725
0	17	1	1	0.1	11	1	0	0	Tr	0.01	0.1	Tr	726
0	14	4	2	0.2	18	2	Tr	Tr	Tr	0.01	Tr	Tr	727
0	10	3	1	0.1	12	2	Tr	Tr	Tr	Tr	Tr	Tr	728
0	13	2	Tr	0.1	16	5	Tr	Tr	Tr	0.01	Tr	1	729
0	10	1	Tr	Tr	13	4	Tr	Tr	Tr	Tr	Tr	1	730
0	18	0	0	Tr	4	11	0	0	0.00	0.00	0.0	0	731
1	30	74	117	1.2	254	285	100	31	0.04	0.17	0.6	Tr	732
Tr	28	119	113	0.3	212	252	Tr	Tr	0.03	0.14	0.4	Tr	733
1	33	79	94	0.2	155	305	Tr	Tr	0.03	0.12	0.6	Tr	734
14	27	130	329	0.3	176	440	130	33	0.04	0.18	0.1	1	735
15	25	146	120	0.2	190	167	140	34	0.05	0.20	0.1	1	736
15	27	133	110	0.5	165	140	140	33	0.10	0.18	0.6	1	737
15	25	131	103	0.1	167	152	140	34	0.04	0.18	0.1	1	738
15	27	129	273	0.1	164	375	140	33	0.04	0.17	0.1	1	739
15	25	132	102	0.1	166	178	140	34	0.04	0.18	0.1	1	740
0	212	187	56	4.8	757	97	0	0	0.02	0.07	0.2	0	741
0	199	3	Tr	0.1	7	5	0	0	0.00	0.00	0.0	0	742
0	12	Tr	Tr	Tr	Tr	Tr	0	0	0.00	0.00	0.0	0	743
0	6	Tr	Tr	Tr	Tr	Tr	0	0	0.00	0.00	0.0	0	744
0	100	1	Tr	Tr	4	2	0	0	0.00	0.00	0.0	0	745
0	22	6	49	0.8	85	36	Tr	Tr	Tr	0.02	0.1	0	746
0	21	38	60	0.5	82	42	40	13	0.02	0.08	0.1	0	747
0	22	274	34	10.1	1,171	38	0	0	0.04	0.08	0.8	0	748
0	32	1	4	Tr	7	19	0	0	0.00	0.00	0.0	0	749
0	1	11	23	0.3	26	2	50	5	0.03	0.04	0.2	3	750
0	12	47	72	1.6	316	79	170	17	0.07	0.06	0.7	9	751
0	8	43	110	1.2	558	7	1,490	149	0.18	0.22	1.9	49	752
0	3	14	37	0.4	186	2	500	50	0.06	0.07	0.6	16	753
0	9	41	99	1.2	392	7	1,470	147	0.12	0.19	1.9	44	754
0	3	14	33	0.4	131	2	490	49	0.04	0.06	0.6	15	755
0	2	11	30	0.5	122	[56]278	380	38	0.04	0.07	0.7	13	756
0	4	10	33	0.4	105	9	10	1	0.03	0.03	0.2	1	757

Item No.	Foods, approximate measures, units, and weight (weight of edible portion only)			Water	Food energy	Protein	Fat	Fatty acids Saturated	Fatty acids Monounsaturated	Fatty acids Polyunsaturated
	Vegetables and Vegetable Products—Con.		Grams	Percent	Calories	Grams	Grams	Grams	Grams	Grams
	Beans:									
	Lima, immature seeds, frozen, cooked, drained:									
758	Thick-seeded types (Fordhooks)	1 cup	170	74	170	10	1	0.1	Tr	0.3
759	Thin-seeded types (baby limas)	1 cup	180	72	190	12	1	0.1	Tr	0.3
	Snap:									
	Cooked, drained:									
760	From raw (cut and French style)	1 cup	125	89	45	2	Tr	0.1	Tr	0.2
761	From frozen (cut)	1 cup	135	92	35	2	Tr	Tr	Tr	0.1
762	Canned, drained solids (cut)	1 cup	135	93	25	2	Tr	Tr	Tr	0.1
	Beans, mature. See Beans, dry (items 527-535) and Black-eyed peas, dry (item 536).									
	Bean sprouts (mung):									
763	Raw	1 cup	104	90	30	3	Tr	Tr	Tr	0.1
764	Cooked, drained	1 cup	124	93	25	3	Tr	Tr	Tr	Tr
	Beets:									
	Cooked, drained:									
765	Diced or sliced	1 cup	170	91	55	2	Tr	Tr	Tr	Tr
766	Whole beets, 2-in diam.	2 beets	100	91	30	1	Tr	Tr	Tr	Tr
767	Canned, drained solids, diced or sliced	1 cup	170	91	55	2	Tr	Tr	Tr	0.1
768	Beet greens, leaves and stems, cooked, drained	1 cup	144	89	40	4	Tr	Tr	0.1	0.1
	Black-eyed peas, immature seeds, cooked and drained:									
769	From raw	1 cup	165	72	180	13	1	0.3	0.1	0.6
770	From frozen	1 cup	170	66	225	14	1	0.3	0.1	0.5
	Broccoli:									
771	Raw	1 spear	151	91	40	4	1	0.1	Tr	0.3
	Cooked, drained:									
	From raw:									
772	Spear, medium	1 spear	180	90	50	5	1	0.1	Tr	0.2
773	Spears, cut into 1/2-in pieces	1 cup	155	90	45	5	Tr	0.1	Tr	0.2
	From frozen:									
774	Piece, 4-1/2 to 5 in long	1 piece	30	91	10	1	Tr	Tr	Tr	Tr
775	Chopped	1 cup	185	91	50	6	Tr	Tr	Tr	0.1
	Brussels sprouts, cooked, drained:									
776	From raw, 7-8 sprouts, 1-1/4 to 1-1/2-in diam.	1 cup	155	87	60	4	1	0.2	0.1	0.4
777	From frozen	1 cup	155	87	65	6	1	0.1	Tr	0.3
	Cabbage, common varieties:									
778	Raw, coarsely shredded or sliced	1 cup	70	93	15	1	Tr	Tr	Tr	0.1
779	Cooked, drained	1 cup	150	94	30	1	Tr	Tr	Tr	0.2
	Cabbage, Chinese:									
780	Pak-choi, cooked, drained	1 cup	170	96	20	3	Tr	Tr	Tr	0.1
781	Pe-tsai, raw, 1-in pieces	1 cup	76	94	10	1	Tr	Tr	Tr	0.1
782	Cabbage, red, raw, coarsely shredded or sliced	1 cup	70	92	20	1	Tr	Tr	Tr	0.1
783	Cabbage, savoy, raw, coarsely shredded or sliced	1 cup	70	91	20	1	Tr	Tr	Tr	Tr

[57] For green varieties; yellow varieties contain 101 IU or 10 RE.
[58] For green varieties; yellow varieties contain 151 IU or 15 RE.
[59] For regular pack; special dietary pack contains 3 mg sodium.

Nutrients in Indicated Quantity

Cho-les-terol	Carbo-hydrate	Calcium	Phos-phorus	Iron	Potas-sium	Sodium	Vitamin A value (IU)	Vitamin A value (RE)	Thiamin	Ribo-flavin	Niacin	Ascorbic acid	Item No.
Milli-grams	Grams	Milli-grams	Milli-grams	Milli-grams	Milli-grams	Milli-grams	Inter-national units	Retinol equiva-lents	Milli-grams	Milli-grams	Milli-grams	Milli-grams	
0	32	37	107	2.3	694	90	320	32	0.13	0.10	1.8	22	758
0	35	50	202	3.5	740	52	300	30	0.13	0.10	1.4	10	759
0	10	58	49	1.6	374	4	[57]830	[57]83	0.09	0.12	0.8	12	760
0	8	61	32	1.1	151	18	[58]710	[58]71	0.06	0.10	0.6	11	761
0	6	35	26	1.2	147	[59]339	[60]470	[60]47	0.02	0.08	0.3	6	762
0	6	14	56	0.9	155	6	20	2	0.09	0.13	0.8	14	763
0	5	15	35	0.8	125	12	20	2	0.06	0.13	1.0	14	764
0	11	19	53	1.1	530	83	20	2	0.05	0.02	0.5	9	765
0	7	11	31	0.6	312	49	10	1	0.03	0.01	0.3	6	766
0	12	26	29	3.1	252	[61]466	20	2	0.02	0.07	0.3	7	767
0	8	164	59	2.7	1,309	347	7,340	734	0.17	0.42	0.7	36	768
0	30	46	196	2.4	693	7	1,050	105	0.11	0.18	1.8	3	769
0	40	39	207	3.6	638	9	130	13	0.44	0.11	1.2	4	770
0	8	72	100	1.3	491	41	2,330	233	0.10	0.18	1.0	141	771
0	10	205	86	2.1	293	20	2,540	254	0.15	0.37	1.4	113	772
0	9	177	74	1.8	253	17	2,180	218	0.13	0.32	1.2	97	773
0	2	15	17	0.2	54	7	570	57	0.02	0.02	0.1	12	774
0	10	94	102	1.1	333	44	3,500	350	0.10	0.15	0.8	74	775
0	13	56	87	1.9	491	33	1,110	111	0.17	0.12	0.9	96	776
0	13	37	84	1.1	504	36	910	91	0.16	0.18	0.8	71	777
0	4	33	16	0.4	172	13	90	9	0.04	0.02	0.2	33	778
0	7	50	38	0.6	308	29	130	13	0.09	0.08	0.3	36	779
0	3	158	49	1.8	631	58	4,370	437	0.05	0.11	0.7	44	780
0	2	59	22	0.2	181	7	910	91	0.03	0.04	0.3	21	781
0	4	36	29	0.3	144	8	30	3	0.04	0.02	0.2	40	782
0	4	25	29	0.3	161	20	700	70	0.05	0.02	0.2	22	783

[60] For green varieties; yellow varieties contain 142 IU or 14 RE.
[61] For regular pack; special dietary pack contains 78 mg sodium.

Item No.	Foods, approximate measures, units, and weight (weight of edible portion only)			Water	Food energy	Protein	Fat	Fatty acids: Saturated	Fatty acids: Monounsaturated	Fatty acids: Polyunsaturated
	Vegetables and Vegetable Products—Con.		Grams	Percent	Calories	Grams	Grams	Grams	Grams	Grams
	Carrots:									
	Raw, without crowns and tips, scraped:									
784	Whole, 7-1/2 by 1-1/8 in, or strips, 2-1/2 to 3 in long	1 carrot or 18 strips	72	88	30	1	Tr	Tr	Tr	0.1
785	Grated	1 cup	110	88	45	1	Tr	Tr	Tr	0.1
	Cooked, sliced, drained:									
786	From raw	1 cup	156	87	70	2	Tr	0.1	Tr	0.1
787	From frozen	1 cup	146	90	55	2	Tr	Tr	Tr	0.1
788	Canned, sliced, drained solids	1 cup	146	93	35	1	Tr	0.1	Tr	0.1
	Cauliflower:									
789	Raw, (flowerets)	1 cup	100	92	25	2	Tr	Tr	Tr	0.1
	Cooked, drained:									
790	From raw (flowerets)	1 cup	125	93	30	2	Tr	Tr	Tr	0.1
791	From frozen (flowerets)	1 cup	180	94	35	3	Tr	0.1	Tr	0.2
	Celery, pascal type, raw:									
792	Stalk, large outer, 8 by 1-1/2 in (at root end)	1 stalk	40	95	5	Tr	Tr	Tr	Tr	Tr
793	Pieces, diced	1 cup	120	95	20	1	Tr	Tr	Tr	0.1
	Collards, cooked, drained:									
794	From raw (leaves without stems)	1 cup	190	96	25	2	Tr	0.1	Tr	0.2
795	From frozen (chopped)	1 cup	170	88	60	5	1	0.1	0.1	0.4
	Corn, sweet:									
	Cooked, drained:									
796	From raw, ear 5 by 1-3/4 in	1 ear	77	70	85	3	1	0.2	0.3	0.5
	From frozen:									
797	Ear, trimmed to about 3-1/2 in long	1 ear	63	73	60	2	Tr	0.1	0.1	0.2
798	Kernels	1 cup	165	76	135	5	Tr	Tr	Tr	0.1
	Canned:									
799	Cream style	1 cup	256	79	185	4	1	0.2	0.3	0.5
800	Whole kernel, vacuum pack	1 cup	210	77	165	5	1	0.2	0.3	0.5
	Cowpeas. See Black-eyed peas, immature (items 769,770), mature (item 536).									
801	Cucumber, with peel, slices, 1/8 in thick (large, 2-1/8-in diam.; small, 1-3/4-in diam.)	6 large or 8 small slices	28	96	5	Tr	Tr	Tr	Tr	Tr
802	Dandelion greens, cooked, drained	1 cup	105	90	35	2	1	0.1	Tr	0.3
803	Eggplant, cooked, steamed	1 cup	96	92	25	1	Tr	Tr	Tr	0.1
804	Endive, curly (including escarole), raw, small pieces	1 cup	50	94	10	1	Tr	Tr	Tr	Tr
805	Jerusalem-artichoke, raw, sliced	1 cup	150	78	115	3	Tr	0.0	Tr	Tr
	Kale, cooked, drained:									
806	From raw, chopped	1 cup	130	91	40	2	1	0.1	Tr	0.3
807	From frozen, chopped	1 cup	130	91	40	4	1	0.1	Tr	0.3
808	Kohlrabi, thickened bulb-like stems, cooked, drained, diced	1 cup	165	90	50	3	Tr	Tr	Tr	0.1
	Lettuce, raw:									
	Butterhead, as Boston types:									
809	Head, 5-in diam	1 head	163	96	20	2	Tr	Tr	Tr	0.2
810	Leaves	1 outer or 2 inner leaves	15	96	Tr	Tr	Tr	Tr	Tr	Tr
	Crisphead, as iceberg:									
811	Head, 6-in diam	1 head	539	96	70	5	1	0.1	Tr	0.5
812	Wedge, 1/4 of head	1 wedge	135	96	20	1	Tr	Tr	Tr	0.1
813	Pieces, chopped or shredded	1 cup	55	96	5	1	Tr	Tr	Tr	0.1
814	Looseleaf (bunching varieties including romaine or cos), chopped or shredded pieces	1 cup	56	94	10	1	Tr	Tr	Tr	0.1

[62]For regular pack; special dietary pack contains 61 mg sodium.
[63]For yellow varieties; white varieties contain only a trace of vitamin A.

Nutrients in Indicated Quantity														
Cholesterol	Carbohydrate	Calcium	Phosphorus	Iron	Potassium	Sodium	Vitamin A value (IU)	Vitamin A value (RE)	Thiamin	Riboflavin	Niacin	Ascorbic acid	Item No.	
Milligrams	Grams	Milligrams	Milligrams	Milligrams	Milligrams	Milligrams	International units	Retinol equivalents	Milligrams	Milligrams	Milligrams	Milligrams		
0	7	19	32	0.4	233	25	20,250	2,025	0.07	0.04	0.7	7	784	
0	11	30	48	0.6	355	39	30,940	3,094	0.11	0.06	1.0	10	785	
0	16	48	47	1.0	354	103	38,300	3,830	0.05	0.09	0.8	4	786	
0	12	41	38	0.7	231	86	25,850	2,585	0.04	0.05	0.6	4	787	
0	8	37	35	0.9	261	[62]352	20,110	2,011	0.03	0.04	0.8	4	788	
0	5	29	46	0.6	355	15	20	2	0.08	0.06	0.6	72	789	
0	6	34	44	0.5	404	8	20	2	0.08	0.07	0.7	69	790	
0	7	31	43	0.7	250	32	40	4	0.07	0.10	0.6	56	791	
0	1	14	10	0.2	114	35	50	5	0.01	0.01	0.1	3	792	
0	4	43	31	0.6	341	106	150	15	0.04	0.04	0.4	8	793	
0	5	148	19	0.8	177	36	4,220	422	0.03	0.08	0.4	19	794	
0	12	357	46	1.9	427	85	10,170	1,017	0.08	0.20	1.1	45	795	
0	19	2	79	0.5	192	13	[63]170	[63]17	0.17	0.06	1.2	5	796	
0	14	2	47	0.4	158	3	[63]130	[63]13	0.11	0.04	1.0	3	797	
0	34	3	78	0.5	229	8	[63]410	[63]41	0.11	0.12	2.1	4	798	
0	46	8	131	1.0	343	[64]730	[63]250	[63]25	0.06	0.14	2.5	12	799	
0	41	11	134	0.9	391	[65]571	[63]510	[63]51	0.09	0.15	2.5	17	800	
0	1	4	5	0.1	42	1	10	1	0.01	0.01	0.1	1	801	
0	7	147	44	1.9	244	46	12,290	1,229	0.14	0.18	0.5	19	802	
0	6	6	21	0.3	238	3	60	6	0.07	0.02	0.6	1	803	
0	2	26	14	0.4	157	11	1,030	103	0.04	0.04	0.2	3	804	
0	26	21	117	5.1	644	6	30	3	0.30	0.09	2.0	6	805	
0	7	94	36	1.2	296	30	9,620	962	0.07	0.09	0.7	53	806	
0	7	179	36	1.2	417	20	8,260	826	0.06	0.15	0.9	33	807	
0	11	41	74	0.7	561	35	60	6	0.07	0.03	0.6	89	808	
0	4	52	38	0.5	419	8	1,580	158	0.10	0.10	0.5	13	809	
0	Tr	5	3	Tr	39	1	150	15	0.01	0.01	Tr	1	810	
0	11	102	108	2.7	852	49	1,780	178	0.25	0.16	1.0	21	811	
0	3	26	27	0.7	213	12	450	45	0.06	0.04	0.3	5	812	
0	1	10	11	0.3	87	5	180	18	0.03	0.02	0.1	2	813	
0	2	38	14	0.8	148	5	1,060	106	0.03	0.04	0.2	10	814	

[64]For regular pack; special dietary pack contains 8 mg sodium.
[65]For regular pack; special dietary pack contains 6 mg sodium.

Item No	Foods, approximate measures, units, and weight (weight of edible portion only)			Water	Food energy	Protein	Fat	Fatty acids: Saturated	Fatty acids: Monounsaturated	Fatty acids: Polyunsaturated
	Vegetables and Vegetable Products—Con.		Grams	Percent	Calories	Grams	Grams	Grams	Grams	Grams
	Mushrooms:									
815	Raw, sliced or chopped	1 cup	70	92	20	1	Tr	Tr	Tr	0.1
816	Cooked, drained	1 cup	156	91	40	3	1	0.1	Tr	0.3
817	Canned, drained solids	1 cup	156	91	35	3	Tr	0.1	Tr	0.2
818	Mustard greens, without stems and midribs, cooked, drained	1 cup	140	94	20	3	Tr	Tr	0.2	0.1
819	Okra pods, 3 by 5/8 in, cooked	8 pods	85	90	25	2	Tr	Tr	Tr	Tr
	Onions:									
	Raw:									
820	Chopped	1 cup	160	91	55	2	Tr	0.1	0.1	0.2
821	Sliced	1 cup	115	91	40	1	Tr	0.1	Tr	0.1
822	Cooked (whole or sliced), drained	1 cup	210	92	60	2	Tr	0.1	Tr	0.1
823	Onions, spring, raw, bulb (3/8-in diam.) and white portion of top	6 onions	30	92	10	1	Tr	Tr	Tr	Tr
824	Onion rings, breaded, par-fried, frozen, prepared	2 rings	20	29	80	1	5	1.7	2.2	1.0
	Parsley:									
825	Raw	10 sprigs	10	88	5	Tr	Tr	Tr	Tr	Tr
826	Freeze-dried	1 tbsp	0.4	2	Tr	Tr	Tr	Tr	Tr	Tr
827	Parsnips, cooked (diced or 2 in lengths), drained	1 cup	156	78	125	2	Tr	0.1	0.2	0.1
828	Peas, edible pod, cooked, drained	1 cup	160	89	65	5	Tr	0.1	Tr	0.2
	Peas, green:									
829	Canned, drained solids	1 cup	170	82	115	8	1	0.1	0.1	0.3
830	Frozen, cooked, drained	1 cup	160	80	125	8	Tr	0.1	Tr	0.2
	Peppers:									
831	Hot chili, raw	1 pepper	45	88	20	1	Tr	Tr	Tr	Tr
	Sweet (about 5 per lb, whole), stem and seeds removed:									
832	Raw	1 pepper	74	93	20	1	Tr	Tr	Tr	0.2
833	Cooked, drained	1 pepper	73	95	15	Tr	Tr	Tr	Tr	0.1
	Potatoes, cooked:									
	Baked (about 2 per lb, raw):									
834	With skin	1 potato	202	71	220	5	Tr	0.1	Tr	0.1
835	Flesh only	1 potato	156	75	145	3	Tr	Tr	Tr	0.1
	Boiled (about 3 per lb, raw):									
836	Peeled after boiling	1 potato	136	77	120	3	Tr	Tr	Tr	0.1
837	Peeled before boiling	1 potato	135	77	115	2	Tr	Tr	Tr	0.1
	French fried, strip, 2 to 3-1/2 in long, frozen:									
838	Oven heated	10 strips	50	53	110	2	4	2.1	1.8	0.3
839	Fried in vegetable oil	10 strips	50	38	160	2	8	2.5	1.6	3.8
	Potato products, prepared:									
	Au gratin:									
840	From dry mix	1 cup	245	79	230	6	10	6.3	2.9	0.3
841	From home recipe	1 cup	245	74	325	12	19	11.6	5.3	0.7
842	Hashed brown, from frozen	1 cup	156	56	340	5	18	7.0	8.0	2.1
	Mashed:									
	From home recipe:									
843	Milk added	1 cup	210	78	160	4	1	0.7	0.3	0.1
844	Milk and margarine added	1 cup	210	76	225	4	9	2.2	3.7	2.5
845	From dehydrated flakes (without milk), water, milk, butter, and salt added	1 cup	210	76	235	4	12	7.2	3.3	0.5
846	Potato salad, made with mayonnaise	1 cup	250	76	360	7	21	3.6	6.2	9.3
	Scalloped:									
847	From dry mix	1 cup	245	79	230	5	11	6.5	3.0	0.5
848	From home recipe	1 cup	245	81	210	7	9	5.5	2.5	0.4

[66] For regular pack; special dietary pack contains 3 mg sodium.
[67] For red peppers; green peppers contain 350 IU or 35 RE.
[68] For green peppers; red peppers contain 4,220 IU or 422 RE.

Nutrients in Indicated Quantity

Cho-les-terol	Carbo-hydrate	Calcium	Phos-phorus	Iron	Potas-sium	Sodium	Vitamin A value (IU)	Vitamin A value (RE)	Thiamin	Ribo-flavin	Niacin	Ascorbic acid	Item No.
Milli-grams	Grams	Milli-grams	Milli-grams	Milli-grams	Milli-grams	Milli-grams	Inter-national units	Retinol equiva-lents	Milli-grams	Milli-grams	Milli-grams	Milli-grams	
0	3	4	73	0.9	259	3	0	0	0.07	0.31	2.9	2	815
0	8	9	136	2.7	555	3	0	0	0.11	0.47	7.0	6	816
0	8	17	103	1.2	201	663	0	0	0.13	0.03	2.5	0	817
0	3	104	57	1.0	283	22	4,240	424	0.06	0.09	0.6	35	818
0	6	54	48	0.4	274	4	490	49	0.11	0.05	0.7	14	819
0	12	40	46	0.6	248	3	0	0	0.10	0.02	0.2	13	820
0	8	29	33	0.4	178	2	0	0	0.07	0.01	0.1	10	821
0	13	57	48	0.4	319	17	0	0	0.09	0.02	0.2	12	822
0	2	18	10	0.6	77	1	1,500	150	0.02	0.04	0.1	14	823
0	8	6	16	0.3	26	75	50	5	0.06	0.03	0.7	Tr	824
0	1	13	4	0.6	54	4	520	52	0.01	0.01	0.1	9	825
0	Tr	1	2	0.2	25	2	250	25	Tr	0.01	Tr	1	826
0	30	58	108	0.9	573	16	0	0	0.13	0.08	1.1	20	827
0	11	67	88	3.2	384	6	210	21	0.20	0.12	0.9	77	828
0	21	34	114	1.6	294	[66]372	1,310	131	0.21	0.13	1.2	16	829
0	23	38	144	2.5	269	139	1,070	107	0.45	0.16	2.4	16	830
0	4	8	21	0.5	153	3	[67]4,840	[67]484	0.04	0.04	0.4	109	831
0	4	4	16	0.9	144	2	[68]390	[68]39	0.06	0.04	0.4	[69]95	832
0	3	3	11	0.6	94	1	[70]280	[70]28	0.04	0.03	0.3	[71]81	833
0	51	20	115	2.7	844	16	0	0	0.22	0.07	3.3	26	834
0	34	8	78	0.5	610	8	0	0	0.16	0.03	2.2	20	835
0	27	7	60	0.4	515	5	0	0	0.14	0.03	2.0	18	836
0	27	11	54	0.4	443	7	0	0	0.13	0.03	1.8	10	837
0	17	5	43	0.7	229	16	0	0	0.06	0.02	1.2	5	838
0	20	10	47	0.4	366	108	0	0	0.09	0.01	1.6	5	839
12	31	203	233	0.8	537	1,076	520	76	0.05	0.20	2.3	8	840
56	28	292	277	1.6	970	1,061	650	93	0.16	0.28	2.4	24	841
0	44	23	112	2.4	680	53	0	0	0.17	0.03	3.8	10	842
4	37	55	101	0.6	628	636	40	12	0.18	0.08	2.3	14	843
4	35	55	97	0.5	607	620	360	42	0.18	0.08	2.3	13	844
29	32	103	118	0.5	489	697	380	44	0.23	0.11	1.4	20	845
170	28	48	130	1.6	635	1,323	520	83	0.19	0.15	2.2	25	846
27	31	88	137	0.9	497	835	360	51	0.05	0.14	2.5	8	847
29	26	140	154	1.4	926	821	330	47	0.17	0.23	2.6	26	848

[69]For green peppers; red peppers contain 141 mg ascorbic acid.
[70]For green peppers; red peppers contain 2,740 IU or 274 RE.
[71]For green peppers; red peppers contain 121 mg ascorbic acid.

Item No.	Foods, approximate measures, units, and weight (weight of edible portion only)			Water	Food energy	Protein	Fat	Fatty acids: Saturated	Fatty acids: Monounsaturated	Fatty acids: Polyunsaturated
	Vegetables and Vegetable Products—Con.		Grams	Percent	Calories	Grams	Grams	Grams	Grams	Grams
849	Potato chips	10 chips	20	3	105	1	7	1.8	1.2	3.6
	Pumpkin:									
850	Cooked from raw, mashed	1 cup	245	94	50	2	Tr	0.1	Tr	Tr
851	Canned	1 cup	245	90	85	3	1	0.4	0.1	Tr
852	Radishes, raw, stem ends, rootlets cut off	4 radishes	18	95	5	Tr	Tr	Tr	Tr	Tr
853	Sauerkraut, canned, solids and liquid	1 cup	236	93	45	2	Tr	0.1	Tr	0.1
	Seaweed:									
854	Kelp, raw	1 oz	28	82	10	Tr	Tr	0.1	Tr	Tr
855	Spirulina, dried	1 oz	28	5	80	16	2	0.8	0.2	0.6
	Southern peas. See Black-eyed peas, immature (items 769,770), mature (item 536).									
	Spinach:									
856	Raw, chopped	1 cup	55	92	10	2	Tr	Tr	Tr	0.1
	Cooked, drained:									
857	From raw	1 cup	180	91	40	5	Tr	0.1	Tr	0.2
858	From frozen (leaf)	1 cup	190	90	55	6	Tr	0.1	Tr	0.2
859	Canned, drained solids	1 cup	214	92	50	6	1	0.2	Tr	0.4
860	Spinach souffle	1 cup	136	74	220	11	18	7.1	6.8	3.1
	Squash, cooked:									
861	Summer (all varieties), sliced, drained	1 cup	180	94	35	2	1	0.1	Tr	0.2
862	Winter (all varieties), baked, cubes	1 cup	205	89	80	2	1	0.3	0.1	0.5
	Sunchoke. See Jerusalem-artichoke (item 805).									
	Sweetpotatoes:									
	Cooked (raw, 5 by 2 in; about 2-1/2 per lb):									
863	Baked in skin, peeled	1 potato	114	73	115	2	Tr	Tr	Tr	0.1
864	Boiled, without skin	1 potato	151	73	160	2	Tr	0.1	Tr	0.2
865	Candied, 2-1/2 by 2-in piece	1 piece	105	67	145	1	3	1.4	0.7	0.2
	Canned:									
866	Solid pack (mashed)	1 cup	255	74	260	5	1	0.1	Tr	0.2
867	Vacuum pack, piece 2-3/4 by 1 in	1 piece	40	76	35	1	Tr	Tr	Tr	Tr
	Tomatoes:									
868	Raw, 2-3/5-in diam. (3 per 12 oz pkg.)	1 tomato	123	94	25	1	Tr	Tr	Tr	0.1
869	Canned, solids and liquid	1 cup	240	94	50	2	1	0.1	0.1	0.2
870	Tomato juice, canned	1 cup	244	94	40	2	Tr	Tr	Tr	0.1
	Tomato products, canned:									
871	Paste	1 cup	262	74	220	10	2	0.3	0.4	0.9
872	Puree	1 cup	250	87	105	4	Tr	Tr	Tr	0.1
873	Sauce	1 cup	245	89	75	3	Tr	0.1	0.1	0.2
874	Turnips, cooked, diced	1 cup	156	94	30	1	Tr	Tr	Tr	0.1
	Turnip greens, cooked, drained:									
875	From raw (leaves and stems)	1 cup	144	93	30	2	Tr	0.1	Tr	0.1
876	From frozen (chopped)	1 cup	164	90	50	5	1	0.2	Tr	0.3
877	Vegetable juice cocktail, canned	1 cup	242	94	45	2	Tr	Tr	Tr	0.1
	Vegetables, mixed:									
878	Canned, drained solids	1 cup	163	87	75	4	Tr	0.1	Tr	0.2
879	Frozen, cooked, drained	1 cup	182	83	105	5	Tr	0.1	Tr	0.1
880	Waterchestnuts, canned	1 cup	140	86	70	1	Tr	Tr	Tr	Tr

[1] Value not determined.
[72] With added salt; if none is added, sodium content is 58 mg.
[73] For regular pack; special dietary pack contains 31 mg sodium.
[74] With added salt; if none is added, sodium content is 24 mg.

Nutrients in Indicated Quantity

Cho-les-terol	Carbo-hydrate	Calcium	Phos-phorus	Iron	Potas-sium	Sodium	Vitamin A value (IU)	Vitamin A value (RE)	Thiamin	Ribo-flavin	Niacin	Ascorbic acid	Item No.
Milli-grams	Grams	Milli-grams	Milli-grams	Milli-grams	Milli-grams	Milli-grams	Inter-national units	Retinol equiva-lents	Milli-grams	Milli-grams	Milli-grams	Milli-grams	
0	10	5	31	0.2	260	94	0	0	0.03	Tr	0.8	8	849
0	12	37	74	1.4	564	2	2,650	265	0.08	0.19	1.0	12	850
0	20	64	86	3.4	505	12	54,040	5,404	0.06	0.13	0.9	10	851
0	1	4	3	0.1	42	4	Tr	Tr	Tr	0.01	0.1	4	852
0	10	71	47	3.5	401	1,560	40	4	0.05	0.05	0.3	35	853
0	3	48	12	0.6	25	66	30	3	0.01	0.04	0.1	([1])	854
0	7	34	33	8.1	386	297	160	16	0.67	1.04	3.6	3	855
0	2	54	27	1.5	307	43	3,690	369	0.04	0.10	0.4	15	856
0	7	245	101	6.4	839	126	14,740	1,474	0.17	0.42	0.9	18	857
0	10	277	91	2.9	566	163	14,790	1,479	0.11	0.32	0.8	23	858
0	7	272	94	4.9	740	[72]683	18,780	1,878	0.03	0.30	0.8	31	859
184	3	230	231	1.3	201	763	3,460	675	0.09	0.30	0.5	3	860
0	8	49	70	0.6	346	2	520	52	0.08	0.07	0.9	10	861
0	18	29	41	0.7	896	2	7,290	729	0.17	0.05	1.4	20	862
0	28	32	63	0.5	397	11	24,880	2,488	0.08	0.14	0.7	28	863
0	37	32	41	0.8	278	20	25,750	2,575	0.08	0.21	1.0	26	864
8	29	27	27	1.2	198	74	4,400	440	0.02	0.04	0.4	7	865
0	59	77	133	3.4	536	191	38,570	3,857	0.07	0.23	2.4	13	866
0	8	9	20	0.4	125	21	3,190	319	0.01	0.02	0.3	11	867
0	5	9	28	0.6	255	10	1,390	139	0.07	0.06	0.7	22	868
0	10	62	46	1.5	530	[73]391	1,450	145	0.11	0.07	1.8	36	869
0	10	22	46	1.4	537	[74]881	1,360	136	0.11	0.08	1.6	45	870
0	49	92	207	7.8	2,442	[75]170	6,470	647	0.41	0.50	8.4	111	871
0	25	38	100	2.3	1,050	[76]50	3,400	340	0.18	0.14	4.3	88	872
0	18	34	78	1.9	909	[77]1,482	2,400	240	0.16	0.14	2.8	32	873
0	8	34	30	0.3	211	78	0	0	0.04	0.04	0.5	18	874
0	6	197	42	1.2	292	42	7,920	792	0.06	0.10	0.6	39	875
0	8	249	56	3.2	367	25	13,080	1,308	0.09	0.12	0.8	36	876
0	11	27	41	1.0	467	883	2,830	283	0.10	0.07	1.8	67	877
0	15	44	68	1.7	474	243	18,990	1,899	0.08	0.08	0.9	8	878
0	24	46	93	1.5	308	64	7,780	778	0.13	0.22	1.5	6	879
0	17	6	27	1.2	165	11	10	1	0.02	0.03	0.5	2	880

[75] With no added salt; if salt is added, sodium content is 2,070 mg.
[76] With no added salt; if salt is added, sodium content is 998 mg.
[77] With salt added.

Miscellaneous Items

Item No.	Foods, approximate measures, units, and weight (weight of edible portion only)			Water	Food energy	Protein	Fat	Fatty acids: Saturated	Fatty acids: Monounsaturated	Fatty acids: Polyunsaturated
			Grams	Percent	Calories	Grams	Grams	Grams	Grams	Grams
	Baking powders for home use:									
	Sodium aluminum sulfate:									
881	With monocalcium phosphate monohydrate	1 tsp	3	2	5	Tr	0	0.0	0.0	0.0
882	With monocalcium phosphate monohydrate, calcium sulfate	1 tsp	2.9	1	5	Tr	0	0.0	0.0	0.0
883	Straight phosphate	1 tsp	3.8	2	5	Tr	0	0.0	0.0	0.0
884	Low sodium	1 tsp	4.3	1	5	Tr	0	0.0	0.0	0.0
885	Catsup	1 cup	273	69	290	5	1	0.2	0.2	0.4
886		1 tbsp	15	69	15	Tr	Tr	Tr	Tr	Tr
887	Celery seed	1 tsp	2	6	10	Tr	1	Tr	0.3	0.1
888	Chili powder	1 tsp	2.6	8	10	Tr	Tr	0.1	0.1	0.2
	Chocolate:									
889	Bitter or baking	1 oz	28	2	145	3	15	9.0	4.9	0.5
	Semisweet, see Candy, (item 715).									
890	Cinnamon	1 tsp	2.3	10	5	Tr	Tr	Tr	Tr	Tr
891	Curry powder	1 tsp	2	10	5	Tr	Tr	([1])	([1])	([1])
892	Garlic powder	1 tsp	2.8	6	10	Tr	Tr	Tr	Tr	Tr
893	Gelatin, dry	1 envelope	7	13	25	6	Tr	Tr	Tr	Tr
894	Mustard, prepared, yellow	1 tsp or individual packet	5	80	5	Tr	Tr	Tr	0.2	Tr
	Olives, canned:									
895	Green	4 medium or 3 extra large	13	78	15	Tr	2	0.2	1.2	0.1
896	Ripe, Mission, pitted	3 small or 2 large	9	73	15	Tr	2	0.3	1.3	0.2
897	Onion powder	1 tsp	2.1	5	5	Tr	Tr	Tr	Tr	Tr
898	Oregano	1 tsp	1.5	7	5	Tr	Tr	Tr	Tr	0.1
899	Paprika	1 tsp	2.1	10	5	Tr	Tr	Tr	Tr	0.2
900	Pepper, black	1 tsp	2.1	11	5	Tr	Tr	Tr	Tr	Tr
	Pickles, cucumber:									
901	Dill, medium, whole, 3-3/4 in long, 1-1/4-in diam.	1 pickle	65	93	5	Tr	Tr	Tr	Tr	0.1
902	Fresh-pack, slices 1-1/2-in diam., 1/4 in thick	2 slices	15	79	10	Tr	Tr	Tr	Tr	Tr
903	Sweet, gherkin, small, whole, about 2-1/2 in long, 3/4-in diam.	1 pickle	15	61	20	Tr	Tr	Tr	Tr	Tr
	Popcorn. See Grain Products, (items 497-499).									
904	Relish, finely chopped, sweet	1 tbsp	15	63	20	Tr	Tr	Tr	Tr	Tr
905	Salt	1 tsp	5.5	0	0	0	0	0.0	0.0	0.0
906	Vinegar, cider	1 tbsp	15	94	Tr	Tr	0	0.0	0.0	0.0
	Yeast:									
907	Baker's, dry, active	1 pkg	7	5	20	3	Tr	Tr	0.1	Tr
908	Brewer's, dry	1 tbsp	8	5	25	3	Tr	Tr	Tr	0.0

[1]Value not determined.

Nutrients in Indicated Quantity													
Cho-les-terol	Carbo-hydrate	Calcium	Phos-phorus	Iron	Potas-sium	Sodium	Vitamin A value (IU)	Vitamin A value (RE)	Thiamin	Ribo-flavin	Niacin	Ascorbic acid	Item No.
Milli-grams	Grams	Milli-grams	Milli-grams	Milli-grams	Milli-grams	Milli-grams	Inter-national units	Retinol equiva-lents	Milli-grams	Milli-grams	Milli-grams	Milli-grams	
0	1	58	87	0.0	5	329	0	0	0.00	0.00	0.0	0	881
0	1	183	45	0.0	4	290	0	0	0.00	0.00	0.0	0	882
0	1	239	359	0.0	6	312	0	0	0.00	0.00	0.0	0	883
0	1	207	314	0.0	891	Tr	0	0	0.00	0.00	0.0	0	884
0	69	60	137	2.2	991	2,845	3,820	382	0.25	0.19	4.4	41	885
0	4	3	8	0.1	54	156	210	21	0.01	0.01	0.2	2	886
0	1	35	11	0.9	28	3	Tr	Tr	0.01	0.01	0.1	Tr	887
0	1	7	8	0.4	50	26	910	91	0.01	0.02	0.2	2	888
0	8	22	109	1.9	235	1	10	1	0.01	0.07	0.4	0	889
0	2	28	1	0.9	12	1	10	1	Tr	Tr	Tr	1	890
0	1	10	7	0.6	31	1	20	2	0.01	0.01	0.1	Tr	891
0	2	2	12	0.1	31	1	0	0	0.01	Tr	Tr	Tr	892
0	0	1	0	0.0	2	6	0	0	0.00	0.00	0.0	0	893
0	Tr	4	4	0.1	7	63	0	0	Tr	0.01	Tr	Tr	894
0	Tr	8	2	0.2	7	312	40	4	Tr	Tr	Tr	0	895
0	Tr	10	2	0.2	2	68	10	1	Tr	Tr	Tr	0	896
0	2	8	7	0.1	20	1	Tr	Tr	0.01	Tr	Tr	Tr	897
0	1	24	3	0.7	25	Tr	100	10	0.01	Tr	0.1	1	898
0	1	4	7	0.5	49	1	1,270	127	0.01	0.04	0.3	1	899
0	1	9	4	0.6	26	1	Tr	Tr	Tr	0.01	Tr	0	900
0	1	17	14	0.7	130	928	70	7	Tr	0.01	Tr	4	901
0	3	5	4	0.3	30	101	20	2	Tr	Tr	Tr	1	902
0	5	2	2	0.2	30	107	10	1	Tr	Tr	Tr	1	903
0	5	3	2	0.1	30	107	20	2	Tr	Tr	0.0	1	904
0	0	14	3	Tr	Tr	2,132	0	0	0.00	0.00	0.0	0	905
0	1	1	1	0.1	15	Tr	0	0	0.00	0.00	0.0	0	906
0	3	3	90	1.1	140	4	Tr	Tr	0.16	0.38	2.6	Tr	907
0	3	[78]17	140	1.4	152	10	Tr	Tr	1.25	0.34	3.0	Tr	908

[78]Value may vary from 6 to 60 mg.

APPENDIX C

CALORIC CONTENT OF FAST FOODS

Arby's

Junior roast beef sandwich	220
Regular roast beef sand.	350
Turkey sand. with dressing	410
without Arby's dressing	345
Ham 'n cheese	380
Super roast beef sandwich	620
Club sandwich	560
Swiss King	660
Beef 'n cheese	450
Turkey deluxe	510
Coleslaw	83

Arthur Treacher's Fish and Chips

Fish (2 pc.)	335
Chips	275
Shrimp (7)	381
Krunch Pups	203
Fish sandwich	440
Chicken (2 pc.)	369
Coleslaw	123
Chowder	112
Chicken sandwich	413

Baskin-Robbins

One scoop (2½ oz.)	
sugar cone	57
chocolate fudge	178
french vanilla	181
rocky road	182
butter pecan	136
jamoca almond fudge	190
chocolate mint	162
jamoca	146
fresh strawberry	141
fresh peach	139
mango sherbet	99
daiquiri ice	84

Burger Chef

Big Chef	542
Cheeseburger	304
Double cheeseburger	434
French fries	240
Regular hamburger	258
Mariner Platter	680
Rancher Platter	640
Shake, chocolate	310
Skipper's Treat	604
Super Chef	530

Burger King

Cheeseburger	350
Hamburger	290
Whopper	630
Whopper with cheese	740
Whaler	744
Double beef Whopper	850
with cheese	950
French fries	214
Large shake	332
Hot dog	291
Onion rings	270
Apple pie	240

Kentucky Fried Chicken

	Original Recipe	Extra Crispy
Wing	136	201
Breast	199	286
Drumstick	117	155
Thigh	257	343
Mashed potatoes		64
Chicken breast filet sandwich		436
French fries		184

Dairy Queen

Small cone	140
chocolate dipped	190
Medium cone	240
chocolate dipped	340
Large cone	340
chocolate dipped	510
Dilly Bar	210
Buster Bar	460
Banana split	540
Small chocolate malt	520
Medium chocolate malt	760
Large chocolate malt	1060
Small chocolate sundae	190
Medium chocolate sundae	310
Large chocolate sundae	440
Hot Fudge Brownie Delight	600
Fiesta sundae	570
Hamburger single	360
Hamburger double	530
with cheese	650
Hamburger triple	710
with cheese	820
Hot dog	280
with cheese	330
with chili	320
Hot dog Super	520
with cheese	580
with chili	570
Brazier onion rings	280
Brazier french fries (2.5 oz.)	200
Brazier french fries (4.0 oz.)	320
Fish sandwich	400
with cheese	440
Dairy Queen Freeze	500
Dairy Queen Sandwich	140
Dairy Queen Float	410
Dairy Queen Parfait	430

Dunkin' Donuts

Cake donuts	
plain cake	240
plain honey dipped	280
plain with white icing	265
with chocolate icing	235
chocolate cake	240
chocolate honey dipped	250

Dunkin' Donuts (continued)

Yeast raised donuts	
sugared	205
honey dipped	225
add 40–50 calories for filling	

Hardee's

Bacon cheeseburger	686
Big Deluxe	546
Big Roast Beef	418
Cheeseburger	335
Chicken fillet	510
Fisherman's Fillet	469
Hamburger	305
Hot dog	346
Hot Ham 'n Cheese	376
Mushroom 'n Swiss	512
Roast Beef Sandwich	377
Turkey Club	426
Apple turnover	282
French fries	239
Milk shake (8 oz.)	320

Long John Silver's

Breaded oysters (6 pc.)	460
Breaded clams (1 order)	526
Chicken planks (4 pc.)	416
Cole slaw (3.5 oz.)	182
Corn on the cob (1 pc.)	176
Fish with batter (2 pc.)	404
Fish with batter (3 pc.)	606
Fries (3 oz.)	247
Hush Puppies (2 pc.)	145
Ocean scallops, fryes, slaw	746
Peg Leg with batter (5 pc.)	703
Treasure Chest (2 pc. fish, 2 Peg Legs, fries, slaw	1015
3-piece dinner	1190
2-piece dinner	995

Pizza Hut

Thin 'n Crispy (half of 10-in. pizza)	
Beef combination	490
Pork combination	520
Cheese	450
Pepperoni	430
Supreme	510

Pizza Hut
(continued)

Thick 'n Chewy (half of 10-in. pizza)	
Beef combination	620
Pork combination	640
Cheese	560
Pepperoni	560
Supreme	640

MacDonald's

Hamburger	255
Cheeseburger	306
Filet of Fish	432
French fries (regular)	220
Big Mac	563
Quarter Pounder	424
with cheese	524
Chocolate shake	383
Strawberry shake	363
Vanilla shake	352
Apple pie	253
Cherry pie	298
Cookies	294
Egg McMuffin	327
English muffin with butter	186
Hotcakes, butter, syrup	500
Sausage	206
Scrambled eggs	180

Taco Bell

Taco	186
Tostada	179
Frijoles	178
Enchirito	454
Burrito	
bean	343
beef	466
Burrito Supreme	457
Combination Burrito	457
Bellbeefer	278
Pintos 'n Cheese	168

White Castle

Hamburger	160
French fries	225
Cheeseburger	185
Fish sandwich	200
Milk shake	213
Onion rings	341
Cinnamon roll	305
Cherry roll	334

Wendy's

Bacon (2 strips)	110
Bacon cheeseburger	460
Breakfast sandwich	320
Chicken sandwich	320
Chili (8 oz.)	260
Danish	360
French fries (reg.)	280
French toast (2 slices)	400
Frosty (12 oz.)	400
Hamburger double	560
Hamburger single	340
Home fries	360
Hot stuffed baked potato	
Bacon and cheese	570
Broccoli and cheese	500
Cheese	590
Chicken a la King	350
Chili and cheese	510
Plain	250
Sour cream w/chives	460
Stroganoff and sour cr.	490
Pickup window side salad	110
Taco salad	390
Toast w/ margarine (2 slices)	250
Omelet #1	250
Omelet #2	290
Omelet #3	280
Omelet #4	210
Sausage (1 patty)	200
Scrambled eggs	190

Adapted from: Carper, J., *The Brand Name Nutrition Counter*. New York: Bantam, 1985; Kraus, B., *Calorie Guide to Brand Name and Basic Foods*. New York: Signet, 1988; Netzer, C., *Brand Name Calorie Counter*. New York: Dell, 1988; and "Diet Digest," *Cosmopolitan's Beauty and Fitness*, Winter, 1985–1986.

APPENDIX

D WHAT DO YOU KNOW ABOUT STRESS?

This is a four-part test.[1] The first three parts are designed to measure your vulnerability to certain types of stress and to increase your awareness of stress and how it affects you. The fourth part will give you some idea of how well you cope with stressful situations.

If you have any concerns or questions about your answers to this assessment you may want to discuss them with a qualified counselor, your family physician, or another professional medical person. For additional information on stress you may wish to write to National Institute of Mental Health, Public Inquiries Section, Rm. 11-A-19, 5600 Fishers Lane, Rockville, MD 20857.

Stress Test, Part One

Read and choose the most appropriate answer for each of the 10 questions as it actually pertains to you.

1. When I can't do something "my way," I simply adjust to do it the easiest way.
   (a) Almost always true, (b) Usually true, (c) Usually false, (d) Almost always false
2. I get upset when someone in front of me drives slowly.
   (a) Almost always true, (b) Usually true, (c) Usually false, (d) Almost always false
3. It bothers me when my plans are dependent upon others.
   (a) Almost always true, (b) Usually true, (c) Usually false, (d) Almost always false

[1]From the Department of Health, Education, and Welfare, Public Health Service, DHEW Publication No. (PHS) 79-50097, Washington, D.C., 1980.

4. Whenever possible, I tend to avoid large crowds.
   (a) Almost always true, (b) Usually true, (c) Usually false, (d) Almost always false
5. I am uncomfortable having to stand in long lines.
   (a) Almost always true, (b) Usually true, (c) Usually false, (d) Almost always false
6. Arguments upset me.
   (a) Almost always true, (b) Usually true, (c) Usually false. (d) Almost always false
7. When my plans don't flow smoothly, I become anxious.
   (a) Almost always true, (b) Usually true, (c) Usually false, (d) Almost always false
8. I require a lot of room (space) to live and work in.
   (a) Almost always true, (b) Usually true, (c) Usually false, (d) Almost always false
9. When I am busy at some task, I hate to be disturbed.
   (a) Almost always true, (b) Usually true, (c) Usually false, (d) Almost always false
10. I believe that "all good things are worth waiting for."
   (a) Almost always true, (b) Usually true, (c) Usually false, (d) Almost always false

To score: 1 and 10, a = 1 pt., b = 2 pts., c = 3 pts., d = 4 pts. 2 through 9, a = 4 pts., b = 3 pts., c = 2 pts., d = 1 pt.

This test measures your vulnerability to stress from being "frustrated," that is, inhibited. Scores in excess of 25 seem to suggest some vulnerability to this source of stress.

Stress Test, Part Two

Circle the letter of the response option that best answers the following 10 questions. How often do you . . .

1. Find yourself with insufficient time to complete your work?
   (a) Almost always, (b) Very often, (c) Seldom, (d) Never
2. Find yourself becoming confused and unable to think clearly because too many things are happening at once?
   (a) Almost always, (b) Very often, (c) Seldom, (d) Never
3. Wish you had help to get everything done?
   (a) Almost always, (b) Very often, (c) Seldom, (d) Never

4. Feel your boss/professor simply expects too much from you?
   (a) Almost always, (b) Very often, (c) Seldom, (d) Never
5. Feel your family/friends expect too much from you?
   (a) Almost always, (b) Very often, (c) Seldom, (d) Never
6. Find your work infringing upon your leisure hours?
   (a) Almost always, (b) Very often, (c) Seldom, (d) Never
7. Find yourself doing extra work to set an example to those around you?
   (a) Almost always, (b) Very often, (c) Seldom, (d) Never
8. Find yourself doing extra work to impress your superiors?
   (a) Almost always, (b) Very often, (c) Seldom, (d) Never
9. Have to skip a meal so that you can get work completed?
   (a) Almost always, (b) Very often, (c) Seldom, (d) Never
10. Feel that you have too much responsibility?
   (a) Almost always, (b) Very often, (c) Seldom, (d) Never

To score: a = 4 pts., b = 3 pts., c = 2 pts., d = 1 pt. Total up your score for this exercise.

This test measures your vulnerability to "overload," that is, having too much to do. Scores in excess of 25 seem to indicate vulnerability to this source of stress.

Stress Test, Part Three

Answer all questions as is *generally* true for you.

1. I hate to wait in lines.
   (a) Almost always true, (b) Usually true, (c) Seldom true, (d) Never true
2. I often find myself racing against the clock to save time.
   (a) Almost always true, (b) Usually true, (c) Seldom true, (d) Never true
3. I become upset if I think something is taking too long.
   (a) Almost always true, (b) Usually true, (c) Seldom true, (d) Never true
4. When under pressure I tend to lose my temper.
   (a) Almost always true, (b) Usually true, (c) Seldom true, (d) Never true
5. My friends tell me that I tend to get irritated easily.
   (a) Almost always true, (b) Usually true, (c) Seldom true, (d) Never true

6. I seldom like to do anything unless I can make it competitive.
   (a) Almost always true, (b) Usually true, (c) Seldom true, (d) Never true
7. When something needs to be done, I'm the first to begin even though the details may still need to be worked out.
   (a) Almost always true, (b) Usually true, (c) Seldom true, (d) Never true
8. When I make a mistake it is usually because I've rushed into something without giving it enough thought and planning.
   (a) Almost always true, (b) Usually true, (c) Seldom true, (d) Never true
9. Whenever possible I will try to do two things at once, like eating while working, or planning while driving or bathing.
   (a) Almost always true, (b) Usually true, (c) Seldom true, (d) Never true
10. When I go on a vacation, I usually take some work along just in case I get a chance.
    (a) Almost always true, (b) Usually true, (c) Seldom true, (d) Never true

To score: a = 4 pts., b = 3 pts., c = 2 pts., d = 1 pt.

This test measures the presence of compulsive, time-urgent, and excessively aggressive behavioral traits. Scores in excess of 25 suggest the presence of one or more of these traits.

Stress Test, Part Four

How do you cope with the stress in your life? There are numerous ways—some are more effective than others—yet some coping strategies may actually be as harmful as the stress they are used to alleviate. This scale was created largely on the basis of results compiled by clinicians and researchers who sought to identify how individuals effectively cope with stress. This scale is an educational tool, not a clinical instrument. Therefore, its purpose is to inform you, thereader, of ways in which you can *effectively* and *healthfully* cope with the stress in your life, while at the same time, through a point system, give you some indication of the relative desirability of the coping strategies you are currently using. Simply follow the instructions given for each of the 14 items listed below. Total your points when you have completed all of the items.

1. Give yourself 10 points if you feel that you have a supportive family around you.
2. Give yourself 10 points if you actively pursue a hobby.
3. Give yourself 10 points if you belong to some social or activity group that meets at least once a month (other than your family).
4. Give yourself 15 points if you are within five pounds of your "ideal" body weight, considering your height and bone structure.
5. Give yourself 15 points if you practice some form of deep relaxation at least three times a week. Deep relaxation exercises include meditation, imagery, yoga, and so on.
6. Give yourself 5 points for each time you exercise thirty minutes or longer during the course of one average week.
7. Give yourself 5 points for each nutritionally balanced and wholesome meal you consume during the course of one average day.
8. Give yourself 5 points if you do something that you really enjoy that is just for you during the course of an average week.
9. Give yourself 10 points if you have some place in your home that you can go in order to relax and/or be alone.
10. Give yourself 10 points if you practice time management techniques in your daily life.
11. Subtract 10 points for each pack of cigarettes you smoke during the course of one average day.
12. Subtract 5 points for each evening during the course of an average week that you take any form of medication or chemical substance (including alcohol) to help you sleep.
13. Subtract 10 points for each day during the course of an average week that you consume any form of medication or chemical substance (including alcohol) to reduce your anxiety or just calm you down.
14. Subtract 5 points for each evening during the course of an average week that you bring work home—work that was meant to be done at your place of employment.

Now calculate your total score. A perfect score would be 115 points. If you scored in the 50–60 range you probably have an adequate collection of coping strategies for most common sources of stress. However, you should keep in mind that the higher your score, the greater your ability to cope with stress in an effective and healthful manner.

INDEX